Colorectal Cancer Screening

Editor

DOUGLAS K. REX

GASTROINTESTINAL ENDOSCOPY CLINICS OF NORTH AMERICA

www.giendo.theclinics.com

Consulting Editor
CHARLES J. LIGHTDALE

July 2020 • Volume 30 • Number 3

ELSEVIER

1600 John F. Kennedy Boulevard ● Suite 1800 ● Philadelphia, Pennsylvania, 19103-2899

http://www.theclinics.com

**GASTROINTESTINAL ENDOSCOPY CLINICS OF NORTH AMERICA Volume 30, Number 3
July 2020 ISSN 1052-5157, ISBN-13: 978-0-323-73338-0**

Editor: Kerry Holland
Developmental Editor: Donald Mumford

Gastrointestinal Endoscopy Clinics of North America (ISSN 1052-5157) is published quarterly by Elsevier Inc., 360 Park Avenue South, New York, NY 10010-1710. Months of issue are January, April, July, and October. Business and Editorial Offices: 1600 John F. Kennedy Blvd., Suite 1800, Philadelphia, PA, 19103-2899. Periodicals postage paid at New York, NY and additional mailing offices. Subscription prices are $359.00 per year for US individuals, $655.00 per year for US institutions, $100.00 per year for US and Canadian students/residents, $399.00 per year for Canadian individuals, $774.00 per year for Canadian institutions, $476.00 per year for international individuals, $774.00 per year for international institutions, and $245.00 per year for international students/residents. To receive student/resident rate, orders must be accompanied by name of affiliated institution, date of term, and the *signature* of program/residency coordinator on institution letterhead. Orders will be billed at individual rate until proof of status is received. Foreign air speed delivery is included in all *Clinics* subscription prices. All prices are subject to change without notice. **POSTMASTER:** Send address change to *Gastrointestinal Endoscopy Clinics of North America*, Elsevier Health Sciences Division, Subscription Customer Service, 3251 Riverport Lane, Maryland Heights, MO 63043. **Customer Service: 1-800-654-2452 (US). From outside the United States, call 1-314-447-8871. Fax: 1-314-447-8029. E-mail: JournalsCustomerService-usa@elsevier.com (for print support) or JournalsOnlineSupport-usa@elsevier.com (for online support).**

Reprints. For copies of 100 or more, of articles in this publication, please contact the Commercial Reprints Department, Elsevier Inc., 360 Park Avenue South, New York, NY 10010-1710. Tel. 212-633-3874; Fax: 212-633-3820; E-mail: reprints@elsevier.com.

Gastrointestinal Endoscopy Clinics of North America is covered in *Excerpta Medica, MEDLINE/PubMed (Index Medicus), and MEDLINE/MEDLARS.*

Contributors

CONSULTING EDITOR

CHARLES J. LIGHTDALE, MD
Professor of Medicine, Division of Digestive and Liver Diseases, Columbia University Medical Center, New York, New York, USA

EDITOR

DOUGLAS K. REX, MD, MACP, MACG, FASGE, AGAF
Division of Gastroenterology/Hepatology, Indiana University School of Medicine, Indianapolis, Indiana, USA

AUTHORS

DENNIS J. AHNEN, MD
Division of Gastroenterology and Hepatology, University of Colorado Hospital, Anschutz Medical Campus, Aurora, Colorado, USA

JOSEPH C. ANDERSON, MD, MHCDS
White River Junction VA Medical Center, Vermont, USA; Dartmouth Geisel School of Medicine, Hanover, New Hampshire, USA; Division of Gastroenterology and Hepatology, University of Connecticut School of Medicine, Farmington, Connecticut, USA

CLEMENT RICHARD BOLAND, MD
Professor of Medicine, University of California, San Diego School of Medicine, La Jolla, California, USA

DURADO BROOKS, MD, MPH
Vice President, Cancer Control Interventions, American Cancer Society, Atlanta, Georgia, USA

LYNN F. BUTTERLY, MD
PI, New Hampshire Colonoscopy Registry, PI, New Hampshire Colorectal Cancer Screening Program, Lebanon, New Hampshire, USA

MICHAEL F. BYRNE, MA, MD (Cantab), FRCPC, MRCP
Clinical Professor of Medicine, Division of Gastroenterology, Vancouver General Hospital, University of British Columbia, Vancouver, British Columbia, Canada

BROOKS D. CASH, MD, AGAF, FACG, FASGE
Professor of Medicine, Division Chief, Division of Gastroenterology, Hepatology, and Nutrition, Houston, Texas, USA

SEUNG WON CHUNG, MD
Department of Internal Medicine, Houston, Texas, USA

JASON A. DOMINITZ, MD, MHS
National Program Director for Gastroenterology, Veterans Health Administration, Professor of Medicine, University of Washington School of Medicine, Seattle, Washington, USA

MARY DOROSHENK, MA
Director of Advocacy and Alliance Relations, Exact Sciences Corporation, Madison, Wisconsin, USA; Exact Sciences Corporation, Arlington, Virginia, USA

JASON D. ECKMANN, MD
Instructor of Medicine, Department of Internal Medicine, Mayo Clinic, Rochester, Minnesota, USA

SEIFELDIN HAKIM, MD
Division of Gastroenterology, Hepatology, and Nutrition, Houston, Texas, USA

ANDREW HAN, MD
Fellow, Department of Medicine, Division of Gastroenterology and Hepatology, Indiana University School of Medicine, Indianapolis, Indiana, USA

THOMAS F. IMPERIALE, MD
Professor, Department of Medicine, Indiana University School of Medicine, Health Services Research and Development, Richard L. Roudebush VA Medical Center, Regenstrief Institute, Inc., Indiana University Melvin and Bren Simon Cancer Center, Indiana University School of Public Health, Indianapolis, Indiana, USA

CHARLES KAHI, MD
Professor, Department of Medicine, Division of Gastroenterology and Hepatology, Indiana University School of Medicine, Richard L. Roudebush VA Medical Center, Indianapolis, Indiana, USA

JOHN B. KISIEL, MD
Associate Professor of Medicine and Consultant, Division of Gastroenterology and Hepatology, Mayo Clinic, Rochester, Minnesota, USA

JENNIFER M. KOLB, MD
Division of Gastroenterology and Hepatology, University of Colorado Hospital, Anschutz Medical Campus, Aurora, Colorado, USA

URI LADABAUM, MD, MS
Professor of Medicine, Director Gastrointestinal Cancer Prevention Program, Division of Gastroenterology and Hepatology, Department of Medicine, Stanford University School of Medicine, Redwood City, California, USA

THEODORE R. LEVIN, MD
Staff Physician, Gastroenterology Department, Kaiser Permanente Medical Group, Research Scientist, Kaiser Permanente Division of Research and Clinical Lead for Colorectal Cancer Screening, The Permanente Medical Group, Inc, Oakland, California, USA

PAUL J. LIMBURG, MD
Professor of Medicine and Consultant, Division of Gastroenterology and Hepatology, Mayo Clinic, Rochester, Minnesota, USA

JENNIFER MARATT, MD
Assistant Professor, Department of Medicine, Division of Gastroenterology and Hepatology, Indiana University School of Medicine, Richard L. Roudebush VA Medical Center, Indianapolis, Indiana, USA

PATRICK O. MONAHAN, PhD
Professor, Department of Biostatistics, Indiana University Melvin and Bren Simon Cancer Center, Indiana University School of Public Health, Health Information and Translational Sciences, Indianapolis, Indiana, USA

SWATI G. PATEL, MD MS
Assistant Professor of Medicine, Division of Gastroenterology and Hepatology, Rocky Mountain Regional VA Medical Center, Aurora, Colorado, USA

DOUGLAS K. REX, MD, MACP, MACG, FASGE, AGAF
Division of Gastroenterology/Hepatology, Indiana University School of Medicine, Indianapolis, Indiana, USA

DOUGLAS J. ROBERTSON, MD, MPH
White River Junction VA Medical Center, Vermont, USA; Dartmouth Geisel School of Medicine, The Dartmouth Institute, Hanover, New Hampshire, USA

N. JEWEL SAMADDER, MD, MSc
Division of Gastroenterology and Hepatology, Department of Clinical Genomics, Mayo Clinic, Phoenix, Arizona, USA

PHILIP SCHOENFELD, MD, MSEd, MSc (Epi)
Chief-Gastroenterology Section, John D. Dingell VA Medical Center, Detroit, Michigan, USA

KEVIN SELBY, MD, MAS
Center for Primary Care and Public Health (Unisanté), University of Lausanne, Lausanne, Switzerland

KATHERINE SHARPE, MTS
Sharpe Consulting, LLC, Decatur, Georgia, USA

DENNIS L. SHUNG, MD
Clinical Fellow, Section of Digestive Diseases, Department of Medicine, Yale School of Medicine, New Haven, Connecticut, USA

SHAHEER SIDDIQUI, MD
Division of Gastroenterology, Hepatology, and Nutrition, Houston, Texas, USA

AMITABH SRIVASTAVA, MD
Brigham and Women's Hospital, Boston, Massachusetts, USA

RICHARD WENDER, MD
Chief Cancer Control Officer, American Cancer Society, Atlanta, Georgia, USA

Contents

> Although colorectal cancer (CRC) can be prevented or detected early through screening and surveillance, barriers that lower adherence to screening significantly limit its effectiveness. Therefore, implementation of interventions that address and overcome adherence barriers is critical to efforts to decrease morbidity and mortality from CRC. This article reviews the current available evidence about interventions to increase adherence to CRC screening.

> Most screening in the United States occurs in an opportunistic fashion, although organized screening occurs in some integrated health care systems. Organized colorectal cancer (CRC) screening consists of an explicit screening policy, defined target population, implementation team, health care team for clinical care delivery, quality assurance infrastructure, and method for identifying cancer outcomes. Implementation of an organized screening program offers opportunities to systematically assess the success of the program and develop interventions to address identified gaps in an effort to optimize CRC outcomes. There is evidence of that organized screening is associated with improvements in screening participation and CRC mortality.

> Colorectal cancer incidence and mortality have decreased in the United States in recent decades, largely through opportunistic screening. Although certain organizations have improved internal screening rates by implementing programmatic screening, most of the United States undergoes opportunistic screening. Much effort and resources have been expended comparing screening tests to determine the most effective; however, deeper analysis of the US population has revealed subsets of ethnicities may be grossly underscreened. The most effective screening test remains the test that is completed and adhered to, and a better question may concern the best method of discussing screening.

Risk stratification is a system by which clinically meaningful separation of risk is achieved in a group of otherwise similar persons. Although parametric logistic regression dominates risk prediction, use of nonparametric and semiparametric methods, including artificial neural networks, is increasing. These statistical-learning and machine-learning methods, along with simple rules, are collectively referred to as "artificial intelligence" (AI). AI requires knowledge of study validity, understanding of model metrics, and determination of whether and to what extent the model can and should be applied to the patient or population under consideration. Further investigation is needed, especially in model validation and impact assessment.

Early onset colorectal cancer (EOCRC) refers to colorectal cancer (CRC) in individuals under age 50. Although the incidence and mortality due to later onset CRC ($\geq$50 years) has been declining over several decades, both are increasing in those under 50. EOCRC is more likely to occur in the distal colon and rectum. There are some unique pathologic and genetic features to these tumors; they are not usually associated with a germline mutation in a gene that predisposes to cancer, and at least some may have a distinct pathogenesis. Initiating CRC screening at an earlier age (40–45 years of age) would presumably detect more early stage and asymptomatic EOCRCs, but this would imply a major additional health care burden. The understanding of EOCRC and the optimal management approach to this problem are unsolved problems.

Serrated polyps are classified into hyperplastic polyps, sessile serrated adenomas/polyps, and traditional serrated adenomas. Although all serrated polyps share characteristic colonic crypts serrations, distinguishing hyperplastic polyps from sessile serrated adenomas/polyps is challenging. Traditional serrated adenomas are cytologically dysplastic lesions; sessile serrated adenomas/polyps develop cytologic dysplasia as they progress to colorectal cancer. A flat and pale appearance of serrated polyps may make detection difficult. Endoscopic mucosal resection has higher rates of complete resection. Close surveillance is recommended for sessile serrated adenomas/polyps, sessile serrated adenomas/polyp with dysplasia, hyperplastic polyps $\geq$10 mm, and traditional serrated adenomas.

Cost-effectiveness analysis compares benefits and costs of different interventions to inform decision makers. Alternatives are compared based on an incremental cost-effectiveness ratio reported in terms of cost per quality-adjusted life-year gained. Multiple cost-effectiveness analyses of colorectal cancer (CRC) screening have been performed. Although regional epidemiology of CRC, relevant screening strategies, regional health system, and applicable medical costs in local currencies differ by country and region, several overarching points emerge from literature on cost-effectiveness of CRC screening. Cost-effectiveness analysis informs decisions in ongoing debates, including preferred age to begin average-risk CRC screening, and implementation of CRC screening tailored to predicted CRC risk.

The National Colorectal Cancer Roundtable (NCCRT) is an organization of organizations with staffing, funding and leadership provided by the American Cancer Society (ACS) and guidance and funding by the Centers for Disease Control and Prevention (CDC). In 2014, ACS, CDC, and the NCCRT launched the 80% by 2018 campaign. This highly successful initiative activated hundreds of organizations to prioritize colorectal cancer screening, disseminated smart, evidence-based interventions, and ultimately led to 9.3 million more Americans being up to date with screening compared with the precampaign rate. It's new campaign, 80% in Every Community, is designed to address persistent screening disparities.

The fecal immunochemical test (FIT) is a tool used for colorectal cancer screening and its use is growing rapidly. FIT, applied as a qualitative or quantitative test, has far better sensitivity for hemoglobin than older, guaiac fecal occult blood tests. This translates into several advantages of FIT, including ability to screen using only 1 stool sample per cycle. This article reviews current understanding of FIT performance as a 1-time test and when applied programmatically. It outlines how to apply the test at the patient level and track performance at the program level. Future prospects for FIT application are highlighted.

Most colorectal cancer screening in the United States occurs in the opportunistic setting, where screening is initiated by a patient-provider interaction. Colonoscopy provides the longest-interval protection, and high-quality colonoscopy is ideally suited to the opportunistic setting. Both detection and colonoscopic resection have improved as a result of intense scientific investigation. Further improvements in detection are expected with the introduction of artificial intelligence programs into colonoscopy platforms. We may expect recommended intervals or colonoscopy after negative examinations performed by high-quality detectors to expand beyond 10 years. Thus, high-quality colonoscopy remains an excellent approach to colorectal cancer screening in the opportunistic setting.

The goal of colorectal cancer (CRC) screening with colonoscopy is to minimize CRC with minimal risk and cost. In order to continuously improve the quality of colonoscopy, different outcomes must be measured. For this topic, the priority indicators to be measured are (1) frequency of scheduling colonoscopy at appropriate interval based on current guidelines; (2) frequency of identifying adenomas in average-risk individuals undergoing their first screening colonoscopy; and, (3) providing guideline-consistent recommendations for repeat colonoscopy after the procedure.

After 2 screen-setting studies showing high sensitivity for colorectal cancer and advanced precancerous lesions, multitarget stool DNA testing was endorsed by the US Preventative Services Task Force as a first-line colorectal cancer screening test. Uptake has increased exponentially since approval by the US Food and Drug Administration and Centers for Medicare and Medicaid Services. Adherence to testing is approximately 70%. Patients with positive results have high diagnostic colonoscopy completion rates in single-center studies. The positive predictive value for colorectal neoplasia in postapproval studies is high. Next-generation test prototypes show promise to extend specificity gains while maintaining high sensitivity.

This article reviews alternative colorectal cancer (CRC) screening tests, including flexible sigmoidoscopy (FS), computed tomography (CT) colonography, and colon capsule endoscopy. FS has abundant and convincing evidence supporting its use for CRC screening and is a commonly used CRC test worldwide. CT colonography has demonstrated convincing results for CRC screening, but concerns regarding cost, accuracy for flat or sessile neoplasia, reproducibility, extracolonic findings, and lack of coverage have limited its use and development. Colon capsule endoscopy has demonstrated encouraging results for polyp detection in average-risk individuals, but is not approved for CRC screening at the current time.

Artificial intelligence may improve value in colonoscopy-based colorectal screening and surveillance by improving quality and decreasing unnecessary costs. The quality of screening and surveillance as measured by adenoma detection rates can be improved through real-time computer-assisted detection of polyps. Unnecessary costs can be decreased with optical biopsies to identify low-risk polyps using computer-assisted diagnosis that can undergo the resect-and-discard or diagnose-and-leave strategy. Key challenges include the clinical integration of artificial intelligence-based technology into the endoscopists' workflow, the effect of this technology on endoscopy center efficiency, and the interpretability of the underlying deep learning algorithms. The future for image-based artificial intelligence in gastroenterology will include applications to improve the diagnosis and treatment of cancers throughout the gastrointestinal tract.

The most commonly recognized high-risk group for colorectal cancer (CRC) is individuals with a positive family history. It is generally recognized that those with a first-degree relative (FDR) with CRC are at a 2-fold or higher risk of CRC or advanced neoplasia. FDRs of patients with advanced adenomas have a similarly increased risk. Accordingly, all major US guidelines recommend starting CRC screening by age 40 in these groups. Barriers to screening this group include patient lack of knowledge on family and polyp history, provider limitations in collecting family history, and insufficient application of guidelines.

GASTROINTESTINAL ENDOSCOPY CLINICS OF NORTH AMERICA

RELATED CLINICS SERIES

Gastroenterology Clinics
Clinics in Liver Disease

THE CLINICS ARE AVAILABLE ONLINE!
Access your subscription at:
www.theclinics.com

Foreword

Colorectal Cancer Screening: Where We Are and Moving Forward

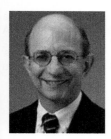

Charles J. Lightdale, MD
Consulting Editor

As I write the foreword to this issue of *Gastrointestinal Endoscopy Clinics of North America* devoted to "Colorectal Cancer Screening," the COVID-19 pandemic continues to rage. Tens of thousands of Americans will die of respiratory complications of the highly contagious coronavirus infection. Mandatory "social distancing" is widely declared in cities and states across the country. In many places, all elective gastrointestinal (GI) endoscopy procedures have been put on hold, including colonoscopies for colorectal cancer screening. This appropriate pause can be taken as an opportunity for GI endoscopists to take some time to ponder what has been achieved and to consider the best strategies for the future.

At some point, the current viral threat will likely be tamed by a combination of public health measures, new treatments, and it is hoped, an effective vaccine. The threat of tens of thousands dying from colorectal cancer, however, will continue, and will have to be addressed with renewed vigor. Yes, colorectal cancer screening has been undoubtedly successful in decreasing incidence and mortality by early detection and by removal of precancerous colorectal polyps. Still, the American Cancer Society projects some 148,000 new cases of colorectal cancer in the United States in 2020 with a mortality of more than 53,000. Colorectal cancer remains the second leading cause of cancer deaths for men and women combined in the United States.

Dr Douglas K. Rex, the Editor of this issue of *Gastrointestinal Endoscopy Clinics of North America*, is widely recognized for his leadership in colorectal cancer screening, and he has crafted a deeply thoughtful list of topics written by an extraordinary group of experts highlighting where we stand with current screening and the challenges as we move forward. How and when to utilize fecal immunochemical testing and multitarget stool DNA testing to extend screening to a greater percent of the population, risk

Gastrointest Endoscopy Clin N Am 30 (2020) xiii–xiv
https://doi.org/10.1016/j.giec.2020.04.002
1052-5157/20/© 2020 Published by Elsevier Inc.

stratification, and the potential for artificial intelligence are among the topics. Dr Rex himself has provided a not-to-be-missed article, "The case for high-quality colonoscopy remaining a premier colorectal cancer screening strategy in the United States." I advise GI endoscopists to take the time to read this important issue now, and to be fully informed and to participate when events allow with new energy in colorectal cancer screening.

Charles J. Lightdale, MD
Department of Medicine
Columbia University Medical Center
161 Fort Washington Avenue
New York, NY 10032, USA

E-mail address:
CJL18@columbia.edu

Preface

Colorectal Cancer Screening

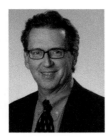

Douglas K. Rex, MD, MACP, MACG, FASGE, AGAF
Editor

Colorectal cancer (CRC) screening is unquestionably effective in reducing CRC mortality. In the United States, CRC incidence rates have been falling for over four decades, and the rate of incidence decline accelerated to 3% to 4% per year in 2000. At least half this decline appears to result from screening.

Despite this success, CRC screening in the United States faces a number of substantial challenges. Greatest among these is that screening rates in the eligible US population have plateaued at just above 60%. Thus, about a third of the US population does not keep up with recommended screenings. Suboptimal adherence is at least partly a function of the US health care system itself, which provides no national organized screening, and which provides only scattered pockets of screening organized by health care plans. Where organized screening is found, adherence rates of about 80% have been documented.

A second phenomenon that remains poorly understood is a steady increase in CRC incidence and mortality in birth cohorts born in the United States and several other countries after about 1970. The drivers of this change have not yet been revealed with any certainty, but the rising incidence is the subject of intense investigation.

Finally, how screening should be done remains the subject of much discussion. In organized screening, the fecal immunochemical test (FIT) seems to nearly always be preferred. In the opportunistic setting, colonoscopy still dominates US screening, and the quality movement in colonoscopy has produced steady gains in overall performance and length of protection from cancer. FIT can be difficult to use in the opportunistic setting, because the resources to achieve adherence to annual testing are usually not present. The FIT-fecal DNA assay has the advantages in this setting of the need to test every three years (rather than every one year with FIT), improved performance over FIT particularly for serrated lesions, and an effective navigation program for persons who have the test ordered. We have also learned the impact of widespread direct-to-consumer marketing on CRC screening from the FIT-fecal DNA test.

Gastrointest Endoscopy Clin N Am 30 (2020) xv–xvi
https://doi.org/10.1016/j.giec.2020.04.001
1052-5157/20/© 2020 Published by Elsevier Inc.

giendo.theclinics.com

All of these issues and many others related to screening are covered in this update. Many thanks to the authors of these articles for their expertise and time in creating this issue of *Gastrointestinal Endoscopy Clinics of North America*. I'm confident you'll find this an excellent update and reference on CRC screening in 2020.

Douglas K. Rex, MD, MACP, MACG, FASGE, AGAF
Division of Gastroenterology/Hepatology
Indiana University School of Medicine
550 North University Boulevard
Suite 4100
Indianapolis, IN 46202, USA

E-mail address:
drex@iu.edu

Proven Strategies for Increasing Adherence to Colorectal Cancer Screening

Lynn F. Butterly, MD*

KEYWORDS

- Colorectal cancer screening • Adherence • Screening interventions
- Patient navigation • Colonoscopy • FOBT • FIT

KEY POINTS

- Colorectal cancer (CRC) is preventable through screening and surveillance, but approximately 35% of eligible individuals in the United States remain unscreened.
- Adherence is critical to the effectiveness of colorectal cancer screening tests.
- Review of extensive literature addressing adherence suggests that patient navigation and direct outreach (active distribution) of fecal occult blood tests are the 2 most promising interventions to increase adherence.
- Many interventions have been shown to offer variable rates of success in improving adherence to CRC screening; it is essential for screening programs and providers to consider and implement those interventions that are feasible and most likely to increase adherence for their specific patient populations.

INTRODUCTION

Despite being one of the few cancers that can be prevented, colorectal cancer (CRC) remains the second most common cause of death from cancer in the United States.[1] Screening and surveillance have been proved to be highly effective in preventing CRC as well as in increasing early detection[2-4]; as a result, CRC screening has received an "A" grade from the evidence-based US Preventive Services Task Force[3] (USPSTF), and worldwide efforts to increase CRC screening rates are underway.

A major factor in the effectiveness of any screening modality is adherence, which measures the proportion of eligible individuals who have complied with recommended testing.[5] Low adherence rates undermine the effectiveness of any screening strategy; this impact becomes increasingly pronounced for modalities requiring more frequent retesting. In addition to its significant impact on clinical outcomes, adherence must be

Geisel School of Medicine at Dartmouth, Dartmouth-Hitchcock Medical Center, Lebanon, NH 03756, USA
* Corresponding author. New Hampshire Colonoscopy Registry, Evergreen Building, Centerra Plaza, Lebanon, NH 03756.
E-mail address: Lynn.Butterly@Hitchcock.org

Gastrointest Endoscopy Clin N Am 30 (2020) 377–392
https://doi.org/10.1016/j.giec.2020.02.003   **giendo.theclinics.com**

considered when assessing the effectiveness of alternative screening modalities in comparison to colonoscopy.[6] The models that support USPSTF recommendations assume 100% adherence, and other modeling studies have suggested that adherence rates of at least 65% to 70% would be required in order for any stool- or blood-based screening modality to match the benefits of colonoscopy.[6] Adherence considerations—and interventions to improve adherence—must be integral to the selection and implementation of test options within any screening program, in order to optimize screening and surveillance outcomes.

The USPSTF has described several strategies for CRC screening.[3] It is estimated that in 2016 approximately 67% of eligible individuals in the United States had been screened for CRC per the recommended intervals,[7] up from 65.5% in 2012.[8] However, an estimated 23 million guideline appropriate adults remain unscreened.[9,10] Screening rates are lower for underserved individuals, such as low-income, uninsured, and minority populations, who face additional barriers with fewer resources through which to overcome those barriers. Socioeconomic factors including degree of education, literacy, income, and ethnicity have all been shown to affect screening uptake.[11–15] Although the United States has seen improvement in access to and utilization of CRC screening over the past few decades, it is clear that adherence remains an issue, one that is even more critical in light of significant disparities that exist throughout the country and the world.

A significant number of CRC deaths in the United States have been attributed to lack of screening.[16] Therefore, to decrease morbidity and mortality from CRC, it is a critical public health imperative to increase adherence, using interventions that address the many known barriers. The following is a review of barriers to adherence, and a description of various interventions to address those barriers, including what is known about the effectiveness of those interventions.

INTERVENTIONS TO INCREASE ADHERENCE

Several barriers affect adherence to CRC screening, including *patient barriers* such as lack of understanding, inaccurate perception of CRC risk, or lack of a provider recommendation,[17–20] as well as difficulties with transportation, language, and cultural issues and cost concerns including time off work; *provider barriers* such as lack of knowledge about CRC screening guidelines, lack of communicating a recommendation to patients, or lack of appropriate individual risk assessment and communication of those risks[21]; and *system barriers* such as scheduling issues and communication gaps that contribute to low rates of return for fecal immunochemical testing (FIT) (eg, lack of patient understanding of the communicated instructions) or lack of appropriate clinical systems (tracking) to ensure follow-up testing after positive results, as well as the frequency of colonoscopy no-shows and poor bowel preps (which consistently undermine successful colonoscopy). All barriers lower adherence and must be addressed to optimize the effectiveness and value of CRC screening and surveillance.

It should be noted that CRC screening is usually not a single event but rather a process that must be repeated at appropriate intervals. Therefore, it is important not only to consider adherence interventions for *first-time screening* but in addition for *ongoing screening* (eg, annual repeat of fecal occult blood tests [FOBT], repeat multitarget stool DNA (mt-sDNA) at 3-year intervals, CTC at 5-year intervals, and repeat colonoscopy at 10-year intervals for average-risk individuals with a negative test, or as per the specific colonoscopy findings and patient risk). Furthermore, a critically important aspect of CRC screening is ensuring that colonoscopy is done for individuals with a *positive test by any other modality*. In terms of decreasing CRC, there is no clinical effectiveness provided to individuals who undergo FOBT, have a positive result, and then do not have a subsequent colonoscopy to find and remove any potential source of occult bleeding.

Multiple interventions to improve adherence have been studied, with variable degrees of success. These interventions include patient navigation, patient reminders, provider reminders, reducing structural barriers such as transportation and language issues, providing assessment and feedback on screening rates to providers, provider education on screening guidelines, ensuring a provider recommendation for screening is given to patients, improving patient education about the procedure (and for colonoscopy, education about the prep as well), active outreach for FOBT for average-risk patients, discussing and providing options (patient choice) for screening when appropriate, financial incentives, and combinations of interventions. Studies have attempted to evaluate these and other interventions, as discussed later. A recent comprehensive systematic review of 73 randomized clinical trials concluded that FOBT outreach and patient navigation, particularly using multicomponent interventions, were associated with increased rates of CRC screening in US trials.[22]

It should be noted that although there may be some cost to most interventions to increase adherence, *effective* strategies will likely be *cost-effective* as well, when accounting for the health care savings derived from lives (and productivity) saved through the prevention of CRC, as well as decreased costs attributable to cancer care. In the United States the cost of treating CRC ranges from $14 to 17 billion dollars per year,[23] with costs continuing to increase as new cancer drugs are developed. Financial cost of lost productivity from CRC was estimated to be an additional $12 billion in 2010.[24]

GENERAL CATEGORIES OF EVIDENCE-BASED INTERVENTIONS APPLICABLE FOR ALL SCREENING MODALITIES
Patient and Provider Reminders

Reminders can be effective interventions to increase adherence for all screening modalities, and are 2 of the evidence-based interventions (EBIs) recommended in the Guide to Community Preventive Services, (the Community Guide) at *https://www.thecommmunityguide.org/topic/cancer*, created by the Department of Health and Human Services supported by the Centers for Disease Control and Prevention (CDC). Other EBIs include *reducing structural barriers* (such as transportation and limited clinic hours) and using *provider assessment and feedback*; small media resources (such as brochures and posters) are also helpful.

Patient reminders (and all EBIs) can be used in many different ways, depending on the screening modality and clinical setting. In addition to opportunistic communication (during in-person visits), mailed reminders, educational contact with patients, inviting patients to call to request screening tests, personal phone calls from staff, videotape and Web-based decision aids, automated patient reminders, and combinations of interventions have also been shown to result in some increase in screening compared with usual care, usually with greater effectiveness for combined strategies.[25–36] Giving patients options (eg, a choice between FOBT and colonoscopy) has been shown to increase adherence[37]; furthermore, specific screening test preferences have been shown to vary among racial/ethnic groups and should be individually evaluated.[11] Studies have also proposed "mHealth" (mobile) apps to increase adherence,[38] with some reported success.

Provider reminders are often provided by office staff processes or EMR notification systems. Implementing provider reminders through EMR systems within integrated systems has been noted to be a promising, low-cost intervention.[39–42] Giving providers a list of their average-risk adult patients who are not up-to-date with CRC screening has also been shown to have a small but significant increase in adherence to FIT screening at 1 year compared with usual care.[43] One study of provider strategies to increase adherence concluded that several individual PCP strategies (such as EMR use, reminders, creating lists, feedback reports, or using designated staff) had little effect, but the use of *multiple* strategies did seem to improve adherence with CRC screening.[44]

INTERVENTIONS TO INCREASE ADHERENCE, BY SCREENING MODALITY

Because barriers to adherence vary by screening option, the following will address barriers and potential solutions for the critical aspects of each of several CRC screening options. Some interventions apply to all screening options. Interventions to address adherence for test options not yet guideline approved[3,45] or not in general use are not discussed due to extremely limited evidence available to inform those assessments.

Colonoscopy

Colonoscopy is the most commonly used CRC screening test in the United States and is used to interrupt the "polyp to cancer sequence." Unlike screening modalities for most other cancers that can only provide early detection of cancer (such as mammography), CRC screening including colonoscopy is one of the few cancer screening options that affords the opportunity for *prevention*. If polyps are discovered and removed within the approximately 10- to 15-year period during which a polyp may undergo multiple mutations and develop into a colorectal cancer, that cancer can potentially be prevented, in addition to earlier discovery if a cancer is already present.

Improving adherence to colonoscopy requires attention to all stages of the screening process, from the provider recommendation through patient education, prep instructions, scheduling, presenting for and undergoing a high-quality colonoscopy, and receiving appropriate recommendations for follow-up; barriers can occur at any of those stages and must be addressed. Interventions for colonoscopy (other than the extensive prep instructions) would also apply to sigmoidoscopy, which is recommended for CRC screening at 10-year intervals (if normal) in conjunction with annual FIT. Potential interventions for each of these stages of the screening process, and overall, are discussed later.

Interventions

Provider recommendation Several studies have demonstrated that lack of a provider recommendation is one of the major reasons patients do not undergo colonoscopy (or other screening).[18,46] Therefore, a focus by both providers and their support staff on techniques to ensure that patients receive a recommendation for screening is a straightforward means to address this issue. EMR and chart reminders or pended orders for testing, "flags" placed by staff on patient charts while rooming patients or review during morning "huddles," meetings, or chart review, as well as posters and other patient education resources suggesting that patients ask their providers about screening can all be effective reminders to ensure a recommendation is made.

Similarly, ensuring provider recommendations for ongoing screening or for follow-up colonoscopy after a positive screening by another modality is key to adherence. Providing PCPs with a (pocket-sized) synopsis of CRC guidelines for screening and surveillance, or having easily accessible links to this information within the EMR, can be helpful in saving PCPs time in ensuring that their recommendations accurately incorporate patient history and individual risks based on current guidelines.

Patient education Patients must be educated about all CRC screening options, particularly colonoscopy, because it is more complex, in order to comply with testing. Although it is difficult for a single provider to comprehensively review all aspects of screening with eligible patients, an approach that includes all or most of the support staff to varying degrees can be highly effective. Small media also may be helpful and cost-effective. Brochures about the importance of screening and cancer prevention that are handed out by receptionists (or available through displays) as patients check in, continuous loop videos or public service announcements (PSAs) about screening displayed in the waiting area, mention of screening by nurses or medical assistants as patients are brought to examination rooms, handouts or prewritten "scripts" that briefly review screening information and can be given out or verbally communicated by medical personnel, posters in waiting rooms, offices, or on the backs of examination room doors, and patient questionnaires that also provide information are all examples of resources that help to educate the patient before contact with the provider, who can reinforce the information provided and help the patient choose and agree to a particular screening modality. Patient education is especially important for colonoscopy, because the patient has to be willing and able to comply with both the prep and the procedure.

Prep information A major barrier to colonoscopy is successful completion of the prep, without which a quality colonoscopy is not possible. Therefore, strategies to effectively communicate prep instructions to patients are essential. These strategies include using prep instructions written at an appropriate educational level, translation into other languages, graphic (cartoon drawings) instructions that do not require reading of text, and video instructions (eg, *https://www.youtube.com Dartmouth-Hitchcock Colonoscopy Prep*) that avoid the need to rely only on written instructions. Several interventions including navigation, patient reminder calls, letters, and EMR reminders, text messaging, and electronic reminder systems have been reported to be variably effective in supporting patients through prep completion.

Scheduling Screening centers and programs must be able to reach patients to schedule. Particularly for disadvantaged people with limited phone minutes, it is important for colonoscopy schedulers to have the correct phone numbers, times to call, and alternative contacts. One aspect of scheduling that is often reported as a barrier is the need for a ride home, which is frequently mandated by endoscopy centers for patients who have received sedation. A helpful distinction is that, although patients should have someone to accompany them home, the companion/escort does not need to be able to drive, have a car, or meet any qualifications other than being older than 18 years and able to responsibly accompany the patient. Other means of transportation may be acceptable to the endoscopy center if the patient is accompanied. Another scheduling barrier negatively affecting adherence is the presence of long delays in scheduling; this issue should be addressed through the implementation of efficiencies within and connecting to the endoscopy unit, which are extensively reviewed elsewhere.

Receiving results and recommendations for follow-up The provision of results and recommendations for appropriate follow-up, to *both* the patient and the PCP is a critical part of the screening process. A major barrier to adherence, particularly for patients served in federally qualified health centers, is lack of this important communication. A PCP may order a colonoscopy and then never know whether the test was actually done, much less what the results and accompanying recommendations are. Clearly, this breakdown in communication has a substantial negative impact on appropriate ongoing CRC screening, especially because tracking down the information can be exceedingly time consuming. Establishing feasible processes to ensure communication with patients and their PCPs is vital to delivery of any effective screening program. Reminder/support processes for providers (PCPs and endoscopists) can also be extremely useful in ensuring ongoing screening and can include, for example, adding specific colonoscopy findings or CRC risk assessment (ie, noting whether the patient is at average, increased, or high risk for CRC) to the patient's problem list (so those assessments can consistently be accessed), or, after a colonoscopy, scheduling future PCP appointments or follow-up colonoscopy at the anticipated interval (if appropriate) will help ensure patient interaction at the appropriate future times.

Other issues All interventions, including those listed earlier, must account for general barriers, such as difficulties with language (phone translation services are often available but require skill to use effectively, written translation may require funding), transportation (many areas have free or shared ride services available), time off work (engaging with employers can help to address this issue), and cultural issues (eg, sex of the provider, which may need to be assessed before scheduling).

Patient navigation The most effective intervention and the only one able to address all or most barriers is patient navigation, which encompasses many of the other interventions discussed earlier. Since its introduction in 1990 by Harold Freeman to improve breast cancer care for low-income women in Harlem, NYC,[47,48] patient navigation has been shown to be effective for several areas of medical care, including access to cancer treatment and screening for cancers, including CRC. As noted earlier, it is 1 of only 2 interventions found to be effective in a recent comprehensive meta-analysis of 73 randomized clinical trials investigating interventions to increase CRC screening.[22] The investigators concluded that FOBT outreach and navigation each substantially increased CRC screening rates in US trials.[22]

Navigation is best defined as individualized assistance to help patients identify and overcome personal and health system barriers to care,[47] which thereby improves adherence to health care processes such as CRC screening. One highly successful navigation model was developed and implemented by the New Hampshire Colorectal Cancer Screening Program (NHCRCSP) in 2009 (https://wwwcdc.gov/cancer/crccp/pdf/nhcrcsp_pn_manual.pdf). Funded through a statewide CDC grant program,[49] over several years the NHCRCSP provided free colonoscopies to low-income, uninsured, or underinsured individuals throughout NH. All patients were navigated, using registered nurses as navigators because medical considerations are involved in assessment and preparation for colonoscopy (eg, comorbid conditions, anticoagulation status, allergies). However, other types of health care professionals, lay individuals, and "peer navigators" can all be used successfully, depending on the *specific outcome and target population* for which the navigation is used. Several, although not all, studies of navigation for CRC screening have shown an increase in completion of screening compared with usual care[50–55]

The NHCRCSP navigated approximately 2000 patients living throughout NH to— and through— colonoscopy, using a 6-topic protocol specifically tailored to ensuring successful completion of colonoscopy. Navigation was delivered telephonically by 2 NHCRCSP navigators (one full time equivalency [FTE] and one 0.2 FTE). All patients were low income (up to 250% of the federal poverty guideline), uninsured, and some were homeless. The prep instructions were translated into 26 languages to serve the ethnically diverse population, and navigators became adept at using telephone language translation services.

Outcomes of the program revealed a high success rate for the navigation intervention. There were only 2 "no-shows" for the approximately 2000 colonoscopies (0.1% no-show rate). Nationally, no-show rates can be as high as 25% to 40%, the latter rate found in underserved populations.[56,57] In addition, less than 1% of patients had an inadequate bowel prep, compared with a reported 25% nationally,[58,59] and 100% of patients *and their PCPs* received results of the colonoscopy as well as recommendations for follow-up and rescreening. Program staff also interacted with endoscopists to ensure that follow-up recommendations were guideline appropriate, and before the start of the program agreement was gained from hospitals associated with the contracted endoscopy centers to provide free cancer care for any patient for whom CRC was identified through the program, as well as for any complications of colonoscopy. These services were also delivered successfully and with ongoing navigation.

In addition to successful completion of colonoscopy, the NHCRCSP navigation program evaluated all patients before entry in the program to ensure that they were actually due for colonoscopy and that it was medically appropriate. All patients were navigated to a PCP visit or to a new PCP in cases where this relationship did not yet exist, to ensure that colonoscopy was medically appropriate for them. Patients were also counseled on how to navigate the health care system beyond simply receiving a screening colonoscopy, in order to ensure better ongoing health care after their interaction with navigation, and additionally were referred to smoking cessation, other cancer screening options, and other services identified as needed by their navigator. Program outcomes highlighted the remarkable potential effectiveness of navigation and were underscored by the universal appreciation of participants for their navigators.

Because of its success, the CDC undertook a formal evaluation of the program, including a comparison study evaluating outcomes for similar patients who underwent colonoscopy with and without navigation at the same center. This study compared patients who were navigated (the subgroup of NHCRCSP patients receiving care at the chosen center) and those not navigated (controls). The comparison evaluation showed that navigated patients were 11 times more likely to complete colonoscopy and almost 6 times more likely to have an adequate bowel preparation than the usual care patients. None of the navigated patients in this comparison study missed an appointment (were "no-shows") versus 15.6% of the usual care control patients, and less than 1% of navigated patients canceled within 24 hours of the scheduled colonoscopy, compared with 16% of the control group patients.[60] Of note, similar to the navigation process, usual care in this setting also consisted of multiple calls with patients (often a higher number of calls than were offered by the navigator) before the procedure. However, the difference in outcomes between the 2 groups demonstrates that it is the *content* of the calls and the *relationship with the patient created by the navigator*—rather than the number of contacts with the patient—that was able to achieve these results.

A subsequent NHCRCSP cost-effectiveness study[61] confirmed the cost-effectiveness of navigation that also has been shown in other studies.[62,63] Navigation can be delivered in a variety of settings; endoscopy centers may be the most *cost-effective* setting for navigation. Endoscopy centers cannot fill a patient colonoscopy slot in the last minute for patients who do not show up (lost revenue), but the medical staff, all equipment, procedure room, cleaning equipment, lights, and all other costs nonetheless remain. The significant decrease in no-show rates and in the need for repeat testing due to inadequate preps that can be achieved by navigation more than makes up for the costs of navigation in terms of the significant loss of billing within endoscopy centers due to both those events.

The CDC and the NHCRCSP also developed a Replication Manual for the NHCRCSP patient navigation model, available through the Dartmouth, CDC,[64] and National Cancer Institute (NCI) Research Tested Intervention Programs (RTIPS) Websites, which can be freely accessed by other navigation programs.

FECAL OCCULT BLOOD TEST

FOBT can be done via guaiac-based testing (gFOBT) or FIT. The former involves an oxidative chemical reaction with hydrogen peroxide (in the developer), for which hemoglobin acts as an enzyme (pseudoperoxidase) to catalyze the reaction (thereby revealing the presence of hemoglobin if the color blue is revealed on the stool card), whereas FIT involves an antibody reaction to the globin moiety of hemoglobin. FIT is specific for human hemoglobin, thereby avoiding the dietary and medication interactions that have made completion of gFOBT more complex, and thereby improving adherence with FIT. Studies have demonstrated a 7% to 10% increase in uptake of FIT over gFOBT due to greater ease of use as well as improved sensitivity.[65,66]

However, not all FITS are alike, and using an evidence-based kit is important to ensuring appropriate sensitivity and specificity, thereby achieving the appropriate outcomes. If FIT sensitivity is higher than optimal, for example, the additional positive results will create the need for colonoscopies that might otherwise have been unnecessary, potentially exposing patients to avoidable risks.

Interventions

Direct mailing
A widely used intervention is mailing information or invitations for screening to patients, which can be very effective in increasing adherence compared with usual care.[67] Electronic invitations when available have been effective as well.[34]

Active distribution
The use of *active distribution of FIT kits*, implemented to overcome access barriers, has been used with reported success.[22,68–70] This intervention involves providing FIT kits to patients either through a mass mailing, during office visits, or in conjunction with another intervention, such as in combination with the provision of flu shots.[6,71] Studies have shown variable degrees of success compared with usual care. An additional consideration for use of active distribution is that FOBT is appropriate for average-risk patients but not for individuals undergoing surveillance (ie, having a personal history of CRC or potentially precancerous polyps) or those with strong family histories of CRC or potentially precancerous polyps. Therefore, any program using mailing or other active distribution of FIT kits should ensure that the appropriate patient groups are the ones receiving this outreach.

Office distribution
FIT kits are often distributed during *office* (provider) visits. Adherence with this screening modality can be improved through the following strategies:

- *Providing options for screening:* offering average-risk patients a choice of options for CRC screening, rather than simply recommending colonoscopy, has been shown to be effective in increasing adherence.[11]
- *Providing adequate instruction for use:* identifying and training specific staff (or laboratory personnel) responsible for providing kits to patients can ensure that patients receive accurate and complete instructions for the use of the FIT kits (or any screening modality). Patients are often reluctant to inquire in detail, and if the written or graphic instructions are not immediately obvious, they may

end up not returning the test simply due to the absence of simple, clear instructions on what to do. Staff interacting with patients should be familiar with all the contents of the FIT kit itself (or the mt-sDNA carton) so that they can accurately explain (and demonstrate) to patients how to use the test kit.

- *Ensuring provision of FITs that are not expired* or due to expire imminently: health centers should have an established process to review expiration dates and ensure that patients are not given kits that are expired or due to expire before the patient is likely to complete them; results from expired kits should be discarded and require repeat testing.
- *Increasing return of FIT kits:* adherence can be increased by *labeling the tube* for the patient, *providing postage* on the return envelope (an important barrier for some patients), *labeling the return envelope* with the return address, *including clear graphic (picture or "cartoon") instructions* with the kits, including a *"return by" date* to create a timeline for compliance, and use of *patient reminders* such as postcards, letters, and/or calls if the kits are not returned within a specified period of time. Tracking and reporting systems (via EMR or other options) should be in place at health centers to ensure reports can be obtained to identify patients with incomplete (unreturned) tests.

Financial incentives

Financial incentives have been shown to have only moderate, if any, effectiveness[72,73]; the potential rewards to patients may need to be quite high (and therefore costly overall) in order to have an effect on adherence. However, the availability of incentives does not seem to lead to an increase in inappropriate screening.[74]

Health fairs/special events

Although available evidence is limited, there is anecdotal and some published evidence to suggest some benefit from these events,[75] especially when held in geographic areas targeting underserved individuals. In addition to providing the opportunity to communicate with people who might otherwise have little or no interaction with medical providers or information, my personal experience having organized dozens of these events is that significant numbers of screening tests (including colonoscopy) follow each of these events, because event personnel are often able to encourage hesitant people by increasing their understanding of the importance of CRC screening and successfully motivate them to comply with testing.

Referral of positive fecal immunochemical testings for colonoscopy

Two critical steps in the FIT screening process are *referral of patients with positive FIT for colonoscopy* and *documenting successful completion of colonoscopy,* both of which are *essential* to prevention and early detection of CRC (the goal of CRC screening). Unfortunately, referral of individuals with positive screening tests for colonoscopy continues to be affected by significant gaps in care, resulting in increased risk of death from CRC.[76] Worldwide, FIT is the most commonly used screening test, but its effectiveness is negated when patients with a positive result fail to successfully complete colonoscopy. It has generally been estimated that nationally only about 50% to 60% of patients with positive FITS complete a colonoscopy. Given the clinical significance conferred by a positive FIT (or other noncolonoscopy screening modality), this is an aspect of health care for which additional interventions must be designed. Specifically, health systems must have tracking systems in place to ensure that data on *completion* of screening (ie, performance of colonoscopy) is captured and adherence increased for those colonoscopies.

Patient and provider reminders as discussed earlier have both been successful in increasing colonoscopy adherence after a positive FIT, together with other strategies as outlined in the colonoscopy section (discussed earlier). A few studies of *provider reminders (eg, electronic reminders)* have noted significant improvement in colonoscopy completion after positive FIT.[39,40,42] Other interventions to address this care gap, including types of navigation and giving performance data to providers, have been investigated.[41] Nonetheless, evidence to guide system-level interventions is limited and currently insufficient.[41] In addition, as with all colonoscopy scheduling, avoidance of long scheduling delays is important both for patient adherence, as well as for the outcome at colonoscopy; delays have been reported to be associated with risk of CRC and more advanced stage at colonoscopy.[77]

Annual repetition of testing

Several studies have investigated strategies to increase adherence to annual repetition of FOBTs, an area known to have high rates of nonadherence. Interventions have included mailed reminders, free FITs, automated phone and text messaging, interactive telephone reminders, and navigation.[27,37,69,78] Although screening with FIT has many appealing features, the fact that annual repetition is key to its effectiveness is a major consideration, because adherence with retesting has often been poor outside of clinical trials.[9,79] A recent trial of annual FIT testing reported a 46% completion of FIT in the first year and 41% in the patients' second year.[80] One outreach intervention for underserved subjects revealed that long-term compliance with FIT tests was lower than the initial uptake for colonoscopy.[81] Patients in a 3-year trial who were given a *choice* between FOBT and colonoscopy continued to have fairly high adherence in subsequent years, whereas adherence for patients randomized to the FOBT group decreased sharply to levels less than that for the choice and colonoscopy groups; patient navigation was noted to be critical to sustaining CRC screening, particularly with FOBT.[82] However, another study reported a very high adherence to FIT over 4 years within their organized health plan.[83] Therefore, screening programs using FIT should prospectively plan for, and maintain implementation of, interventions to improve ongoing annual adherence (such as offering choices and using reminders) as part of their screening policies and processes, in order to avoid this major clinical pitfall as much as possible.

COLOGUARD

The use of mt-sDNA (Cologuard) has increased significantly in the past few years. Testing involves several molecular markers that are shed into the stool by CRC and polyps, as well as fecal immunochemical testing, and is repeated every 3 years if negative. Patients with positive results must be referred for colonoscopy.

Interventions

Ordering process

Health systems and practices must have *an established process* in place to provide the PCP order (and patient insurance or other information) to Exact Sciences, because all kits are sent to patients from, and are developed by, Exact Sciences Corporation in Madison, Wisconsin. It is not uncommon for PCPs to believe that writing an order for Cologuard is sufficient to ensure its completion at their health center; this may not be the case if there is no established process to reliably communicate the request to Exact Sciences. A process for transmitting the information confidentially to Exact Sciences and identification and training of individuals responsible for that transmission are necessary. Similarly, a process must be established for test results (which are reported as positive or negative) to be provided to the health center/providers by Exact Sciences.

Return reminders
Exact Sciences uses navigators to contact patients who have not returned kits mailed to them by Exact Sciences; these navigators have been effective in increasing the return rates. Nonetheless, providers or health centers can expand this intervention through the addition of their own patient reminders. Provider reminders are essential to recognizing and improving adherence for patients with incomplete testing, both in terms of return of the mt-sDNA kit and, critically, in terms of referral to colonoscopy for those with positive results.

Rescreening and follow-up of positive test
Similarly, patient and provider reminders may be helpful for repeat testing in 3 years if the initial test is negative; ordering a PCP visit and/or a repeat mt-sDNA at a 3-year interval may also improve adherence to screening. As with FIT, it is critically important for all positive tests to be followed by a colonoscopy in a reasonable time interval; the interventions to increase adherence noted earlier also apply to this screening modality.

COMPUTED TOMOGRAPHIC COLONOGRAPHY

Computed tomographic colonography (CTC), also known as "virtual colonoscopy" is another CRC screening test recommended by the USPSTF for average-risk patients. Although issues such as cost-effectiveness have limited its use to some degree, CTC has been shown to have high sensitivity and is preferred by some patients over optical colonoscopy.[84,85] As with other screening modalities, however, a positive test must be followed by a colonoscopy to remove lesions reported on CTC. Therefore, adherence to both the initial test and either follow-up rescreening (in 5 years for normal examinations) or colonoscopy for positive tests should be a focus of care for patients screened by CTC, and adherence interventions described earlier would be useful.

In summary, interventions to increase adherence to CRC screening have been extensively reported, including multiple randomized trials. The 2 methodologies that have most clearly been shown to be effective are active outreach for FOBT and patient navigation. Although navigation has been variably defined and implemented, it is clear that navigation models exist that can achieve remarkable success in improving adherence to screening. It will be important to expand on these successes and to recognize that adherence to CRC screening is a goal that *can* be realized, thereby leading to decreased morbidity and mortality from CRC and improved public health.

ACKNOWLEDGMENTS

Many thanks to Christina M. Robinson, M.S. for her review and editing of the article and to Gail Sullivan, R.N. for her review.

REFERENCES

1. National Cancer Institute. Cancer stat facts: colorectal cancer. 2017. Available at: https://seer.cancer.gov/statfacts/html.colorect.html.
2. Zauber AG, Winawer SJ, O'Brien MJ, et al. Colonoscopic polypectomy and long-term prevention of colorectal-cancer deaths. N Engl J Med 2012;366: 687–96.

3. Bibbins-Domingo K, Grossman DC, Curry SJ, et al. Screening for colorectal cancer: US preventive services task force recommendation statement. JAMA 2016; 315:2564–75.
4. Brenner H, Stock C, Hoffmeister M. Effect of screening sigmoidoscopy and screening colonoscopy on colorectal cancer incidence and mortality: systematic review and meta-analysis of randomised controlled trials and observational studies. BMJ 2014;348:g2467.
5. Hassan C, Kaminski MF, Repici A. How to ensure patient adherence to colorectal cancer screening and surveillance in your practice. Gastroenterology 2018;155: 252–7.
6. D'Andrea E, Ahnen DJ, Sussman DA, et al. Quantifying the impact of adherence to screening strategies on colorectal cancer incidence and mortality. Cancer Med 2019;9(2):824–36.
7. Joseph DA, King JB, Richards TB, et al. Use of colorectal cancer screening tests by state. Prev Chronic Dis 2018;15:E80.
8. Smith RA, Andrews KS, Brooks D, et al. Cancer screening in the United States, 2017: a review of current American Cancer Society guidelines and current issues in cancer screening. CA Cancer J Clin 2017;67:100–21.
9. Winawer SJ, Fischer SE, Levin B. Evidence-based, reality-driven colorectal cancer screening guidelines: the critical relationship of adherence to effectiveness. Jama 2016;315:2065–6.
10. Centers for Disease Control and Prevention (CDC). Vital signs: colorectal cancer screening test use–United States, 2012. MMWR Morb Mortal Wkly Rep 2013;62: 881–8.
11. Inadomi JM, Vijan S, Janz NK, et al. Adherence to colorectal cancer screening: a randomized clinical trial of competing strategies. Arch Intern Med 2012;172: 575–82.
12. Liss DT, Baker DW. Understanding current racial/ethnic disparities in colorectal cancer screening in the United States: the contribution of socioeconomic status and access to care. Am J Prev Med 2014;46:228–36.
13. May FP, Bromley EG, Reid MW, et al. Low uptake of colorectal cancer screening among African Americans in an integrated Veterans Affairs health care network. Gastrointest Endosc 2014;80:291–8.
14. Seibert RG, Hanchate AD, Berz JP, et al. National disparities in colorectal cancer screening among obese adults. Am J Prev Med 2017;53:e41–9.
15. Senore C, Armaroli P, Silvani M, et al. Comparing different strategies for colorectal cancer screening in Italy: predictors of patients' participation. Am J Gastroenterol 2010;105:188–98.
16. Meester RG, Doubeni CA, Lansdorp-Vogelaar I, et al. Colorectal cancer deaths attributable to nonuse of screening in the United States. Ann Epidemiol 2015; 25:208–13.e1.
17. Boguradzka A, Wiszniewski M, Kaminski MF, et al. The effect of primary care physician counseling on participation rate and use of sedation in colonoscopy-based colorectal cancer screening program–a randomized controlled study. Scand J Gastroenterol 2014;49:878–84.
18. Bromley EG, May FP, Federer L, et al. Explaining persistent under-use of colonoscopic cancer screening in African Americans: a systematic review. Prev Med 2015;71:40–8.
19. Hong YR, Tauscher J, Cardel M. Distrust in health care and cultural factors are associated with uptake of colorectal cancer screening in Hispanic and Asian Americans. Cancer 2018;124:335–45.

20. Klabunde CN, Vernon SW, Nadel MR, et al. Barriers to colorectal cancer screening: a comparison of reports from primary care physicians and average-risk adults. Med Care 2005;43:939–44.

21. Kinney AY, Boonyasiriwat W, Walters ST, et al. Telehealth personalized cancer risk communication to motivate colonoscopy in relatives of patients with colorectal cancer: the family CARE Randomized controlled trial. J Clin Oncol 2014;32: 654–62.

22. Dougherty MK, Brenner AT, Crockett SD, et al. Evaluation of interventions intended to increase colorectal cancer screening rates in the United States: a systematic review and meta-analysis. JAMA Intern Med 2018;178:1645–58.

23. Mariotto AB, Yabroff KR, Shao Y, et al. Projections of the cost of cancer care in the United States: 2010-2020. J Natl Cancer Inst 2011;103:117–28.

24. Elkin EB, Shapiro E, Snow JG, et al. The economic impact of a patient navigator program to increase screening colonoscopy. Cancer 2012;118:5982–8.

25. Cameron KA, Persell SD, Brown T, et al. Patient outreach to promote colorectal cancer screening among patients with an expired order for colonoscopy: a randomized controlled trial. Arch Intern Med 2011;171:642–6.

26. Coronado GD, Rivelli JS, Fuoco MJ, et al. Effect of reminding patients to complete fecal immunochemical testing: a comparative effectiveness study of automated and live approaches. J Gen Intern Med 2018;33:72–8.

27. Green BB, Wang CY, Anderson ML, et al. An automated intervention with stepped increases in support to increase uptake of colorectal cancer screening: a randomized trial. Ann Intern Med 2013;158:301–11.

28. Menon U, Belue R, Wahab S, et al. A randomized trial comparing the effect of two phone-based interventions on colorectal cancer screening adherence. Ann Behav Med 2011;42:294–303.

29. Miller DP Jr, Spangler JG, Case LD, et al. Effectiveness of a web-based colorectal cancer screening patient decision aid: a randomized controlled trial in a mixed-literacy population. Am J Prev Med 2011;40:608–15.

30. Mosen DM, Feldstein AC, Perrin N, et al. Automated telephone calls improved completion of fecal occult blood testing. Med Care 2010;48:604–10.

31. Pignone M, Harris R, Kinsinger L. Videotape-based decision aid for colon cancer screening. A randomized, controlled trial. Ann Intern Med 2000;133:761–9.

32. Reuland DS, Brenner AT, Hoffman R, et al. Effect of combined patient decision aid and patient navigation vs usual care for colorectal cancer screening in a vulnerable patient population: a randomized clinical trial. JAMA Intern Med 2017;177: 967–74.

33. Schroy PC 3rd, Emmons KM, Peters E, et al. Aid-assisted decision making and colorectal cancer screening: a randomized controlled trial. Am J Prev Med 2012;43:573–83.

34. Sequist TD, Zaslavsky AM, Colditz GA, et al. Electronic patient messages to promote colorectal cancer screening: a randomized controlled trial. Arch Intern Med 2011;171:636–41.

35. Weinberg DS, Keenan E, Ruth K, et al. A randomized comparison of print and web communication on colorectal cancer screening. JAMA Intern Med 2013; 173:122–9.

36. Mankaney G, Rizk M, Sarvepalli S, et al. Patient-initiated colonoscopy scheduling effectively increases colorectal cancer screening adherence. Dig Dis Sci 2019; 64:2497–504.

37. Wong MC, Ching JY, Huang J, et al. Effectiveness of reminder strategies on cancer screening adherence: a randomised controlled trial. Br J Gen Pract 2018;68: e604–11.

38. Griffin L, Lee D, Jaisle A, et al. Creating an mHealth App for colorectal cancer screening: user-centered design approach. JMIR Hum Factors 2019;6:e12700.

39. Larson MF, Ko CW, Dominitz JA. Effectiveness of a provider reminder on fecal occult blood test follow-up. Dig Dis Sci 2009;54:1991–6.

40. Murphy DR, Wu L, Thomas EJ, et al. Electronic trigger-based intervention to reduce delays in diagnostic evaluation for cancer: a cluster randomized controlled trial. J Clin Oncol 2015;33:3560–7.

41. Selby K, Baumgartner C, Levin TR, et al. Interventions to improve follow-up of positive results on fecal blood tests: a systematic review. Ann Intern Med 2017; 167:565–75.

42. Myers RE, Turner B, Weinberg D, et al. Impact of a physician-oriented intervention on follow-up in colorectal cancer screening. Prev Med 2004;38:375–81.

43. Rat C, Pogu C, Le Donne D, et al. Effect of physician notification regarding nonadherence to colorectal cancer screening on patient participation in fecal immunochemical test cancer screening: a randomized clinical trial. JAMA 2017;318: 816–24.

44. Baxter NN, Sutradhar R, Li Q, et al. Do primary care provider strategies improve patient participation in colorectal cancer screening? Am J Gastroenterol 2017; 112:622–32.

45. Rex DK, Boland CR, Dominitz JA, et al. Colorectal cancer screening: recommendations for physicians and patients from the U.S. Multi-society task force on colorectal cancer. Gastroenterology 2017;153:307–23.

46. Robinson CM, Cassells AN, Greene MA, et al. Barriers to colorectal cancer screening among publicly insured urban women: no knowledge of tests and no clinician recommendation. J Natl Med Assoc 2011;103:746–53.

47. Freeman HP. The origin, evolution, and principles of patient navigation. Cancer Epidemiol Biomarkers Prev 2012;21:1614–7.

48. Freeman HP, Muth BJ, Kerner JF. Expanding access to cancer screening and clinical follow-up among the medically underserved. Cancer Pract 1995;3:19–30.

49. Joseph DA, DeGroff AS, Hayes NS, et al. The Colorectal Cancer Control Program: partnering to increase population level screening. Gastrointest Endosc 2011;73: 429–34.

50. Chen LA, Santos S, Jandorf L, et al. A program to enhance completion of screening colonoscopy among urban minorities. Clin Gastroenterol Hepatol 2008;6:443–50.

51. Honeycutt S, Green R, Ballard D, et al. Evaluation of a patient navigation program to promote colorectal cancer screening in rural Georgia, USA. Cancer 2013;119: 3059–66.

52. Jandorf L, Gutierrez Y, Lopez J, et al. Use of a patient navigator to increase colorectal cancer screening in an urban neighborhood health clinic. J UrbanHealth 2005;82:216–24.

53. Lasser KE, Murillo J, Lisboa S, et al. Colorectal cancer screening among ethnically diverse, low-income patients: a randomized controlled trial. Arch Intern Med 2011;171:906–12.

54. Lasser KE, Murillo J, Medlin E, et al. A multilevel intervention to promote colorectal cancer screening among community health center patients: results of a pilot study. BMC Fam Pract 2009;10:37.

55. Percac-Lima S, Grant RW, Green AR, et al. A culturally tailored navigator program for colorectal cancer screening in a community health center: a randomized, controlled trial. J Gen Intern Med 2009;24:211–7.
56. Berg BP, Murr M, Chermak D, et al. Estimating the cost of no-shows and evaluating the effects of mitigation strategies. Med Decis Making 2013;33:976–85.
57. Kazarian ES, Carreira FS, Toribara NW, et al. Colonoscopy completion in a large safety net health care system. Clin Gastroenterol Hepatol 2008;6:438–42.
58. Harewood GC, Sharma VK, de Garmo P. Impact of colonoscopy preparation quality on detection of suspected colonic neoplasia. Gastrointest Endosc 2003; 58:76–9.
59. Johnson DA, Barkun AN, Cohen LB, et al. Optimizing adequacy of bowel cleansing for colonoscopy: recommendations from the US multi-society task force on colorectal cancer. Gastroenterology 2014;147:903–24.
60. Rice K, Gressard L, DeGroff A, et al. Increasing colonoscopy screening in disparate populations: results from an evaluation of patient navigation in the New Hampshire Colorectal Cancer Screening Program. Cancer 2017;123:3356–66.
61. Rice K, Sharma K, Li C, et al. Cost-effectiveness of a patient navigation intervention to increase colonoscopy screening among low-income adults in New Hampshire. Cancer 2019;125:601–9.
62. Ladabaum U, Mannalithara A, Jandorf L, et al. Cost-effectiveness of patient navigation to increase adherence with screening colonoscopy among minority individuals. Cancer 2015;121:1088–97.
63. De Mil R, Guillaume E, Guittet L, et al. Cost-effectiveness analysis of a navigation program for colorectal cancer screening to reduce social health inequalities: a french cluster randomized controlled trial. Value Health 2018;21:685–91.
64. Available at: https://www.cdc.gov/cancer/crccp/pdf/nhcrcsp_pn_manual.pdf.
65. Chambers JA, Callander AS, Grangeret R, et al. Attitudes towards the Faecal Occult Blood Test (FOBT) versus the Faecal Immunochemical Test (FIT) for colorectal cancer screening: perceived ease of completion and disgust. BMC Cancer 2016;16:96.
66. Moss S, Mathews C, Day TJ, et al. Increased uptake and improved outcomes of bowel cancer screening with a faecal immunochemical test: results from a pilot study within the national screening programme in England. Gut 2017;66: 1631–44.
67. Gupta S, Halm EA, Rockey DC, et al. Comparative effectiveness of fecal immunochemical test outreach, colonoscopy outreach, and usual care for boosting colorectal cancer screening among the underserved: a randomized clinical trial. JAMA Intern Med 2013;173:1725–32.
68. Giorgi Rossi P, Grazzini G, Anti M, et al. Direct mailing of faecal occult blood tests for colorectal cancer screening: a randomized population study from Central Italy. J Med Screen 2011;18:121–7.
69. Green BB, Anderson ML, Chubak J, et al. Impact of continued mailed fecal tests in the patient-centered medical home: year 3 of the systems of support to increase colon cancer screening and follow-up randomized trial. Cancer 2016; 122:312–21.
70. Van Roosbroeck S, Hoeck S, Van Hal G. Population-based screening for colorectal cancer using an immunochemical faecal occult blood test: a comparison of two invitation strategies. Cancer Epidemiol 2012;36:e317–24.
71. Potter MB, Ackerson LM, Gomez V, et al. Effectiveness and reach of the FLU-FIT program in an integrated health care system: a multisite randomized trial. Am J PublicHealth 2013;103:1128–33.

72. Gupta S, Miller S, Koch M, et al. Financial incentives for promoting colorectal cancer screening: a randomized, comparative effectiveness trial. Am J Gastroenterol 2016;111:1630–6.

73. Kullgren JT, Dicks TN, Fu X, et al. Financial incentives for completion of fecal occult blood tests among veterans: a 2-stage, pragmatic, cluster, randomized, controlled trial. Ann Intern Med 2014;161:S35–43.

74. Morland TB, Synnestvedt M, Honeywell S Jr, et al. Effect of a financial incentive for colorectal cancer screening adherence on the appropriateness of colonoscopy orders. Am J Med Qual 2017;32:292–8.

75. Escoffery C, Rodgers KC, Kegler MC, et al. A systematic review of special events to promote breast, cervical and colorectal cancer screening in the United States. BMC Public Health 2014;14:274.

76. Doubeni CA, Fedewa SA, Levin TR, et al. Modifiable failures in the colorectal cancer screening process and their association with risk of death. Gastroenterology 2019;156:63–74.e6.

77. Corley DA, Jensen CD, Quinn VP, et al. Association between time to colonoscopy after a positive fecal test result and risk of colorectal cancer and cancer stage at diagnosis. JAMA 2017;317:1631–41.

78. Baker DW, Brown T, Buchanan DR, et al. Comparative effectiveness of a multifaceted intervention to improve adherence to annual colorectal cancer screening in community health centers: a randomized clinical trial. JAMA Intern Med 2014; 174:1235–41.

79. Gellad ZF, Stechuchak KM, Fisher DA, et al. Longitudinal adherence to fecal occult blood testing impacts colorectal cancer screening quality. Am J Gastroenterol 2011;106:1125–34.

80. Nielson CM, Vollmer WM, Petrik AF, et al. Factors affecting adherence in a pragmatic trial of annual fecal immunochemical testing for colorectal cancer. J Gen Intern Med 2019;34:978–85.

81. Singal AG, Gupta S, Skinner CS, et al. Effect of colonoscopy outreach vs fecal immunochemical test outreach on colorectal cancer screening completion: a randomized clinical trial. JAMA 2017;318:806–15.

82. Liang PS, Wheat CL, Abhat A, et al. Adherence to competing strategies for colorectal cancer screening over 3 years. Am J Gastroenterol 2016;111:105–14.

83. Jensen CD, Corley DA, Quinn VP, et al. Fecal immunochemical test program performance over 4 rounds of annual screening: a retrospective cohort study. Ann Intern Med 2016;164:456–63.

84. Sali L, Mascalchi M, Falchini M, et al. Reduced and full-preparation CT colonography, fecal immunochemical test, and colonoscopy for population screening of colorectal cancer: a randomized trial. J Natl Cancer Inst 2016;108 [pii:djv319].

85. Stoop EM, de Haan MC, de Wijkerslooth TR, et al. Participation and yield of colonoscopy versus non-cathartic CT colonography in population-based screening for colorectal cancer: a randomised controlled trial. Lancet Oncol 2012;13:55–64.

What Is Organized Screening and What Is Its Value?

Jason A. Dominitz, MD, MHS[a],*, Theodore R. Levin, MD[b,c]

KEYWORDS

- Colorectal neoplasms • Cancer screening • Mass screening • Colonoscopy
- Occult blood • Patient navigation

KEY POINTS

- Colorectal cancer (CRC) screening is widely recommended and underused. Up to one-third of age-eligible adults in the United States remain unscreened for CRC.
- Organized screening offers the opportunity to invite all eligible adults, through mailed reminders, leveraging other providers (medical assistants, nurses, and pharmacists).
- Organized screening also offers a platform to measure and improve quality of screening, through tracking of follow-up of positive tests and measuring colonoscopy quality.
- Organized screening, by offering screening to all eligible adults, also offers a means to address the observed disparity in screening uptake in underserved and underinsured communities.

INTRODUCTION

Despite the proved effectiveness of colorectal cancer (CRC) screening to reduce cancer incidence and mortality,[1] fewer than two-thirds of screen-eligible adults in the United States currently are up to date with CRC screening.[2] Each step in the cascade of events in effective CRC screening is associated with specific barriers to completion **(Table 1)**.[3,4] For example, with colonoscopic screening, the necessary steps include identification of eligible individuals, offering and acceptance of colonoscopy, bowel preparation, performance of high-quality colonoscopy (including adequate polypectomy, as needed), safe transportation after sedation, accurate interpretation of pathology results, determination of appropriate postcolonoscopy screening or surveillance

T.R. Levin's work was supported by The Permanente Medical Group Delivery Science and Physician Researcher Program, and National Institute of Health/National Cancer Institute grant #UM1CA222035.

[a] Veterans Health Administration, University of Washington School of Medicine, Seattle, WA, USA; [b] Gastroenterology Department, Kaiser Permanente Medical Center, The Permanente Medical Group, 1425 South Main Street, Walnut Creek, CA 94596, USA; [c] The Kaiser Permanente Division of Research, Oakland, CA 94612, USA

* Corresponding author. VA Puget Sound Health Care System, 1660 South Columbian Way, 111-S-Gastro, Seattle, WA 98108.
E-mail address: Jason.dominitz@va.gov

Table 1
Barriers to colorectal cancer screening and surveillance

Health system/facility level	1. Lack of screening policy 2. Lack of an organized screening program 3. Financial barriers to offering screening 4. Providing a limited choice of screening tests 5. Inadequate data systems for tracking individuals through the screening and surveillance process 6. Inability to offer reminders to providers and participants

Provider level	1. Limited access
	  A. Long wait times
	  B. Long travel distances
	2. Insufficient counseling about screening
	3. Lack of facilitation through the screening process
	  A. Lack of reminders
	  B. Lack of navigation

Participant level	1. Lack of awareness of CRC screening and its benefits
	2. Aversion/negative views of cancer
	  A. Fear of cancer
	  B. Fatalism (eg, no benefit of screening)
	3. Negative attitudes toward screening tests
	  A. Embarrassment
	  B. Questioning the efficacy of the test
	4. Lack of motivation
	  A. Other health concerns dominate
	  B. Competing life demands and scheduling challenges
	5. Cultural
	  A. Natural remedies can conquer CRC
	  B. Ethic food protects from CRC
	6. Gender
	  A. Perceived as a male disease
	  B. Screening tests are viewed as offensive to masculinity
	7. Socioeconomic
	  A. Inability to take off time from work
	  B. Lack of transportation and/or locating an escort
	  C. Low health literacy
	  D. Language barriers

Adapted from Honein-AbouHaidar GN, Kastner M, Vuong V, et al. Systematic review and meta-study synthesis of qualitative studies evaluation facilitators and barriers to participation in colorectal cancer screening. Cancer, Epidemiology, Biomarkers and Prevention 2015;25(6);907-17 and Hassan C, Kaminski MF, Repici A. How to ensure patient adherence to colorectal cancer screening and surveillance in your practice. Gastroenterology 2018;155:252-257; with permission.

recommendations, and, ultimately, appropriate performance of that next test at the recommended interval. Effective fecal immunochemical test (FIT) or fecal DNA screening requires the additional step of timely colonoscopic follow-up of those testing positive. Likewise, for those found with cancer, timely and high-quality surgery as well as medical oncology and/or radiation oncology care is necessary to maximize the benefits of screening.

Each of these steps can occur in the opportunistic health care setting, such as independent private practices, group practices, or individual hospitals. There are abundant empirical and trial data, however, demonstrating that implementation of programmatic or organized screening for population health management can result in improved adherence with CRC screening and downstream benefits for CRC outcomes.[5–7] There are multiple implementation strategies that have been demonstrated to be effective at addressing gaps in this screening cascade, such as use of clinical reminders, outreach, navigators, and quality assurance programs. There is no 1 best organized screening approach; health care settings may use 1 or more strategies to move along a continuum toward organized screening. This article discusses some of the key steps and implementation strategies for an effective CRC screening program.

ORGANIZED SCREENING DEFINED

The International Agency for Research on Cancer defines an organized screening program as having the following features: (1) an explicit policy with specified age categories, method, and interval for screening; (2) a defined target population; (3) a management team responsible for implementation; (4) a health care team for decisions and care; (5) a quality assurance structure; and (6) a method for identifying cancer occurrence in the population.[8] A conceptual model that outlines the steps in the screening process has been developed by the National Cancer Institute–funded Population-based Research Optimizing Screening through Personalized Regimens (PROSPR) consortium in an effort to improve the screening process in the United States (**Fig. 1**).[9] In contrast, opportunistic screening is conducted outside of an organized screening program (**Table 2**). Compared with opportunistic screening, organized screening focuses on the quality of the screening process, including follow-up of participants.[10]

IDENTIFYING THE POPULATION AT RISK

Although current guidelines from the US Preventive Services Task Force recommend screening for average-risk adults, ages 50 to 75, they also suggest that individuals

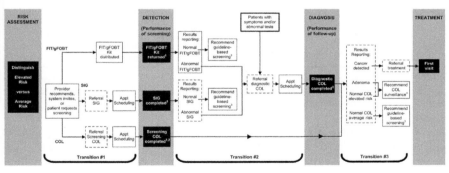

Fig. 1. PROSPR process model for CRC screening. Appt, appointment; COL, colonoscopy; FIT, fecal immunochemical test; gFOBT, guaiac-based fecal occult blood test; SIG, flexible sigmoidoscopy. [a] Potential for inconclusive Screening test result. [b] Excisional treatment of precancerous lesions usually occurs during the colonoscopy procedure. [c] U.S. Multi-Society Task Force on Colorectal Cancer recommends FIT or gFOBT every year, SIG every 5 years with FIT/gFOBT every 3 years, or COL every 10 years. [d] Timing of surveillance regimen depends on size, number, and histology of polyps detected. (*From* Tiro, J.A. et al. Cancer Epidemiol Biomarkers Prev 2014;23:1147-1158, with permission.)

Table 2
Comparing and contrasting opportunistic screening with organized screening

Characteristic	Opportunistic Screening[a]	Organized Screening
Who to screen?	Individual provider decides for each patient.	Program defines screening cohort inclusion and exclusion criteria.
When is screening offered?	During clinic visits	May be dependent or independent of clinic visits • Clinical reminders may display in an EHR during clinic visits • Outreach of screening can occur between clinic visits
What screening test is offered?	Shared decision making between patient and provider. Some may offer a choice, whereas others may offer sequential screening.	Program typically determines approach to screening. Shared decision making is still possible but typically is secondary to the programmatic approach. Most organized screening programs offer noninvasive screening.
How is follow-up of positive tests arranged?	Individual provider is responsible for arranging diagnostic evaluation.	Tracking registries are used to augment provider action.
Quality assurance	Variable	The program establishes benchmarks for screening (eg, participation, diagnostic evaluation of abnormal results, and colonoscopy quality) and monitors clinical outcomes.
Adoption of new technology	Variable	The program may establish criteria for adoption of new technology, such as changes in FIT products, thresholds for quantitative hemoglobin, and adoption of new biomarker tests.

[a] Note that, in practice, opportunistic screening often includes some components of an organized screening program. For example, an individual provider may maintain a log of patients due for screening and send reminders to their patients.

ages 76 to 84 may benefit from screening.[1] Recently, based on data showing a rising incidence of cancer in younger adults, the American Cancer Society offered a "qualified recommendation" for screening to begin at age 45.[11] Although these recommendations offer a starting point for identifying the population at risk, there are challenges in operationalizing these recommendations in a CRC screening program. The primary challenge is in the definition of average risk in order to identify the target population (**Box 1**). Ideally, a screening program has access to all information required to determine the risk of the population, including age, family history, and the dates and results of all prior screening tests. Unfortunately, this information often is incomplete, especially in health care systems where patients may receive care both within and outside of the health care system that is delivering the screening program.

A key advantage of organized screening is that it provides greater protection against the harms of screening—including underuse, overuse, and misuse. Underuse of screening can occur when individuals with a personal or family history of colorectal neoplasia are offered an inappropriate screening test (eg, a stool-based test instead of colonoscopy) or are offered screening at an inappropriate initiation age or interval

---

Box 1
Identifying the target population

- Define inclusion criteria for screening, such as age range
- Define exclusion criteria, such as
  - Normal colonoscopy in the past 10 years
  - Flexible sigmoidoscopy in the past 5 years
  - FIT in the past 12 months
  - FIT-DNA in the past 3 years
  - CT colonography in the past 5 years
  - Clinical criteria (eg, limited life expectancy and hospice)
- Build processes to avoid underscreening
  - Assess prior history of colorectal neoplasia
  - Assess family history of CRC
  - Assess for symptoms that warrant diagnostic evaluation
- Build processes to avoid overscreening
  - Assess prior screening history and results
  - Assess for comorbidity and exclude, as appropriate

---

eg, offering FIT screening at age 50 to someone with a strong family history of CRC). Conversely, overuse of screening can occur when a program offers screening to individuals who are not yet due (eg, offering screening to an individual who had a normal, high-quality colonoscopy <10 years ago), who have limited life expectancy and are unlikely to benefit from screening, or who may experience harm from screening due to comorbid conditions.[12] For example, it has been estimated that overuse occurs in up to 24% of Medicare beneficiaries, 14% of veterans undergoing screening colonoscopy, and 26% of veterans undergoing fecal occult blood testing.[13,14] Screening is misused when it is done in a way that achieves no benefits—for example, fecal testing done using in-office stool samples rather than the recommended home technique or repeating a FIT after it is positive, rather than proceeding to colonoscopy.[15]

Ultimately, an organized screening program takes a population health approach and tries to improve overall CRC screening practice. Rather than aiming for perfect screening for all individuals, the program strives to maximize benefit while minimizing harm. With respect to minimizing underscreening and overscreening, there are several approaches that can be used. First and foremost is the use of an electronic health record (EHR) to capture key risk factor information. With a sophisticated EHR, individuals who are appropriate for CRC screening can be identified through an automated process to generate screening invitations directly to the population (eg, by mail or personal or automated phone calls) or clinical reminders for providers to see when they access the medical record. Although age is universally documented, family history, prior screening results, and other exclusions may not be documented in the EHR or are not recorded in a format that allows for automated extraction.[16] The performance of a colonoscopy or FIT often can be determined through billing codes (eg, current procedural terminology) or review of laboratory results, assuming the test occurred within the health care system. But identifying colonoscopy surveillance recommendations requires creation of a formal process for tracking the recommended intervals and due dates.

It is critically important to craft the invitation for screening to minimize underscreening and overscreening. For example, mailed letters or telephone calls should explicitly state that individuals with worrisome signs or symptoms (eg, rectal bleeding), a prior history of colon polyps, or a family history of CRC should talk to their doctor (or call the screening center) to determine what testing is appropriate for them. In addition, standardized checklists should be utilized for all staff who talk with these individuals to confirm the appropriateness of the screening test. For example, prior to a screening colonoscopy, the staff should inquire about the most recent colonoscopy date and findings.

HOW TO OFFER SCREENING AND INTERVENTIONS TO IMPROVE UPTAKE OF SCREENING

Organized screening programs use a variety of evidence-based approaches to improve CRC screening uptake by members of the target population (**Table 3**). These include interventions to increase patient demand for screening, increase the reliable offer of screening, and remove barriers to screening.[17,18] Demand for screening can be increased through population-based public awareness campaigns,[19] employing pharmacists to promote screening or deliver FIT kits,[20] distributing educational materials via mailed outreach (small media: letters, postcards, and newsletters),[21] or clinic-based decision aids[22] (**Table 4**). Recommendation and offer of screening can be increased by employing office-based reminders (either paper chart–based stickers or EHR reminders),[5,23–25] using office support or other staff members as navigators,[22,26–29] mailed outreach with FIT[5,25,29–36] or invitations to schedule colonoscopy,[30,31,34] and delivering provider assessment and feedback on performance.[24,32,37] Many of these approaches have been demonstrated as effective strategies among underserved populations,[30,31,35,36,38,39] which may help organized screening programs address disparities in CRC screening. Structural and economic

Table 3 Increase demand for screening		
Approach	**Details**	**Considerations**
Public awareness campaign	• Television advertisements • Web site with program info • Phone information line • Print advertisements • Posters • Information pamphlets • Street teams distributing program literature and information	• Increases awareness and social acceptability of screening • Increases demand for screening • Office visit with PCP is still required to get test kit or referral for colonoscopy.

Patient-facing or client-facing materials	• Small media
	  ○ Letters
	  ○ Postcards
	  ○ Newsletters
	• Decision aids
		• Requires identification of the target population
		• May be linked to screening up to date status or just a generic reminder to increase screening

Provide information and possibly testing in pharmacies	• Provide information about the importance of screening for CRC. • Refer individuals at increased risk. • Open communication with primary care physicians is essential. • Dispense screening kits to eligible participants, where allowed.	• Has been used in Canada, but not reported in the United States

Table 4
Increase the recommendation and offer of screening

Intervention	Examples	Comments
Primary care physician awareness campaign	• Information kits • Patient counseling materials • Journal articles • Dedicated Web site • Continuing education events • Academic detailing	• Increases awareness among primary care physicians, who are essential to the process • Not tied to an individual patient completion
Provider reminders	• Paper chart stickers • Electronic chart reminders	• Requires previsit chart review or programming of EHR data
Using support staff and other patient navigators	• Address barriers by linking patients to existing resources, not by creating new resources or services. • Improve follow-up with colonoscopy. • Improve FIT completion. • May be nurses or trained unlicensed staff • May be office-based (when rooming patients) • At other preventive services events (eg, FluFIT) • Phone navigation another option	• Requires a team approach: • Administrators to champion the program • Supervisors to provide clinical and administrative support • Navigators with a defined role within the health care team
Mailed outreach	• Mailed outreach allows consistent invitations to all eligible patients, including those not attending office visits. • Stool-based screening is better suited to mailed invitation.	• Start-up costs to using a third-party vendor, only justified by a relatively large target population • If done by clinic staff, can be hard to sustain with competing priorities
Provider assessment and feedback	• Regular reporting of practice or physician-based screening rates informs physicians of performance identification of bright spots and adaptation of best practices. • Reinforces the importance of screening	• Reporting can be challenging for small practices.

barriers to screening also can be decreased through making screening more convenient by offering rides and expanding hours[21] and tying screening to other visits, such as a flu shot clinic (**Table 5**).[28,40] In addition, expanding insurance coverage has had a demonstrable effect on increasing screening rates and improving the cancer stage at diagnosis.[41,42] Finally, offering a choice between colonoscopy and FIT is effective at increasing screening participation, either as an active choice between the two[34,43] or by sequentially offering colonoscopy first followed by FIT for those who decline colonoscopy.[44] Screening choice can be managed by primary care physicians during office visits[43] or through mailed invitation.[34] Over time, however, the early benefit of having a choice of FIT versus colonoscopy can be lost if screening

Table 5
Removing barriers to screening

Intervention	Examples	Comments
Improve insurance coverage	• Medicaid expansion in the Affordable Care Act has been associated with increased screening participation.	• Colonoscopy follow-up to a positive FIT still is not covered without copayment.
Reduce structural barriers	• Screening tied to other visits • Providing transportation to screening visit • Expanded hours • Reduced out-of-pocket costs • Screening centers closer to where patients live and work	• May be challenging in areas with limited resources • Insurance rules not under the control of health care providers
Provide a choice of screening tests	• Can be delivered by mail or in office • Sequential (offer colonoscopy first) • Active (offer colonoscopy and FIT simultaneously)	• When offered a choice, more people complete screening. • Active choice may lead to better adherence. • Continued adherence with FIT can erode in the absence of a program of active reminding.

is not offered consistently and reminded each year.[45,46] A recent review of multilevel interventions quantified the benefit for several interventions that have been formally tested in randomized controlled trials, demonstrating that direct outreach and patient navigation were the most effective interventions to improve screening, leading to a 2-fold increase in screening (**Table 6**).[18]

Table 6
Summary of single-component interventions to increase colorectal cancer screening

Intervention	Definition	Effectiveness
Outreach	Disseminating screening outside the primary care setting	Odds ratio 2.26 (95% CI, 1.81–2.81)
Navigation	Assisting individuals to complete the screening process	Odds ratio 2.01 (95% CI, 1.64–2.46)
Patient education	Delivering screening information via multimedia or in-person modalities	Odds ratio 1.20 (95% CI, 1.06–1.36)
Academic detailing	Educating providers and giving feedback on screening completion rates	3%–10% absolute increase
Inreach	Reminding providers to screen	10% absolute increase
Financial incentives	Giving monetary rewards to individuals to complete screening	Variable effectiveness
Preference	Allowing individuals a choice of screening strategies	10% absolute increase

From Inadomi JM, Issaka RB, Green BB. What Multi-Level Interventions Do We Need to Increase the Colorectal Cancer Screening Rate to 80%? Clin Gastroenterol Hepatol 2019 [epub ahead of print], with permission.

SPECIAL CONSIDERATIONS FOR FECAL IMMUNOCHEMICAL TEST: ADJUSTING CUTOFFS AND ENSURING FOLLOW-UP

The potentially high positivity rate for FIT can strain colonoscopy resources. Most large-scale screening programs that use FIT use the quantitative form of the test, even though the fixed cutoff used for reporting may cause it to appear qualitative.[5,32,47] The quantitative FIT has the advantage of allowing the cutoff for a positive test to be adjusted to target test positivity to available colonoscopy resources. In the Dutch national CRC screening program, initial estimates of uptake and test positivity were based on several pilot studies.[47] Once the program was launched, however, uptake of screening was higher than expected. In addition, the FIT brand was changed for the national program to a version with a higher positivity rate.[47] These 2 factors led to a higher than expected number of positive tests, straining available colonoscopy capacity. In response, the organizers elected to adjust the cutoff for a positive test to a more manageable level.[47] Organized screening program are well positioned for tracking the volume of positive tests and available colonoscopy capacity in order to adjust, by policy, the cutoff of a positive test. In the United States, lowering the screening cutoff to improve sensitivity of FIT for cancer and decrease false-negative tests would require an off-label change to tests that are Food and Drug Administration cleared at a specific level. The small increase in cancer detection at lower positivity thresholds is counterbalanced by a substantial increase in positive tests.[48]

The effectiveness of FIT screening is dependent on timely and consistent colonoscopy follow-up of positive tests.[49] Delay of follow-up colonoscopy longer than 6 months to 9 months is associated with an increased risk for advanced CRC.[50,51] Examples of effective evidence-based interventions to improve colonoscopy follow-up are few. In a recent systematic review, moderate evidence supports the use of patient navigators, provider reminders, and data driven feedback on performance.[52] In the Kaiser Permanente Northern California (KPNC) program, more than 83% of those testing positive with FIT receive a diagnostic colonoscopy.[53] This relatively high adherence is achieved through a combination of strategies, including health insurance coverage treating a FIT-positive follow-up colonoscopy as a preventive ($0 copay) procedure, setting a goal of colonoscopy follow-up within 4 weeks of a positive FIT, tracking FIT-positive patients through to completion of colonoscopy, early telephone contact to directly schedule follow-up colonoscopies, assigning the responsibility for follow-up tracking and scheduling to gastroenterology departments (vs primary care), and increasing colonoscopy capacity.[53] In the Veterans Health Administration (VA) system, similar organizational factors were effective at increasing colonoscopy follow-up, including notifying gastroenterology providers directly about patients with positive tests, providing feedback to primary care about referral timeliness, and ensuring adequate capacity to perform colonoscopy.[54]

ASSURING APPROPRIATE SURVEILLANCE

Colonoscopic surveillance recommendations, based on the findings of index and subsequent colonoscopies, strive to minimize patient risk and assure appropriate utilization of health care resources.[55,56] The literature is rife, however, with studies documenting both overuse and underuse of colonoscopic surveillance. Underuse and overuse may result from inappropriate surveillance recommendations or postcolonoscopy events, such as new symptoms or patient nonadherence to the recommendations. A recent meta-analysis found that 42.6% of colonoscopies were earlier and 7.9% were later than recommended by the relevant guideline for that population.[57]

Cohort studies of colonoscopic surveillance tell a similar story. For example, among Medicare patients with a negative screening colonoscopy, 46.2% underwent a repeated colonoscopy within 7 years, and 42.5% of these patients (23.5% of the total) had no clear indication.[13] Within the VA health care system, Murphy and colleagues[58] found that 16% of patients with no adenomas and 26% of those with low-risk adenomas had overuse of colonoscopy, whereas 52% of those with high risk adenomas either underwent colonoscopy after the recommended interval or failed to have surveillance colonoscopy. Data from the Prostate, Lung, Colorectal and Ovarian cancer screening trial also demonstrated significant overuse of surveillance colonoscopy among low-risk individuals and underuse of surveillance among those with advanced adenomas.[59] For example, 46.7% of those with only 1 to 2 nonadvanced adenomas and 26.5% of those with no adenomas underwent surveillance colonoscopy within 5 years, whereas only 58.4% of those with advanced adenomas underwent surveillance within that timeframe.

There can be valid reasons for shortening the surveillance recommendation, such as after colonoscopy with an inadequate bowel preparation.[60] But studies have demonstrated many other reasons for guideline nonadherence, including disagreement with or lack of awareness of the guideline, concerns about missed neoplasia or malpractice, and reimbursement or financial reasons.[57] There are several steps that an organized screening program can undertake to try to address this issue. First, education of endoscopists, including distribution and discussion of guidelines, educational letters, wallet cards, and posters, has been demonstrated to improve guideline adherence.[61,62] Second, many modern endoscopy reporting systems include data fields to record surveillance recommendations at the completion of the procedure or after review of the pathology results. These systems can generate reports in order to assess compliance with guidelines as part of an organizational quality improvement program. Establishing formal expectations for adherence to guidelines (eg, as part of the ongoing professional practice evaluation) can exert pressure on providers to counteract other influences. These systems also can generate lists or even recall letters for patients who are due for surveillance in order to minimize underuse of screening. These systems do require the endoscopist or other staff to input the surveillance recommendation manually, although use of decision support systems and artificial intelligence may facilitate this process in the future.[63,64] Currently, all VA medical centers utilize a set of CRC clinical reminders embedded within the EHR to help assure that (1) a recommendation is documented after every colonoscopy, (2) a clinical reminder is activated when colonoscopy is due, and (3) reports can be generated to identify those veterans who are due for surveillance. A similar system is in place at KNPC.

QUALITY ASSURANCE IN SCREENING PROGRAMS

Each step in the CRC screening program offers opportunities for quality assurance, irrespective of what screening test is used. Organized screening programs can take advantage of the systems inherent in their program to continually monitor screening performance, clinical outcomes (eg, interval cancers[65]), and test interventions designed to address any gaps in the process. For example, all VA facilities have deployed a new system of CRC screening and surveillance reminders, including (1) an average-risk screening reminder, (2) a diagnostic colonoscopy reminder (for those who have a positive FIT result), (3) a gap reminder for veterans who had a colonoscopy but do not have a documented plan for future screening or surveillance, and (4) a surveillance colonoscopy due reminder. These reminders are supplemented by a collection of reports that can be produced at the level of the individual provider, provider team, facility, region, or nation. These reports include potential gaps in care, such as veterans who have been given a FIT kit but have not yet returned it. The VA has used this reminder and report system to identify other quality gaps, such as the proportion of veterans with a positive FIT who have undergone diagnostic colonoscopy. Through analysis of documented reasons for lack of colonoscopy, the VA can identify targets for intervention, such as provider education about appropriate follow-up and other efforts to discourage overuse of FIT screening.

There also are abundant examples of quality assurance programs related to the performance of colonoscopy, especially because the adenoma detection rate (ADR) has been shown associated with a subsequent risk of CRC incidence and mortality.[66,67] After identifying a problem with ADR and interval cancers in Poland, Kaminski and colleagues[68] tested a quality assurance program to educated endoscopy leaders from low performing facilities and demonstrated improvements in the ADR not only of the trained provider but also of the facility overall. Moreover, they have shown that improvement in the ADR are associated with decreasing risk of interval cancer and cancer death.[69] Guidelines for quality assurance in endoscopy for CRC screening have been published within North America and Europe[70,71] In the United Kingdom, the establishment of a quality assurance program for colonoscopy, including endoscopic training, accreditation of endoscopy services, and accreditation of screening endoscopists, has been associated with significant improvements in key colonoscopy performance indicators.[72]

KPNC has studied the association between the timeliness of diagnostic colonoscopy after positive FIT and CRC outcomes, leading to evidence to guide policy on this issue.[51] In KPNC, those testing positive on FIT are tracked using an EHR-linked database, and colonoscopy follow-up is a shared responsibility between the primary care and gastroenterology departments,[52,53] which, along with maintaining adequate colonoscopy access, has been shown associated with colonoscopy follow-up rates above 80%.[53] KPNC also regularly reports ADRs for endoscopists. In 2014, all colonoscopists were required to complete a Web-based training. Over the past 5 years, KPNC has seen substantial increases in ADRs across the entire program.[73]

TESTING NEW SCREENING MODALITIES

The past decade has demonstrated the marketing of several new and innovative approaches to CRC screening.[74–77] Unfortunately, the evidence to support the population health benefits of these novel screening tests falls short of that available for more established tests, such as fecal occult blood testing/FIT, sigmoidoscopy, and colonoscopy, leading to varying levels of endorsement for their use.[78–81] One of the major advantages of an organized screening program is the ability to not only offer these new screening modalities but also study variations in different components of the screening program. These studies help understand the real-world effectiveness of screening tests, as opposed to the efficacy reported from clinical trials that often include highly selected expert clinicians and study participants. For example, after Atkin and colleagues[82] reported results from a randomized controlled trial demonstrating that 1-time flexible sigmoidoscopy resulted in a significant reduction in CRC mortality compared with controls, a flexible sigmoidoscopy screening program was announced in England in late 2010.[83] Three pilot sites were used, with testing of different invitations strategies, and a simple invitation was found more effective than an interactive approach. In another example, several European countries are studying colonoscopy versus no-screening or FIT.[84–86] The Dutch CRC screening program has evaluated many aspects of FIT, including comparison of different kits,[87] varying cutoff levels for determining a positive FIT,[47] the number of FITs,[88] and screening at different 1-year to 3-year intervals.[89] Finally, the Dutch have programmatically compared computed tomography (CT) colonography to colonoscopy, finding that CT colonography was associated with greater participation but that colonoscopy had greater yield for neoplasia, especially sessile serrated lesions.[90,91]

VALUE OF ORGANIZED SCREENING

Value in health care can be defined as health outcomes relative to cost.[92] With respect to CRC screening, the health outcomes sought are reductions in CRC incidence, morbidity, and mortality. Organized screening programs aim to maximize this benefit while controlling the cost of the interventions. In the setting of opportunistic screening, the individual provider and patient select the screening test based on a variety of factors, such as convenience, invasiveness, perceived efficacy, and cost to the patient. A patient's decision also may be influenced by other factors, such as direct-to-consumer advertising, which has become ubiquitous in the United States. For providers, the decision may be influenced by performance metrics, because many providers are financially rewarded for achieving high CRC screening rates for their population. Given that the current CRC screening quality metrics give credit for any colonoscopy within the past 10 years, there is benefit for the provider if a patient undergoes colonoscopy. Organized screening programs also are subject to these influences, although they may exert more control over which tests are recommended or covered by the screening program, and these recommendations generally consider the cost to the health care system.

So, what is the value of organized screening? Most (63%–76%) of the current CRC deaths have been attributed to nonuse of screening.[49,93] Although there will never be a randomized trial comparing organized to opportunistic screening, there is considerable empirical evidence that the initiation of an organized screening program is associated with improvements in both process and outcome measures related to CRC. An early indicator of the value of organized screening can be found in process measures, such as adherence with CRC screening. For example, in 2005 the VA launched the Colorectal Cancer Care Collaborative (C4) in an effort to address a variety of recognized gaps in care, including screening, diagnostic evaluation, and treatment of CRC.[94] Through the efforts of C4 and other VA interventions, the VA has seen adherence with CRC screening exceed 80% every year since 2009, although challenges remain with overuse of screening and diagnostic evaluation of positive screening results.[14,58,95–97] Organized screening programs also offer tremendous opportunities for quality assurance programs, as discussed previously.

Ultimately, it is hoped that CRC incidence and mortality are reduced, which have been declining in the United States since the 1980s, around the time that CRC screening was first recommended, with 53% of the decline in CRC mortality from 1975-2000 estimated to be attributable to the benefits of screening.[98] Most of the screening in the United States, however, occurs in the opportunistic setting. Empirical evidence that organized screening is superior to opportunistic screening is lacking.[99] Organized CRC screening is more common in Europe than in the United States, which has facilitated the development of quality assurance programs.[100] Earlier adoption of opportunistic screening in the United States and generous reimbursement for colonoscopy have led to more than 60% of the US population reporting having been screened for CRC,[2] higher rates than have been reported in Europe.[100] At least 1 organized screening program in the United States has reported CRC screening rates above 80%.[5] The implementation of screening outreach and subsequent rise in screening participation were associated with a significant decrease in CRC mortality

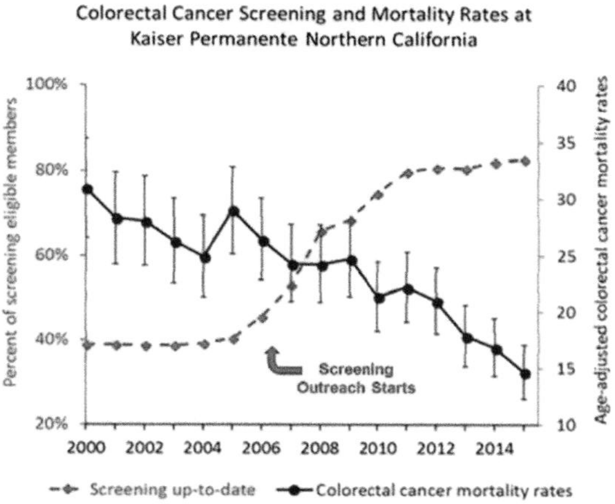

Fig. 2. Association between increase in screening participation and decrease in CRC mortality in KPNC. (*From* Levin TR, Corley DA, Jensen CD, et al. Effects of Organized Colorectal Cancer Screening on Cancer Incidence and Mortality in a Large Community-Based Population. Gastroenterology 2018;155:1383–1391.e5; with permission.)

Fig. 2). In addition, underuse, overuse, and misuse of CRC screening remain significant problems in the United States,[101] and an organized approach to screening provides a way to address each of these problems. Furthermore, organized screening favors the broad adoption of evidence-based interventions to address disparities in CRC screening access and uptake.[102]

SUMMARY

Organized CRC screening consists of (1) an explicit policy with specified age categories, method, and interval for screening; (2) a defined target population; (3) a management team responsible for implementation; (4) a health care team for decisions and care; (5) a quality assurance structure; and (6) a method for identifying cancer occurrence in the population.[8] Implementation of an organized screening program offers opportunities to ensure that all eligible adults receive screening and systematically assess the success of the program and develop interventions to address any identified gaps in an ongoing effort to optimize CRC outcomes.

ACKNOWLEDGMENTS

This material is the result of work supported in part by resources from the Veterans Health Administration. The views expressed in this article are those of the authors and do not necessarily represent the views of the Department of Veterans Affairs.

DISCLOSURE

The authors have nothing to disclose.

REFERENCES

1. US Preventive Services Task Force, Bibbins-Domingo K, Grossman DC, Krist AH, et al. Screening for colorectal cancer: US preventive services task force recommendation statement. JAMA 2016;315:2564–75.

2. White A, Thompson TD, White MC, et al. Cancer screening test use — United States, 2015. MMWR Morb Mortal Wkly Rep 2017;66:201–6.

3. Honein-AbouHaidar GN, Kastner M, Vuong V, et al. Systematic review and meta-study synthesis of qualitative studies evaluating facilitators and barriers to participation in colorectal cancer screening. Cancer Epidemiol Biomarkers Prev 2016;25:907–17.

4. Hassan C, Kaminski MF, Repici A. How to ensure patient adherence to colorectal cancer screening and surveillance in your practice. Gastroenterology 2018;155:252–7.

5. Levin TR, Corley DA, Jensen CD, et al. Effects of organized colorectal cancer screening on cancer incidence and mortality in a large community-based population. Gastroenterology 2018;155:1383–91.e5.

6. Chiu HM, Chen SL, Yen AM, et al. Effectiveness of fecal immunochemical testing in reducing colorectal cancer mortality from the One Million Taiwanese Screening Program. Cancer 2015;121:3221–9.

7. Zorzi M, Hassan C, Capodaglio G, et al. Long-term performance of colorectal cancerscreening programmes based on the faecal immunochemical test. Gut 2018;67:2124–30.

8. International Agency for Research on Cancer. Cervix cancer screening. IARC Handbook of Cancer Prevention, vol. 10. Lyon, France: IARC Press; 2005. p. 117–62.

9. Tiro JA, Kamineni A, Levin TR, et al. The colorectal cancer screening process in community settings: a conceptual model for the population-based research optimizing screening through personalized regimens consortium. Cancer Epidemiol Biomarkers Prev 2014;23:1147–58.

10. Miles A, Cockburn J, Smith RA, et al. A perspective from countries using organized screening programs. Cancer 2004;101:1201–13.

11. Wolf AMD, Fontham ETH, Church TR, et al. Colorectal cancer screening for average-risk adults: 2018 guideline update from the American Cancer Society. CA Cancer J Clin 2018;68(4):250–81.

12. Walter LC, Lindquist K, Nugent S, et al. Impact of age and comorbidity on colorectal cancer screening among older veterans. Ann Intern Med 2009;150:465–73.

13. Goodwin JS, Singh A, Reddy N, et al. Overuse of screening colonoscopy in the Medicare population. Arch Intern Med 2011;171:1335–43.

14. Powell AA, Saini SD, Breitenstein MK, et al. Rates and correlates of potentially inappropriate colorectal cancer screening in the Veterans Health Administration. J Gen Intern Med 2015;30:732–41.

15. Steinwachs D, Allen JD, Barlow WE, et al. National Institutes of Health state-of-the-science conference statement: enhancing use and quality of colorectal cancer screening. Ann Intern Med 2010;152:663–7.

16. Petrik AF, Green BB, Vollmer WM, et al. The validation of electronic health records in accurately identifying patients eligible for colorectal cancer screening in safety net clinics. Fam Pract 2016;33:639–43.

17. The Community Preventive Services Task Force. Guide to community preventive services. cancer screening: multicomponent interventions—colorectal cancer, vol. 2017, 2017. Available at: https://www.thecommunityguide.org/findings/cancer-screening-multicomponent-interventions-colorectal-cancer. Accessed March 4, 2020.

18. Inadomi JM, Issaka RB, Green BB. What multi-level interventions do we need to increase the colorectal cancer screening rate to 80%? Clin Gastroenterol Hepatol 2019 [pii:S1542-3565(19)31495-8].
19. Rabeneck L, Tinmouth JM, Paszat LF, et al. Ontario's ColonCancerCheck: results from Canada's First Province-wide colorectal cancer screening program. Cancer Epidemiol Biomarkers Prev 2014;23:508–15.
20. Havlicek AJ, Mansell H. The community pharmacist's role in cancer screening and prevention. CPJ 2016;149:274–82.
21. Baron RC, Rimer BK, Coates RJ, et al. Client-directed interventions to increase community access to breast, cervical, and colorectal cancer screening a systematic review. Am J Prev Med 2008;35:S56–66.
22. Reuland DS, Brenner AT, Hoffman R, et al. Effect of combined patient decision aid and patient navigation vs usual care for colorectal cancer screening in a vulnerable patient population: a randomized clinical trial. JAMA Intern Med 2017;177:967–74.
23. Sarfaty M, Wender R. How to increase colorectal cancer screening rates in practice. CA Cancer J Clin 2007;57:354–66.
24. Feldman J, Davie S, Kiran T. Measuring and improving cervical, breast, and colorectal cancer screening rates in a multi-site urban practice in Toronto, Canada. BMJ Qual Improv Rep 2017;6 [pii: u213991.w5531].
25. Green BB, Wang C-Y, Anderson ML, et al. An automated intervention with stepped increases in support to increase uptake of colorectal cancer screening: a randomized trial. Ann Intern Med 2013;158:301–11.
26. Escoffery C, Fernandez ME, Vernon SW, et al. Patient navigation in a colorectal cancer screening program. J Public Health Manag Pract 2015;21:433–40.
27. Ritvo P, Myers RE, Serenity M, et al. Taxonomy for colorectal cancer screening promotion: lessons from recent randomized controlled trials. Prev Med 2017; 101:229–34.
28. Potter MB, Walsh JM, Yu TM, et al. The effectiveness of the FLU-FOBT program in primary care a randomized trial. Am J Prev Med 2011;41:9–16.
29. Yu C, Skootsky S, Grossman M, et al. A multi-level fit-based quality improvement initiative to improve colorectal cancer screening in a managed care population. Clin Transl Gastroenterol 2018;9:177.
30. Singal AG, Gupta S, Skinner CS, et al. Effect of colonoscopy outreach vs fecal immunochemical test outreach on colorectal cancer screening completion: a randomized clinical trial. JAMA 2017;318:806–15.
31. Gupta S, Halm EA, Rockey DC, et al. Comparative effectiveness of fecal immunochemical test outreach, colonoscopy outreach, and usual care for boosting colorectal cancer screening among the underserved: a randomized clinical trial. JAMA Intern Med 2013;173:1725–32.
32. Levin TR, Jamieson L, Burley DA, et al. Organized colorectal cancer screening in integrated health care systems. Epidemiol Rev 2011;33:101–10.
33. Coronado GD, Petrik AF, Vollmer WM, et al. Effectiveness of a mailed colorectal cancer screening outreach program in community health clinics: the STOP CRC cluster randomized clinical trial. JAMA Intern Med 2018;178:1174–81.
34. Mehta SJ, Induru V, Santos D, et al. Effect of sequential or active choice for colorectal cancer screening outreach: a randomized clinical trial. JAMA Netw Open 2019;2:e1910305.
35. Issaka RB, Avila P, Whitaker E, et al. Population health interventions to improve colorectal cancer screening by fecal immunochemical tests: a systematic review. Prev Med 2019;118:113–21.

36. Jager M, Demb J, Asghar A, et al. Mailed outreach is superior to usual care alone for colorectal cancer screening in the USA: a systematic review and meta-analysis. Dig Dis Sci 2019;64:2489–96.

37. Sabatino SA, Habarta N, Baron RC, et al. Interventions to increase recommendation and delivery of screening for breast, cervical, and colorectal cancers by healthcare providers systematic reviews of provider assessment and feedback and provider incentives. Am J Prev Med 2008;35:S67–74.

38. Singal AG, Gupta S, Tiro JA, et al. Outreach invitations for FIT and colonoscopy improve colorectal cancer screening rates: A randomized controlled trial in a safety-net health system. Cancer 2016;122:456–63.

39. Coronado GD, Golovaty I, Longton G, et al. Effectiveness of a clinic-based colorectal cancer screening promotion program for underserved Hispanics. Cancer 2011;117:1745–54.

40. Potter MB, Somkin CP, Ackerson LM, et al. The FLU-FIT program: an effective colorectal cancer screening program for high volume flu shot clinics. Am J Manag Care 2011;17:577–83.

41. Hendryx M, Luo J. Increased cancer screening for low-income adults under the affordable care act medicaid expansion. Med Care 2018;56:944–9.

42. Gross CP, Andersen MS, Krumholz HM, et al. Relation between Medicare screening reimbursement and stage at diagnosis for older patients with colon cancer. JAMA 2006;296:2815–22.

43. Inadomi JM, Vijan S, Janz NK, et al. Adherence to colorectal cancer screening: a randomized clinical trial of competing strategies. Arch Intern Med 2012;172:575–82.

44. Senore C, Ederle A, Benazzato L, et al. Offering people a choice for colorectal cancer screening. Gut 2013;62:735–40.

45. Liang PS, Wheat CL, Abhat A, et al. Adherence to competing strategies for colorectal cancer screening over 3 years. Am J Gastroenterol 2016;111:105–14.

46. Green BB, Anderson ML, Cook AJ, et al. A centralized mailed program with stepped increases of support increases time in compliance with colorectal cancer screening guidelines over 5 years: a randomized trial. Cancer 2017;123:4472–80.

47. Toes-Zoutendijk E, van Leerdam ME, Dekker E, et al. Real-time monitoring of results during first year of dutch colorectal cancer screening program and optimization by altering fecal immunochemical test cut-off levels. Gastroenterology 2017;152:767–75.e2.

48. Selby K, Jensen CD, Lee JK, et al. Influence of varying quantitative fecal immunochemical test positivity thresholds on colorectal cancer detection: a community-based cohort study. Ann Intern Med 2018;169:439–47.

49. Doubeni CA, Fedewa SA, Levin TR, et al. Modifiable failures in the colorectal cancer screening process and their association with risk of death. Gastroenterology 2019;156:63–74.e6.

50. Lee YC, Fann JC, Chiang TH, et al. Time to colonoscopy and risk of colorectal cancer in patients with positive results from fecal immunochemical tests. Clin Gastroenterol Hepatol 2019;17:1332–40.e3.

51. Corley DA, Jensen CD, Quinn VP, et al. Association between time to colonoscopy after a positive fecal test result and risk of colorectal cancer and cancer stage at diagnosis. JAMA 2017;317:1631–41.

52. Selby K, Baumgartner C, Levin TR, et al. Interventions to improve follow-up of positive results on fecal blood tests: a systematic review. Ann Intern Med 2017;167:565–75.

53. Selby K, Jensen CD, Zhao WK, et al. Strategies to improve follow-up after positive fecal immunochemical tests in a community-based setting: a mixed-methods study. Clin Transl Gastroenterol 2019;10:e00010.
54. Partin MR, Burgess DJ, Burgess JF Jr, et al. Organizational predictors of colonoscopy follow-up for positive fecal occult blood test results: an observational study. Cancer Epidemiol Biomarkers Prev 2015;24:422–34.
55. Lieberman DA, Rex DK, Winawer SJ, et al. Guidelines for colonoscopy surveillance after screening and polypectomy: a consensus update by the US multi-society task force on colorectal cancer. Gastroenterology 2012;143:844–57.
56. Hassan C, Quintero E, Dumonceau JM, et al. Post-polypectomy colonoscopy surveillance: European Society of Gastrointestinal Endoscopy (ESGE) Guideline. Endoscopy 2013;45:842–51.
57. Djinbachian R, Dube AJ, Durand M, et al. Adherence to post-polypectomy surveillance guidelines: a systematic review and meta-analysis. Endoscopy 2019; 51:673–83.
58. Murphy CC, Sandler RS, Grubber JM, et al. Underuse and overuse of colonoscopy for repeat screening and surveillance in the veterans health administration. Clin Gastroenterol Hepatol 2016;14:436–44.e1.
59. Schoen RE, Pinsky PF, Weissfeld JL, et al. Utilization of surveillance colonoscopy in community practice. Gastroenterology 2010;138:73–81.
60. Johnson DA, Barkun AN, Cohen LB, et al. Optimizing adequacy of bowel cleansing for colonoscopy: recommendations from the US multi-society task force on colorectal cancer. Am J Gastroenterol 2014;109:1528–45.
61. Sanaka MR, Super DM, Feldman ES, et al. Improving compliance with postpolypectomy surveillance guidelines: an interventional study using a continuous quality improvement initiative. Gastrointest Endosc 2006;63:97–103.
62. Gessl I, Waldmann E, Britto-Arias M, et al. Surveillance colonoscopy in Austria: are we following the guidelines? Endoscopy 2018;50:119–27.
63. Magrath M, Yang E, Ahn C, et al. Impact of a clinical decision support system on guideline adherence of surveillance recommendations for colonoscopy after polypectomy. J Natl Compr Canc Netw 2018;16:1321–8.
64. Hou JK, Imler TD, Imperiale TF. Current and future applications of natural language processing in the field of digestive diseases. Clin Gastroenterol Hepatol 2014;12:1257–61.
65. Rutter MD, Beintaris I, Valori R, et al. World endoscopy organization consensus statements on post-colonoscopy and post-imaging colorectal cancer. Gastroenterology 2018;155:909–25.e3.
66. Corley DA, Jensen CD, Marks AR, et al. Adenoma detection rate and risk of colorectal cancer and death. N Engl J Med 2014;370:1298–306.
67. Kaminski MF, Regula J, Kraszewska E, et al. Quality indicators for colonoscopy and the risk of interval cancer. N Engl J Med 2010;362:1795–803.
68. Kaminski MF, Anderson J, Valori R, et al. Leadership training to improve adenoma detection rate in screening colonoscopy: a randomised trial. Gut 2016; 65:616–24.
69. Kaminski MF, Wieszczy P, Rupinski M, et al. Increased rate of adenoma detection associates with reduced risk of colorectal cancer and death. Gastroenterology 2017;153:98–105.
70. Rex DK, Schoenfeld PS, Cohen J, et al. Quality indicators for colonoscopy. Gastrointest Endosc 2015;81:31–53.
71. Valori R, Rey JF, Atkin WS, et al. European guidelines for quality assurance in colorectal cancer screening and diagnosis. First Edition–Quality assurance in

endoscopy in colorectal cancer screening and diagnosis. Endoscopy 2012 44(Suppl 3):SE88–105.

72. Siau K, Green JT, Hawkes ND, et al. Impact of the Joint Advisory Group on Gastrointestinal Endoscopy (JAG) on endoscopy services in the UK and beyond. Frontline Gastroenterol 2019;10:93–106.

73. Corley DA, Jensen C, Lee JK, et al. Increasing physician adenoma detection rate is associated with a reduced risk of post-colonoscopy colorectal cancer. Gastroenterology 2019;156:S-1-51.

74. Johnson CD, Chen M-H, Toledano AY, et al. Accuracy of CT colonography for detection of large adenomas and cancers. N Engl J Med 2008;359:1207–17 [Erratum appears in N Engl J Med 2008;359(26):2853].

75. Imperiale TF, Ransohoff DF, Itzkowitz SH, et al. Multitarget stool DNA testing for colorectal-cancer screening. N Engl J Med 2014;370:1287–97.

76. Church TR, Wandell M, Lofton-Day C, et al. Prospective evaluation of methylated SEPT9 in plasma for detection of asymptomatic colorectal cancer. Gut 2014;63: 317–25.

77. Rex DK, Adler SN, Aisenberg J, et al. Accuracy of capsule colonoscopy in detecting colorectal polyps in a screening population. Gastroenterology 2015;148: 948–57.e2.

78. Rex DK, Boland CR, Dominitz JA, et al. Colorectal cancer screening: recommendations for physicians and patients from the U.S. multi-society task force on colorectal cancer. Gastroenterology 2017;153:307–23.

79. Canadian Task Force on Preventive Health Care. Recommendations on screening for colorectal cancer in primary care. CMAJ 2016;188:340–8.

80. Lauby-Secretan B, Vilahur N, Bianchini F, et al. The IARC perspective on colorectal cancer screening. N Engl J Med 2018;378:1734–40.

81. Qaseem A, Crandall CJ, Mustafa RA, et al. Screening for colorectal cancer in asymptomatic average-risk adults: a guidance statement from the American College of Physicians. Ann Intern Med 2019;171:643–54.

82. Atkin WS, Edwards R, Kralj-Hans I, et al. Once-only flexible sigmoidoscopy screening in prevention of colorectal cancer: a multicentre randomised controlled trial. Lancet 2010;375:1624–33.

83. Bevan R, Rubin G, Sofianopoulou E, et al. Implementing a national flexible sigmoidoscopy screening program: results of the English early pilot. Endoscopy 2015;47:225–31.

84. Quintero E, Castells A, Bujanda L, et al. Colonoscopy versus fecal immunochemical testing in colorectal-cancer screening. N Engl J Med 2012;366: 697–706.

85. Bretthauer M, Kaminski MF, Loberg M, et al. Population-based colonoscopy screening for colorectal cancer: a randomized clinical trial. JAMA Intern Med 2016;176:894–902.

86. SCREESCO - Screening of Swedish Colons. Available at: https://clinicaltrials.gov/ct2/show/NCT02078804, Accessed March 8, 2020.

87. Grobbee EJ, van der Vlugt M, van Vuuren AJ, et al. A randomised comparison of two faecal immunochemical tests in population-based colorectal cancer screening. Gut 2017;66:1975–82.

88. Schreuders EH, Grobbee EJ, Nieuwenburg SAV, et al. Multiple rounds of one sample versus two sample faecal immunochemical test-based colorectal cancer screening: a population-based study. Lancet Gastroenterol Hepatol 2019; 4:622–31.

89. van Roon AH, Goede SL, van Ballegooijen M, et al. Random comparison of repeated faecal immunochemical testing at different intervals for population-based colorectal cancer screening. Gut 2013;62:409–15.

90. Ijspeert JEG, Tutein Nolthenius CJ, Kuipers EJ, et al. CT-colonography vs. colonoscopy for detection of high-risk sessile serrated polyps. Am J Gastroenterol 2016;111:516–22.

91. Stoop EM, de Haan MC, de Wijkerslooth TR, et al. Participation and yield of colonoscopy versus non-cathartic CT colonography in population-based screening for colorectal cancer: a randomised controlled trial. Lancet Oncol 2012;13:55–64.

92. Porter ME. What is value in health care? N Engl J Med 2010;363:2477–81.

93. Meester RGS, Doubeni CA, Lansdorp-Vogelaar I, et al. Colorectal cancer deaths attributable to nonuse of screening in the United States. Ann Epidemiol 2015;25:208–13.e1.

94. Jackson GL, Powell AA, Ordin DL, et al. Developing and sustaining quality improvement partnerships in the VA: the colorectal cancer care collaborative. J Gen Intern Med 2010;25(Suppl 1):38–43.

95. Saini SD, Powell AA, Dominitz JA, et al. Developing and testing an electronic measure of screening colonoscopy overuse in a large integrated healthcare system. J Gen Intern Med 2016;31(Suppl 1):53–60.

96. Johnson MR, Grubber J, Grambow SC, et al. Physician non-adherence to colonoscopy interval guidelines in the veterans affairs healthcare system. Gastroenterology 2015;149:938–51.

97. May F, Yano EM, Provenzale D, et al. Barriers to follow-up colonoscopies for patients with positive results from fecal immunochemical tests during colorectal cancer screening. Clin Gastroenterol Hepatol 2019;17(3):469–76.

98. Edwards BK, Ward E, Kohler BA, et al. Annual report to the nation on the status of cancer, 1975-2006, featuring colorectal cancer trends and impact of interventions (risk factors, screening, and treatment) to reduce future rates. Cancer 2010;116:544–73.

99. Madlensky L, Goel V, Polzer J, et al. Assessing the evidence for organised cancer screening programmes. Eur J Cancer 2003;39:1648–53.

100. Hoff G, Dominitz JA. Contrasting US and European approaches to colorectal cancer screening: which is best? Gut 2010;59:407–14.

101. Holden DJ. Systematic review: enhancing the use and quality of colorectal cancer screening. Ann Intern Med 2010;152:668.

102. Joseph DA, Meester RG, Zauber AG, et al. Colorectal cancer screening: estimated future colonoscopy need and current volume and capacity. Cancer 2016;122:2479–86.

Colorectal Cancer Screening Decisions in the Opportunistic Setting

Andrew Han, MD[a,*], Jennifer Maratt, MD[a,b], Charles Kahi, MD[a,b]

KEYWORDS

- Colorectal • Cancer • Screening • Opportunistic

KEY POINTS

- Colorectal cancer incidence and mortality are declining the in the United States, but overall screening rates have stagnated.
- In the opportunistic setting, 3 frameworks for discussing screening are (1) multiple options, (2) sequential, and (3) risk stratified.
- Colonoscopy is currently the gold standard for screening, but noninvasive options, especially fecal immunochemical testing, can provide effective alternatives when colonoscopy is not desired.
- More detailed analysis of demographics may suggest that certain ethnicities are being severely overlooked, despite the overall high rates of screening.

INTRODUCTION

The primary goal of colorectal cancer (CRC) screening is to identify cancer in its early stages and precancerous lesions in individuals who are asymptomatic and have no history of CRC or polyps. Studies since the early 1990s have shown the value of screening,[1] leading to guidelines for CRC screening being introduced in the mid-1990s.[2] Since then, multiple guidelines from various organizations such as the US Multi-Society Task Force, which represents the 3 largest gastroenterology societies, and the US Preventive Services Task Force (USPSTF) have provided recommendations for screening average-risk individuals aged 50 to 75 years.[3,4] Through robust efforts to improve CRC screening, such as National Colorectal Cancer Roundtable's 80% by 2018 initiative, which represented a collaborative effort by more than 1000 organizations to reach 80% of Americans screened for CRC by the year 2018, CRC-related incidence and mortality, among those more than 50 years of age, has been

[a] Department of Medicine, Division of Gastroenterology and Hepatology, Indiana University School of Medicine, 702 Rotary Circle, Suite 225, Indianapolis, IN 46202, USA; [b] Richard L. Roudebush VA Medical Center, 1481 West 10th Street, 111G, Indianapolis, IN 46202, USA
* Corresponding author.
E-mail address: anhan@iu.edu

Gastrointest Endoscopy Clin N Am 30 (2020) 413–422
https://doi.org/10.1016/j.giec.2020.02.012
1052-5157/20/© 2020 Elsevier Inc. All rights reserved.

declining in the United States over the past several decades.[5] These results were achieved largely through opportunistic screening, which refers to provider-initiated screening when seeing a patient in the office. In the context of opportunistic screening, 3 broad strategies exist: multiple options, sequential, and risk stratified (**Table 1**).[4]

FRAMEWORKS FOR DISCUSSING SCREENING

The multiple options strategy consists of discussing the risks and benefits of 2 or more screening options, from which the patient selects a screening test. There are currently 9 different tests or test combinations available in the United States that have been reviewed and discussed in major guidelines: colonoscopy, fecal immunochemical test (FIT), FIT–fecal DNA stool test, guaiac fecal occult blood test (gFOBT), sigmoidoscopy, sigmoidoscopy plus fecal occult blood test, computed tomography (CT) colonography, barium enema, and the Septin9 serum assay.[3,4] Detailed discussion of the pros and cons of 9 tests within 1 office visit is highly impractical and unlikely to be sustainable in clinical practice. In addition, although 9 tests are available, in practice, 3 tests receive widespread use in the United States: colonoscopy, FIT, and the FIT–fecal DNA stool test. Focusing discussion to 2 or 3 preferred testing options seems to be ideal,[6] because offering more options has not been found to improve adherence to screening.[7–10] If patients decline all offered options, then an additional option may be offered.

With the sequential approach to screening, the provider's preferred screening option is offered to the patient, which is typically colonoscopy in the United States.[3] Colonoscopy remains the gold standard for CRC screening in the United States for several reasons. No other screening test approaches the sensitivity of colonoscopy for precancerous lesions, because colonoscopy has sensitivity rates 4 times higher than the next closest test, which is the FIT–fecal DNA test.[11] In addition, no other test can provide the immediate benefit of preventing colon cancer by removing precancerous lesions during the same session.[12,13] If the patient declines colonoscopy, then the next test is offered, usually FIT, and so forth. For any other screening, a positive result would need to be followed up with diagnostic colonoscopy. One consideration to keep in mind is that, although most insurance companies cover costs of screening, diagnostic colonoscopy following other positive testing may incur costs to the patient.

The risk-stratified strategy seeks to direct those patients with a higher predicted risk of having precancerous lesions directly to colonoscopy, whereas noninvasive tests would be offered to individuals with lower pretest probability. Average risk represents a wide spectrum, and, along with family history, several lifestyle factors, including

Table 1
Strategies for discussing screening in the opportunistic setting

Approach	Description
Risk stratified	Colonoscopy is offered to patients with high pretest probability; other tests are offered to patients with lower perceived risk
Multiple options	Pros and cons of multiple (2 or more) screening tests are presented
Sequential	Provider's preferred test is offered first. If the patient declines, another option is offered, and so on

From Force, U.S.P.S.T., et al., Screening for Colorectal Cancer: US Preventive Services Task Force Recommendation Statement. JAMA, 2016. **315**(23): p. 2564-2575; with permission.

history of cigarette smoking, obesity, sedentary lifestyle, or diabetes, have been implicated in higher risk of CRC.[14,15] Risk indices can assist with identifying which patients would most benefit from colonoscopy as opposed to noninvasive testing, thereby preventing unnecessary exposure to the potential harms of invasive testing.[16] By the same token, older patients, given their higher rates of background methylation, could be cautioned that FIT–fecal DNA stool tests are more likely to produce false-positive results compared with younger patients, and therefore be offered different tests to avoid triggering unnecessary endoscopy.

There are currently no comparative trials to identify 1 method as superior to the others, and the USPSTF does not recommend 1 approach more than the others. However, a recent randomized clinical trial by Mehta and colleagues[10] investigated effects on response rates to sequential choice and what the investigators named "active choice," which correlates with multiple options as described by the USMSTF. In the trial, average-risk patients aged 50 to 74 years who showed good adherence to primary care visits and were not up to date on CRC screening were assigned to 1 of 3 mailed outreach options for CRC screening: (1) direct phone number to schedule colonoscopy; (2) direct phone number to schedule colonoscopy, followed by a mailed FIT kit if no response received within 4 weeks; and (3) direct phone number to schedule colonoscopy as well as a FIT kit simultaneously. Four-hundred and thirty-eight patients with a median age of 56 years of age (interquartile range, 52–63 years) were included in the intention-to-treat analysis, and screening rates for the choice arms did not achieve statistically significant increases compared with the colonoscopy-alone group. Of the patients who did complete screening, 90.5% (95% confidence interval [CI], 78.0%–103.0%) chose colonoscopy in the colonoscopy-only arm, 52.0% (95% CI, 32.4%–71.6%; $P = .005$) chose colonoscopy in the sequential choice arm, and only 37.9% (95% CI, 20.2%–55.6%; $P<.001$) opted for colonoscopy in the active choice cohort.[10]

OVERVIEW OF WIDELY USED SCREENING TESTS IN THE UNITED STATES

Although there are 9 tests currently available in the United States, in practice, only 3 receive widespread use: colonoscopy, FIT, and FIT–fecal DNA stool testing. The specific breakdown of recommended screening modalities and intervals vary based on guideline, but, overall, the United States–based guideline recommendations are generally congruent (**Table 2**). Most guidelines endorse initiating screening at age 50 years for average-risk individuals; however, the American Cancer Society (ACS) guidelines published in 2018 endorsed a qualified recommendation to begin screening in all comers at age 45 years based on data that the incidence of CRC was increasing in the younger population.[17] No other organization has yet corroborated starting screening at age 45 years, except in the African American population.[3]

FLEXIBLE SIGMOIDOSCOPY

Randomized controlled trials showed that flexible sigmoidoscopy reduces CRC incidence and mortality,[18] and long-term follow-up from the Prostate, Lung, Colorectal, and Ovarian Cancer (PLCO) screening trial showed sustained reductions in CRC incidence and mortality.[19] Positive results from trials involving flexible sigmoidoscopy form the foundations for endorsement of colonoscopy as an effective screening test. Although still in use in Europe, flexible sigmoidoscopy has fallen out of use in the United States.[20] Although flexible sigmoidoscopy has shown reproducible benefits in reducing distal CRC, the procedure is by definition unable to examine the entire colon. In an era when right-sided colon cancers arising from serrated lesions are

Table 2
Screening recommendations for average-risk individuals by major United States guideline

Organization	Year of Publication	Age to Initiate Screening (y)	Age to Stop Screening (y)	Recommended Screening Tests/Interval (y)	Preferred Test Modality	References
ACP	2019	50	75 (or when life expectancy ≤10 y)	FIT (2) HSgFOBT (2) FS (10) + FIT (2) Colonoscopy (10)	Unspecified	White et al,[20] 2017
ACS	2018	45	75	FIT (1) HSgFOBT (1) Multitarget fecal DNA (3) Colonoscopy (10) CT colonography (5) FS (5)	Unspecified	Wolf et al,[17] 2018
United States Multi-Society Task Force	2017	50; 45 if African American	75 or life expectancy <10 y	Colonoscopy (10) FIT (1) CT colonography (5) FIT + fecal DNA (3) FS (10) Capsule colonoscopy (5) Septin9 not recommended	Tier 1: colonoscopy, FIT Tier 2: CT colonography, FIT + fecal DNA, FS Tier 3: capsule colonography Tiers beyond tier 1 offered only if all tests from preceding tiers declined	Rex et al,[3] 2017
USPSTF	2016 (update pending)	50	75	gFOBT (1) FIT (1) FIT + fecal DNA (1–3) Colonoscopy (10) CT colonography (5) FS (5) FS (10) + FIT (1)	Unspecified	USPSTF et al,[4] 2016

Abbreviations: ACP, American College of Physicians; ACS, American Cancer Society; FS, flexible sigmoidoscopy; HSgFOBT, high-sensitivity gFOBT.

becoming more prevalent, the concept of intentionally not examining the entire colon has not been comfortable with patients or providers in the United States. If used as a screening modality, the American College of Physicians (ACP) guidelines endorse combining flexible sigmoidoscopy with FIT, whereas the USPSTF recommend either flexible sigmoidoscopy alone or combined with FIT.[3,21]

COLONOSCOPY

No discussion involving CRC screening can escape mention of colonoscopy, because colonoscopy remains the gold standard for screening. Although there are no completed randomized controlled studies directly investigating the benefits of colonoscopy, several case-control, observational studies, and models extrapolating from flexible sigmoidoscopy, have shown benefits on CRC incidence and CRC-related mortality.[19,22–25] The impact of colonoscopy on CRC incidence and mortality can also be gleaned from a concomitant decrease in incidence over the same time period that colonoscopy became widely adopted.[26] Colonoscopy is consistently shown to have the highest efficacy for preventing CRC deaths in network meta-analyses comparing different screening modalities.[18,27] Of all the CRC screening options, only colonoscopy is recommended at 10-year intervals. Quality measures in colonoscopy have been of immense interest, and the adenoma detection rate (ADR), first proposed in 2002,[28] has since been effectively validated to show an inverse relationship between ADR and risk of CRC diagnosed after colonoscopy, or postcolonoscopy CRC (PCCRC).[29,30] PCCRC within 5 years has been blamed for missed lesions at baseline colonoscopy,[31] once again driving the point that not all colonoscopies are equal.

In addition to the risk of missed lesions, colonoscopy has other notable drawbacks. Colonoscopy requires bowel preparation, which can itself be prohibitive to obtaining colonoscopy for patients. A meta-analysis of 9 studies reviewing more than 1600 patients showed no difference in preparation quality while improving tolerability by patients and subsequent willingness to undergo repeat preparation.[32] Adverse events related to colonoscopy are small but real, estimated at 4 colonic perforations per 10,000 colonoscopies; 8 major bleeding episodes (typically related to polypectomy) per 10,000 colonoscopies; and smaller risks of aspiration pneumonitis, typically when screening colonoscopy is performed with deep sedation.[33]

FECAL IMMUNOCHEMICAL TEST

Much like colonoscopy and flexible sigmoidoscopy, FIT was preceded by a similar but distinct test in the form of gFOBT. gFOBT relied on the oxidation reaction of heme to cause a change in color on a test card. Randomized controlled trials evaluating the use of gFOBT showed reduction in CRC-related mortality.[1] A significant limitation of gFOBT is that any substrate that can cause oxidation, including heme from red meat, other dietary peroxidases from plants, and ascorbic acid, could trigger a false-positive reaction. Predictably, the gFOBT showed a very low positive predictive value of 3% to 10%, and has been replaced in the United States by use of FIT.

By definition, FIT is composed of an immunochemical component. FIT is an antibody that reacts specifically to human globin. As a result, other substrates with peroxidase activity, such as red meat, do not need to be avoided before undergoing FIT. gFOBT required patients to smear stool samples onto 3 test cards. Although varied kits are commercially in use in the United States, FIT generally comprises an applicator and a tube where the applicator is inserted. The FIT collection process requires no preparation in the form of modified diets or special medications, and sample collection is much more convenient because only 1 sample is needed. For these reasons, as well as its cheaper cost compared with other screening tests, FIT is the preferred test for most organized screening programs in the world. Meta-analyses estimate FIT sensitivity and specificity to be 79% and 94%, respectively, for CRC.[34,35] One important point to note with FIT tests is that the cutoff points for hemoglobin, when adjusted, can affect the sensitivity and specificity dramatically. A recent meta-analysis reported a boost in sensitivity and specificity to 91% and 90% by reducing the cutoff from 20 μg/g feces to 10 μg/g feces, but with a subsequent increase in the false-positive rate to 10%.[36]

FECAL IMMUNOCHEMICAL TEST–FECAL DNA STOOL TEST

FIT–fecal DNA stool testing is a new test on the market, and currently only 1 is available, under the brand name Cologuard (Exact Sciences, Madison, WI). The FIT–fecal DNA stool test consists of 2 tests: a DNA test assessing for mutations and methylation, and a proprietary FIT. FIT-DNA testing has roughly double the sensitivity for advanced adenomas compared with FIT, but with slightly lower specificity at 87% to 90%.[37] However, the FIT-DNA test is recommended once every 3 years,[3,4] compared with yearly for FIT (or biennially in other guidelines), which can be enticing for patients wishing to forego frequent testing. Pertinent barriers to FIT-DNA becoming more widely popular are higher cost compared with FIT ($600 vs $25). With the data from the meta-analysis of FIT using a lower hemoglobin cutoff potentially matching the performance characteristics of FIT-DNA, FIT-DNA may be further relegated if those results are corroborated by more studies.

BIG PICTURE FOR OPPORTUNISTIC SCREENING

Regardless of the inherent characteristics of each screening test, the true, real-world values are determined ultimately by patient adherence. Colonoscopy is more invasive, costly, and time-consuming than noninvasive testing but can potentially confer up to a decade of protection. FIT is easy to obtain, but multiple studies have shown drop-off in adherence after 3 to 4 rounds.[38,39] Screening is the package process of initial testing, continued adherence, and follow-up with colonoscopy for any positive tests. Even if a hypothetical CRC screening test were to reach 100% sensitivity and specificity, the benefits would only be seen based on continued adherence. This point becomes even more important when noting that an analysis performed in Houston, Texas, found that, of new CRC cases, more than half were attributed to being overdue on screening, or otherwise nonadherent.[40] In that sense, the question arises, is the method of screening as important as the delivery? Namely, should clinicians be analyzing different populations to determine why they have been unable to meet national goals for CRC screening?

ISLANDS OF RESISTANCE

After a remarkable increase in screening rates from 2000 to 2008, overall rates of screening in the United States seem to be plateauing at a little more than 60% for the past several years.[20,26,41] The previously mentioned 80% by 2018 initiative, despite impressive buy-in including local health departments, failed to meet its target and has since been rebranded as the 80% Pledge by removing the target date. The US Preventive Services Task Force's ongoing initiative called Healthy People 2020 has set its target of reaching 70.5% screened by the year 2020. The "elephant in the room" is that large health organizations such as Kaiser Permanente in Northern California and the Veterans Health Administration (VA) have had remarkable success in achieving rates of around 80% for colon cancer screening through implementation of organized screening.[42,43] The VA specifically showed that patients with veteran status–related health care coverage showed higher rates of CRC screening compared with veterans with alternate sources of health care,[43] possibly because of patients with veteran status–related health care being confined to the VA system. However, the United States, like many large nations, lacks the necessary infrastructure to roll out programmatic screening at a national level.

HOW TO MAXIMIZE OPPORTUNISTIC SCREENING

Breaking down the details of successful screening in the United States, although the overall total reached 61.3% in 2015, investigating the demographics reveals stark disparities in screening among minorities and those with low socioeconomic status.[20,41,44] Complicating analysis even further, broad ethnic categorizations such as Asian American and Pacific Islander, which represents the single fastest-growing minority population in the United States, are insufficient; subgroup analysis showed that, when divided into ethnicities such as Korean, Japanese, and Chinese, Koreans had remarkably lower rates of screening (32.7%) compared with the highest group, which were the Japanese (59.8%).[45] Different ethnic groups reflected cultural preferences for CRC screening tests. African Americans, a group recommended to initiate CRC screening at lower age because of higher risk, had significantly lower rates of overall screening as well as uptake of colonoscopy compared with non-Hispanic white people.[46] Barriers to CRC screening, such as distrust in health care, unwillingness to undergo colon prep, financial instability precluding ability to take time off work for colonoscopy, or lack of understanding regarding risks of CRC, have all been implicated.[6,20,45]

As the lens for evaluating CRC screening shifts away from comparing the tests to the people being screened (or not screened), limitations of opportunistic screening rapidly become apparent. Aids such as systematic reminders, the physical action of mailing out test kits for FIT, and mechanisms for following up on positive tests, all of which are present to some degree in organized screening, all on already burdened clinical providers with a limited amount of time to spend per patient. However, until an integrated health care system can be achieved in the United States, the benefits of improving CRC screening are real, and worth fighting for.

DISCLOSURE

The authors have nothing to disclose.

REFERENCES

1. Mandel JS, Bond JH, Church TR, et al. Reducing mortality from colorectal cancer by screening for fecal occult blood. Minnesota Colon Cancer Control Study. N Engl J Med 1993;328(19):1365–71.

2. Winawer SJ, Fletcher RH, Miller L, et al. Colorectal cancer screening: clinical guidelines and rationale. Gastroenterology 1997;112(2):594–642.

3. Rex DK, Boland CR, Dominitz JA, et al. Colorectal cancer screening: recommendations for physicians and patients from the U.S. multi-society task force on colorectal cancer. Gastroenterology 2017;153(1):307–23.

4. US Preventive Services Task Force, Bibbins-Domingo K, Grossman DC, Curry SJ, et al. Screening for colorectal cancer: US preventive services task force recommendation statement. JAMA 2016;315(23):2564–75.
5. Siegel RL, Miller KD, Jemal A. Cancer statistics, 2019. CA Cancer J Clin 2019; 69(1):7–34.
6. Inadomi JM, Vijan S, Janz NK, et al. Adherence to colorectal cancer screening: a randomized clinical trial of competing strategies. Arch Intern Med 2012;172(7): 575–82.
7. Scott RG, Edwards JT, Fritschi L, et al. Community-based screening by colonoscopy or computed tomographic colonography in asymptomatic average-risk subjects. Am J Gastroenterol 2004;99(6):1145–51.
8. Multicentre Australian Colorectal-neoplasia Screening (MACS) Group. A comparison of colorectal neoplasia screening tests: a multicentre community-based study of the impact of consumer choice. Med J Aust 2006;184(11):546–50.
9. Griffith JM, Lewis CL, Brenner AR, et al. The effect of offering different numbers of colorectal cancer screening test options in a decision aid: a pilot randomized trial. BMC Med Inform Decis Mak 2008;8:4.
10. Mehta SJ, Induru V, Santos D, et al. Effect of sequential or active choice for colorectal cancer screening outreach: a randomized clinical trial. JAMA Netw Open 2019;2(8):e1910305.
11. Zauber AG, Lansdorp-Vogelaar I, Knudsen AB, et al. Evaluating test strategies for colorectal cancer screening: a decision analysis for the U.S. Preventive Services Task Force. Ann Intern Med 2008;149(9):659–69.
12. Rex DK. Colonoscopy: the current king of the hill in the USA. Dig Dis Sci 2015; 60(3):639–46.
13. Zauber AG, Winawer SJ, O'Brien MJ, et al. Colonoscopic polypectomy and long-term prevention of colorectal-cancer deaths. N Engl J Med 2012;366(8):687–96.
14. Rangul V, Sund ER, Mork PJ, et al. The associations of sitting time and physical activity on total and site-specific cancer incidence: results from the HUNT study, Norway. PLoS One 2018;13(10):e0206015.
15. Nguyen LH, Liu PH, Zheng X, et al. Sedentary behaviors, TV viewing time, and risk of young-onset colorectal cancer. JNCI Cancer Spectr 2018;2(4):pky073.
16. Imperiale TF, Monahan PO, Stump TE, et al. Derivation and validation of a scoring system to stratify risk for advanced colorectal neoplasia in asymptomatic adults: a cross-sectional study. Ann Intern Med 2015;163(5):339–46.
17. Wolf AMD, Fontham ETH, Church TR, et al. Colorectal cancer screening for average-risk adults: 2018 guideline update from the American Cancer Society. CA Cancer J Clin 2018;68(4):250–81.
18. Elmunzer BJ, Singal AG, Sussman JB, et al. Comparing the effectiveness of competing tests for reducing colorectal cancer mortality: a network meta-analysis. Gastrointest Endosc 2015;81(3):700–709 e3.
19. Miller EA, Pinsky PF, Schoen RE, et al. Effect of flexible sigmoidoscopy screening on colorectal cancer incidence and mortality: long-term follow-up of the randomised US PLCO cancer screening trial. Lancet Gastroenterol Hepatol 2019; 4(2):101–10.
20. White A, Thompson TD, White MC, et al. Cancer screening test use - United States, 2015. MMWR Morb Mortal Wkly Rep 2017;66(8):201–6.
21. Qaseem A, Crandall CJ, Mustafa RA, et al. Screening for colorectal cancer in asymptomatic average-risk adults: a guidance statement from the American College of Physicians. Ann Intern Med 2019;171(9):643–54.

22. Lee JK, Jensen CD, Levin TR, et al. Long-term risk of colorectal cancer and related death after adenoma removal in a large, community-based population. Gastroenterology 2020;158(4):884–94.e5.

23. Fitzpatrick-Lewis D, Ali MU, Warren R, et al. Screening for colorectal cancer: a systematic review and meta-analysis. Clin Colorectal Cancer 2016;15(4): 298–313.

24. Brenner H, Chang-Claude J, Seiler CM, et al. Protection from colorectal cancer after colonoscopy: a population-based, case-control study. Ann Intern Med 2011;154(1):22–30.

25. Kahi CJ, Imperiale TF, Juliar BE, et al. Effect of screening colonoscopy on colorectal cancer incidence and mortality. Clin Gastroenterol Hepatol 2009;7(7): 770–5 [quiz: 711].

26. Siegel RL, Fedewa SA, Anderson WF, et al. Colorectal cancer incidence patterns in the United States, 1974-2013. J Natl Cancer Inst 2017;109(8).

27. Zhang J, Cheng Z, Ma Y, et al. Effectiveness of screening modalities in colorectal cancer: a network meta-analysis. Clin Colorectal Cancer 2017;16(4):252–63.

28. Rex DK, Bond JH, Winawer S, et al. Quality in the technical performance of colonoscopy and the continuous quality improvement process for colonoscopy: recommendations of the U.S. Multi-Society Task Force on Colorectal Cancer. Am J Gastroenterol 2002;97(6):1296–308.

29. Corley DA, Levin TR, Doubeni CA. Adenoma detection rate and risk of colorectal cancer and death. N Engl J Med 2014;370(26):2541.

30. Kaminski MF, Wieszczy P, Rupinski M, et al. Increased rate of adenoma detection associates with reduced risk of colorectal cancer and death. Gastroenterology 2017;153(1):98–105.

31. Robertson DJ, Lieberman DA, Winawer SJ, et al. Colorectal cancers soon after colonoscopy: a pooled multicohort analysis. Gut 2014;63(6):949–56.

32. Nguyen DL, Jamal MM, Nguyen ET, et al. Low-residue versus clear liquid diet before colonoscopy: a meta-analysis of randomized, controlled trials. Gastrointest Endosc 2016;83(3):499–507.e1.

33. Cooper GS, Kou TD, Rex DK. Complications following colonoscopy with anesthesia assistance: a population-based analysis. JAMA Intern Med 2013;173(7): 551–6.

34. Lee JK, Liles EG, Bent S, et al. Accuracy of fecal immunochemical tests for colorectal cancer: systematic review and meta-analysis. Ann Intern Med 2014; 160(3):171.

35. Lin JS, Piper MA, Perdue LA, et al. Screening for colorectal cancer: updated evidence report and systematic review for the US preventive services task force. JAMA 2016;315(23):2576–94.

36. Imperiale TF, Gruber RN, Stump TE, et al. Performance characteristics of fecal immunochemical tests for colorectal cancer and advanced adenomatous polyps: a systematic review and meta-analysis. Ann Intern Med 2019;170(5):319–29.

37. Imperiale TF, Ransohoff DF, Itzkowitz SH. Multitarget stool DNA testing for colorectal-cancer screening. N Engl J Med 2014;370(14):1287–97.

38. Kapidzic A, Grobbee EJ, Hol L, et al. Attendance and yield over three rounds of population-based fecal immunochemical test screening. Am J Gastroenterol 2014;109(8):1257–64.

39. Jensen CD, Corley DA, Quinn VP, et al. Fecal immunochemical test program performance over 4 rounds of annual screening: a retrospective cohort study. Ann Intern Med 2016;164(7):456–63.

40. Tau A, Bernica J, Thrift AP, et al. Changing trends in colorectal cancers (detected by screening, during screening intervals, or associated with nonadherence) identify possible health care system quality measures. Gastroenterology 2019;156(3): 809–11.
41. Hall IJ, Tangka FKL, Sabatino SA, et al. Patterns and trends in cancer screening in the United States. Prev Chronic Dis 2018;15:E97.
42. Levin TR, Corley DA, Jensen CD, et al. Effects of organized colorectal cancer screening on cancer incidence and mortality in a large community-based population. Gastroenterology 2018;155(5):1383–91.e5.
43. May FP, Yano EM, Provenzale D, et al. The association between primary source of healthcare coverage and colorectal cancer screening among US veterans. Dig Dis Sci 2017;62(8):1923–32.
44. de Moor JS, Cohen RA, Shapiro JA, et al. Colorectal cancer screening in the United States: trends from 2008 to 2015 and variation by health insurance coverage. Prev Med 2018;112:199–206.
45. Jackson CS, Oman M, Patel AM, et al. Health disparities in colorectal cancer among racial and ethnic minorities in the United States. J Gastrointest Oncol 2016;7(Suppl 1):S32–43.
46. May FP, Bromley EG, Reid MW, et al. Low uptake of colorectal cancer screening among African Americans in an integrated Veterans Affairs health care network. Gastrointest Endosc 2014;80(2):291–8.

Risk Stratification Strategies for Colorectal Cancer Screening

From Logistic Regression to Artificial Intelligence

Thomas F. Imperiale, MD[a,c,d,e,*], Patrick O. Monahan, PhD[b,e,f]

KEYWORDS

- Risk stratification • Colorectal cancer screening • Risk prediction models
- Cancer prevention • Multivariate methods • Machine learning methods

KEY POINTS

- Risk stratification in colorectal cancer (CRC) screening involves using factors associated with CRC or advanced neoplasia to estimate individual patient risk. It requires a decision or question, a risk and its timeframe, risk factors, and a system or method for integrating them.
- Among the methods for integrating risk factors (collectively referred to as artificial intelligence), 2 distinguishing features are (1) whether the system uses clinical pre-processing or instead a ground-up approach in which the machine explores unfiltered categories of candidate predictor variables, and (2) the flexibility-interpretability tradeoff inherent in the method.
- Several risk prediction models/risk stratification schemes predict current risk of advanced neoplasia, whereas far fewer predict future risk of CRC. The models use various performance metrics, which include calibration, discrimination, and risk separation.
- Risk stratification in CRC screening has the potential to improve the uptake, efficiency, and effectiveness of screening. This area requires further research on model validation and impact assessment.

[a] Department of Medicine, Indiana University School of Medicine, Indianapolis, IN, USA; [b] Department of Biostatistics, Indiana University School of Medicine and Richard M. Fairbanks School of Public Health, Indianapolis, IN, USA; [c] Health Services Research and Development, Richard L. Roudebush VA Medical Center, Indianapolis, IN, USA; [d] Regenstrief Institute, Inc., 1101 West 10th Street, Indianapolis, IN 46202, USA; [e] Indiana University Melvin and Bren Simon Cancer Center, Indiana University School of Medicine, Indianapolis, IN, USA; [f] Health Information and Translational Sciences, 410 West 10th Street Suite 3000, Indianapolis, IN 46202, USA
* Corresponding author. Regenstrief Institute, Inc., 1101 West 10th Street, Indianapolis, IN 46202.
E-mail address: timperia@iu.edu

Gastrointest Endoscopy Clin N Am 30 (2020) 423–440
https://doi.org/10.1016/j.giec.2020.02.004
1052-5157/20/Published by Elsevier Inc.

INTRODUCTION

Risk stratification is an important tool in both clinical medicine and population health. In the current era of precision/personalized medicine, risk stratification may be used to tailor preventive, diagnostic, and therapeutic strategies for individual patients or for subgroups of a population. For more than a half century, parametric regression modeling (mainly logistic regression) has been the dominant statistical technique used for creation of risk models and subsequent risk stratification tools. However, within the past decade, more automated (ie, "ground-up") approaches, and nonparametric methods such as neural networks, have established a presence in risk prediction; these newer methods promise to have a larger role going forward. To most, these are considered "black box" methods; however, they have an understandable and underlying theoretical and statistical foundation. Although these methods have flexibility to fit nuances in relationships, making their results more difficult to interpret, ad hoc techniques are emerging to help improve interpretability.

The aim of this article is to define and discuss the current and emerging methods of risk prediction and risk stratification, and to do so within the clinical and population health context of colorectal cancer (CRC) screening. This article discusses the what, how, and why of risk stratification as it applies to CRC screening, along with consideration of barriers to using risk prediction models for CRC screening. We also describe an agenda for research.

RISK STRATIFICATION

The need to understand, estimate, and incorporate risks into decision-making is omnipresent in both clinical medicine and public health. Risk is used in diagnosis ("What is the likelihood of this patient having disease X?"), prognosis ("What is this patient's chance of surviving 5 years with condition X?"), response to treatment ("How likely is this patient to respond to Drug X?"), and disease prevention ("Is screening this patient for X required at this time?"). We may begin the process of risk estimation in each of these settings with a general sense of the risk in the population under consideration or in the particular clinical setting. We then use risk factors (demographics, signs, symptoms, and other test results) to revise the risk estimate. The estimate moves up or down until it crosses a threshold for further testing, treating, or no further consideration of a particular diagnosis.

Risk stratification is an extension of the process of risk estimation, consisting of a system or process by which clinically meaningful separation of risk is achieved in a group of otherwise similar persons. It is a tool used in both clinical medicine and in population health to estimate risk for a particular outcome, for either an individual person or a group of individuals, and to separate individuals into different levels of risk, generally low, intermediate, and high risk. The separation is usually achieved based on specific demographic, lifestyle, clinical, and more recently, genetic, features of each member of the group. Risk stratification enables providers and policy makers to identify an appropriate level of health care and health services for the distinct subgroups ("strata"). It has the potential to improve the quality, appropriateness, and efficiency of health care provided.

One of the first and best-known examples of risk stratification is the Framingham Risk Score, created to estimate a person's 10-year risk of developing coronary heart disease (CHD).[1] It was created from a large cohort study of disease-free residents of Framingham, MA, who were followed for 20 years, during which time some residents experienced clinical events of CHD. Six factors were independently related to CHD risk in both gender-stratified analyses: age, blood pressure, total cholesterol level, high-density lipoprotein level, diabetes, and cigarette smoking.[2] Gender-specific risk scores were subsequently developed, for which "plugged-in" patient-specific values provide an estimate of the 10-year risk of a CHD event.[3]

In the areas of gastroenterology and hepatology, risk prediction models and risk scores are available for a myriad of diagnoses. Best known are the prognostic models for acute upper gastrointestinal bleeding (the Blatchford and Rockall scores,[4,5] among several), acute pancreatitis (Acute Physiology and Chronic Health Evaluation [APACHE-II] and Bedside Index of Severity in Acute Pancreatitis [BISAP] scores[6,7]), and progression of cirrhosis (Child-Turcotte-Pugh, MELD[8,9]), to name a few. In the domain of disease prevention, risk scores are less prevalent due to the challenges of risk prediction for conditions such as cancer, which are uncommon if not rare at the population level. Nevertheless, there are risk prediction models for breast cancer that are used in decision-making about when and how to screen women for breast cancer.[10] Below, we discuss the ones created for risk prediction of CRC and its precursor lesion, the advanced adenoma. We first want to consider the "why" of risk prediction models for CRC.

Why Risk Stratification?

There are many reasons, both individual patient-wise and societal, to use risk stratification in general. An overarching reason is that more and more people expect it. They hear the terms "personalized medicine," "precision medicine," and "providing the right care to the right patient at the right time," and want this for their own health care. Risk stratification may be used to tailor whether, when, and how to screen, test, or treat for a specific condition. Tailoring involves adjusting the intensity of management based on an individual's risk for a particular diagnosis. For patients, the adjustment is intended to optimize the balance between benefits and harms; for society, it is intended to improve efficiency: the use of current health care resources while minimizing waste and cost of unnecessary, low-yield, or low-value tests and treatments.

These principles are readily applied to CRC screening. From the individual patient perspective, there are at least a few reasons why CRC screening should be tailored more aggressively toward those at high risk. First, CRC is common among cancers (the second most common cancer and cancer death in men and women combined). Second, screening is effective in reducing CRC incidence and mortality, and does so cost-effectively. Third, screening is underutilized; current adherence rates are 60% to 65%.[11] In the same way, there are reasons to use risk stratification to tailor screening away from low-risk persons. Screening has risks. For example, false-positive test results can lead to unnecessary procedures with their more significant risks. These risks are of greater concern and relatively greater magnitude when the potential benefit is small or none. Further, when it comes to prevention of a uncommon or rare condition such as CRC, the great majority of persons do not benefit from screening.

From a societal perspective, using risk stratification to tailor CRC screening toward high-risk persons should be done to minimize lost productivity and downstream economic effects. Further, care of the patient with cancer is expensive, particularly for advanced-stage disease, with cost of some of the newer "personalized" agents exceeding $100,000 per year.[12] Similarly, reducing screening intensity for low-risk persons has the favorable effects of reducing the total cost of screening (ie, CRC screening may be cost-effective, but costs in the tens of billions of dollars annually)[13] and making resources available for other patients and other societal needs.

What Is Required for Risk Stratification?

Any use of risk stratification requires 4 elements. The first is the clinical or public health decision or question under consideration; for example, "What is this patient's prognosis given condition X?" or "How should this patient (or the population) be screened for CRC?" The second element is the condition or outcome. For CRC, the most relevant clinical outcomes are CRC itself and advanced neoplasia (AN; the combination of CRC and advanced precancerous polyps). Because advanced precancerous polyps nearly always lend themselves to definitive treatment at the time of colonoscopy, they are an attractive outcome. Further, because of their higher prevalence (vs CRC), AN has driven the great majority of studies on risk factors for CRC. The third element is identifying the risk of interest. What is the best overall estimate for risk? Part of considering this element is to identify factors affecting the risk under consideration, as well as its timeframe: is it a current risk or future risk? Regardless of whether a future or current risk is chosen, there needs to be factors associated with that risk. Under current implementation of CRC screening, only age and family history are considered in decision-making about whether, when, and how to screen. Depending on the specific guideline and family history, age is dichotomized at 50, 45, 40, or 10 years earlier than the youngest first-degree relative was at the time of CRC diagnosis. For average-risk persons, CRC risk nearly doubles for each decade between ages 50 and 80,[14] yet this information is not used in decision-making. We know much more about the factors related to risks of CRC and AN, yet we do not use them currently. These factors include cigarette smoking history, diet, physical activity, body mass index (BMI), metabolic syndrome, diabetes, and regular use of nonsteroidal anti-inflammatory drugs and aspirin, to name a few.[15] One reason these factors are usually not considered is the lack of a way to readily integrate or combine these factors to estimate risk. This shortcoming leads us to the final element required for risk estimation/stratification: a statistical method that allows simultaneous consideration of several risk factors to measure individual patient risk and place that risk into a stratum (or provide an estimated probability of risk). Let us now consider some of the current as well as up-and-coming methods for risk estimation and risk stratification. All of these methods are considered to perform both "machine learning" and "statistical learning" in that they use computers to generate algorithms using parametric or nonparametric methods that have a statistical foundation.[16]

SELECTED MODELING TECHNIQUES FOR RISK PREDICTION
Overview

"Artificial intelligence" (AI) can refer to either simple rules or to "identifying patterns in the data" using specific machine-learning and statistical-learning methods (**Fig. 1**). Two important features distinguish artificial learning methods. The first is whether the analyst applies clinical judgment to pre-process the data or instead applies a purely "ground-up" approach in which the machine explores the unfiltered or uncombined categories of the original predictors (called "features" in machine learning). The clinical pre-processing approach is often used in the biostatistical community, and involves understanding the modeling process in context of the underlying science. This process includes making decisions about how to categorize continuous or multi-category predictors into more clinically meaningful categories, such as pack-years for smoking or intervals for BMI. In the ground-up approach, the analyst purposely attempts to minimize clinical pre-processing to reduce analyst time (and thereby increase scalability) and to increase the potential to uncover potential relationships that are not preconceived. Nevertheless, the ground-up approach often involves data pre-processing decisions,

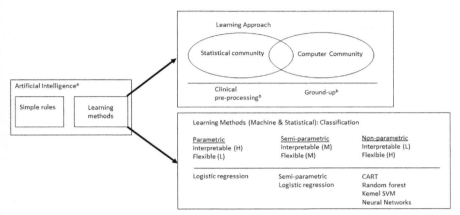

Fig. 1. Overview of AI methods. [a] AI = any technique that enables computers to mimic human behavior and perform tasks that normally require human intelligence. [b] Both approaches involve data science pre-processing decisions. H, high; L, low; M, moderate; SVM, support vector machine. An example of a simple rule is: start CRC screening at age 50.

such as how to handle missing data. The second important feature is the flexibility-interpretability tradeoff of the specific method used. The salient distinction between methods is their flexibility (and consequently their interpretability), not their terminology or their origins (eg, machine vs statistical learning).

For example, regarding origins, logistic regression is a traditional statistical method but is included in machine-learning text books. Neural network analysis is commonly used in the machine-learning community, but has a statistical foundation, is included in statistical-learning text books, and is similar to the statistical methods of project pursuit regression[16] and polynomial logistic regression.[17]

We will now explain how the salient difference among these methods is the extent of their flexibility[16] by focusing on methods for classifying or predicting a categorical response variable, such as CRC or AN. These methods are called "supervised" learning in the computer science community because training is supervised by known values of the dependent variable. In unsupervised learning, the analysis of a set of variables is not connected to an outcome variable. Examples of unsupervised learning include variable-based factor analysis, or person-based cluster analysis, of a set of CRC risk factors, performed to understand whether risk factors can be represented by a fewer number of factors (ie, dimensionality reduction) or whether there are groups of persons (ie, clusters) with similar combinations of risk factors, respectively. We will not discuss unsupervised methods further because they are less relevant for risk stratification. Supervised parametric models such as logistic regression provide (1) a test and an estimate of the magnitude of association (ie, odds ratio [OR]) between each predictor and the response (also known as the outcome or dependent variable); (2) easily interpretable results because a single regression coefficient describes the relationship between the feature and the response; and (3) an estimate of the probability of the response variable at the subject level. In logistic regression, the shape of the relationship between a continuous predictor (independent) variable and the response (dependent) variable is not very flexible because it assumes linearity between continuous features and the log odds of the response variable. Models with this restriction usually perform very well, and are preferred for their parsimony, if the true population relationship is reasonably linear.

If the population relationship between the predictor and outcome variables is markedly nonlinear, more accurate learning can be achieved by using semiparametric and nonparametric methods that attain greater flexibility. These nonparametric and semiparametric methods include classification tree analysis, support vector, random forest with bagging and boosting, neural networks, and semiparametric logistic regression, to name a few of the popular methods. In addition, "ensemble" methods incorporate results from more than one learning method or from more than one resampled data set within a learning method. Increased flexibility in these methods is generally attained through 1 or both of 2 general avenues: incorporating nonlinear relationships and/or interactions. Interactions allow the relationship between one feature and the response to depend on 1 or more other features, resulting in identifying subgroups. These subgroups are defined by combinations of features and can be illustrated by branches of trees, such as in the classification tree methods. Classification tree methods also conveniently automate the data-driven search for thresholds for categorizing continuous features when forming these subgroups. Nonlinear relationships between features and the response are incorporated in methods such as neural networks and generalized additive models.

Generalized additive models, such as nonparametric and semiparametric logistic regression, have origins in the statistical community. They incorporate nonlinear relationships between continuous predictors and the response variable by using scatterplot smoothers, while retaining a high degree of interpretability through the ability to provide probability estimates and tests of association.[16]

Although some flexible methods do not routinely provide probability estimates or tests of association and therefore have lower interpretability, their process for classification does have a probabilistic foundation. For example, the artificial neural network method was inspired by brain neural networks but can be demystified by realizing that it essentially involves creating new variables (ie, hidden layers), derived from weighted combinations of features, which are then used to predict the response through nonlinear (eg, sigmoid [or S-shaped]) functions. Furthermore, these "activation" functions are not deterministic or binary as mistakenly thought by some practitioners; they assume values ranging from 0 to 1, which are then categorized into a 0 versus 1 response classification, and the neural network's "cost function" is similar to the sum of squared residuals between observed and fitted values. Partial derivatives from calculus are used to iteratively update and estimate weights that minimize the cost function. Although calculus is used in neural networks, no learning method is inherently deterministic. Even if probabilities are not explicitly represented in formulas, all learning about complex phenomena, by definition, is affected by statistical sampling error. Sampling error is captured in the validation process, explained later in this article, making validation one of the most important aspects of evaluating model performance.

It is necessary to understand the metrics by which models are evaluated. The 2 most common measures for model evaluation are calibration and discrimination, both of which are statistical measures. Calibration conveys how well the model "fits" the data, and is measured by comparing the difference between observed and expected values for each observation in the sample. A small difference indicates a good-fitting model. Discrimination refers to how well a model can discriminate between an observation with the outcome and one without it. In logistic regression, a popular discrimination measure is the area under the receiver operating characteristic curve (AUROC; estimated with the c-statistic), which plots sensitivity (true-positive fraction) versus (1 − specificity) (or false-positive fraction) (**Fig. 2**). The diagonal bisecting line in **Fig. 2** represents no discrimination (as good as tossing a coin). The AUROC

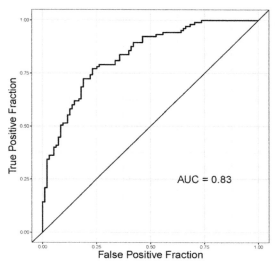

True Positive Fraction

AUC = 0.83

False Positive Fraction

Fig. 2. AUROC curve.

for the model in **Fig. 2** is 0.83, representing very good discrimination. Calibration and discrimination are "statistical" aspects of model performance. There is a third measure that is more "clinical"; it is the risk separation between strata or categories. This measure is more of a judgment about whether the difference(s) in estimated risk between or among categories is meaningful enough to affect decision-making about management. For example, if the respective risks for AN in the low-risk, intermediate-risk, and high-risk groups are 1%, 3%, and 6%, it is questionable whether these differences are "important" enough to affect which test is used for screening: a noninvasive test or lower endoscopy. On the other hand, if the respective risks for AN are 2%, 7%, and 25%, most persons in the high-risk group might best consider colonoscopy, whereas those in the low-risk group could safely and efficiently choose noninvasive screening.

For any model, the proof of how "good" it is requires testing it, a process known as validation. If allowed by larger sample sizes, the validation and test process can be separated into a validation data set used for evaluating particular "tuning" parameters and model building steps, and a test data set reserved for the final test of competing models. Some degree of model validation should be expected by potential adopters of the model. Indeed, the lack of literature on robust validation of models may be one reason limiting their more widespread use in clinical practice and public health settings. The rigor of testing determines the robustness of the model. Internal methods rely on a single data set and involve submitting it to resampling (eg, bootstrap) or multi-split-sample cross-validation methods. A more robust test of a model is a prospective evaluation by independent investigators in another setting from the one(s) in which the model was developed.

Among the internal methods, an estimate of the out-of-training sample prediction error can be obtained either indirectly and approximately through statistical indices such as the Akaike Information Criterion or Mallow's C, or directly through cross-validation.[16] The most commonly used internal cross-validation method is the "split-sample" technique, in which a portion of the dataset (typically 67%–80%) is used for model development, and the remaining portion is used to test the model's performance. However, an alternative, the k-fold cross-validation procedure, commonly performed with 5 or 10 folds, has several advantages.[16] First, its results have less bias than those of the split-sample procedure and lower variability (ie, better precision) than those of the leave-one-out procedure.[16] Second, unlike the split-sample procedure, the k-fold procedure provides an estimate of the mean and standard error of the cross-validation prediction error across the (eg, 5 or 10) hold-out validation samples.[16] Third, nonstatisticians tend to find split-sample and k-fold cross-validation more intuitive and easier to understand than the "leave-one-out" or bootstrap resampling procedures.

Validation is crucial because more flexible methods, by definition, usually fit data and classify responses in training (or derivation) samples better than less flexible methods. More flexible models have more parameters, more nonparametric "smoothing" (and therefore more nonlinearity), and more interaction terms. In cross-validation, more flexible, and therefore more complex, methods may fit a validation or test set poorly compared with less flexible methods. For example, age as a continuous variable will perfectly classify the outcome (eg, presence or absence of AN) in a training sample of 100 persons if 99 polynomial terms for age are entered into logistic regression. However, this high-degree-polynomial model would perform poorly on cross-validation metrics (and probably worse than a simple linear model) because the 98 nuanced bends in the curves between age and the logit of the outcome will be very different in one sample versus another sample due to statistical sampling error.

Logistic Regression

Among the several commonly used parametric regression techniques, logistic regression is most frequently used for risk stratification. What is being modeled is the logarithm of the odds of the outcome (or dependent) variable. The underlying assumptions are that the outcome variable has a binomial distribution, and that the relationship between the log odds of the outcome and the predictors is linear.

Logistic regression is the appropriate method when the dependent variable is binary or dichotomous (eg, presence or absence of disease); it explains the relationship between this single dependent dichotomous variable and one or more independent variables. It allows development of a predictive equation based on the probability of the outcome (such as present/absent, dead/alive). As with all modeling methods, the goal of logistic regression is to maximize the number of correct predictions of outcome for individual observations in the sample dataset using the most parsimonious model, meaning the simplest model that satisfies the underlying assumptions with the fewest variables and greatest explanatory power. The output of logistic regression is a set of estimated coefficients for an equation in the following format:

$$\text{Log}_e (p/1-p) = \beta_0 + \beta_1 x_1 + \beta_2 x_2 + ...+ \beta_n x_n,$$

where p is the probably of a binary event (eg, death, or presence/absence of AN), x_1, x_2, and x_n are the independent (or predictor) variables, and $\beta_{1 \to n}$ are the regression coefficients associated with reference group and the $x_{1 \to n}$ variables. The reference group, β_0, is derived from those individuals who have the reference level for all of the independent variables.

Even though the outcome for each observation in an existing dataset is known to be present or absent, the estimated probability for any single observation in the dataset is calculated by plugging in the specific values for the predictor variables (for example, age, sex, a first-degree relative with CRC), multiplying by its respective coefficient, summing the products (which will yield a log odds value between -1 and $+1$), and exponentiating that value, which provides the odds of the outcome for an individual. The odds may be converted to a probability using the following formula:

p(robability) = odds/(odds + 1), and provides the probability (or risk) of the outcome for that individual based on parameter estimates from the entire sample.

As an alternative to providing an odds or probability, the regression coefficients may be used to create a risk score for each individual. Each independent variable's contribution to the risk score depends on the value of its coefficient.[18] The coefficients can be rescaled, using a clinically meaningful metric such as the risk associated with a 5-year age interval, to produce a risk score that has a manageable point range (eg, 0–10 points instead of 0–158 points).[18] For a risk prediction model from our group,[19] we developed a risk score by re-scaling the log odds coefficients. Consistent with the Framingham approach, we prefer to derive risk scores using log odds coefficients instead of ORs, because the former are symmetric around their null value of 0, whereas the latter are asymmetric around their null value of 1.[18]

Nearly all of the "CRC" risk prediction models use current risk of AN as the outcome (present/absent); only a few predict a future risk of CRC.[20,21] Peng and colleagues[22] recently reviewed risk scores for predicting AN, finding 22 studies of 17 original risk scores that include a median number of 5 independent risk factors. The models most commonly include age, sex, BMI, cigarette smoking, and a first-degree relative with CRC. The AUROCs ranged from 0.62 to 0.77, representing fair-to-good discrimination.

There are fewer risk prediction models for estimating future risk of CRC because CRC is a much less common outcome than is AN, making model development more challenging. The National Cancer Institute's Risk Assessment Tool for Colorectal Cancer (http://www.cancer.gov/colorectalcancerrisk/) surveys the user for demographic features, personal and family medical history, diet and lifestyle information, and over-the-counter medication use. The risk assessment tool estimates 5-year and lifetime risks of CRC, and compares them with the average risk for the same age, gender, and race/ethnicity. In addition to future CRC risk, the model also estimates current risk for AN,[21,23] demonstrating its versatility in predicting 2 outcomes in 2 different timeframes.

There are other risk prediction models that use logistic regression to predict future CRC risk. Using cohort data from the Physicians' Health Study, Driver and colleagues[24] developed a model predicting 20-year risk of CRC among male physicians, identifying age by decade, smoking history, alcohol use, and BMI as independent risk factors. Using the ORs from these variables, the investigators created a risk score that ranged from 0 to 10, collapsing the scores to form 3 risk groups: low risk (scores of 0–3), intermediate risk (scores of 4–6), and high risk (scores of 7–10), in which the respective 20-year risks of CRC were 1%, 3%, and 6%. The model demonstrated good calibration (goodness-of-fit P value of 0.91) and fair discrimination (c-statistic by bootstrap validation of 0.69). However, the clinical importance of the risk separation is questionable. Further, the generalizability of the model and risk score, beyond US male physicians, is uncertain. A recent model was created to determine the starting age for CRC screening. Jeon and colleagues[25] used 2 large case-control studies, the GRECC (Geriatric Research, Education, and Clinical Centers) Consortium and the Colorectal Transdisciplinary study, with nearly 10,000 CRC cases and just over 10,000 controls, to estimate whether a person's 10-year CRC risk exceeded a threshold of 1%, which was based on the average 10-year risk for 50-year old men and women combined. Four models were created: Model I used family history alone; Model II used family history and an "E" score, the latter measuring risk based on 19 environmental (ie, phenotypic) factors; Model III used family history and a "G" score, which measured genetic risk based on 63 CRC-associated single-nucleotide polymorphisms; and Model IV used family history, "E" score and "G" score combined. Model metrics indicated that adding either "E" or "G" score to family history provided fair discrimination, with little improvement shown by Model IV, the combined model. Interestingly, the "E" and "G" components appeared to result in the same degree of risk prediction.

Classification and Regression Trees

Introduced in 1984, CART (Classification and Regression Trees) was first used in the clinical setting to identify patients at high risk of myocardial infarction within the first 24 hours of hospitalization. CART is a method of risk stratification that uses decision-tree algorithms for classification or regression predictive modeling. The tree is constructed through a method known as binary recursive partitioning, an iterative process that splits the data into branches with the goals of (1) identifying which factors are most important in a model predicting the dependent (or "target") outcome, and (2) dividing the study population or dataset into smaller and more homogeneous subgroups. Classification trees are used when the target variable is categorical (race/ethnicity, gender, marital status, eye color, or findings on colonoscopy, such as no neoplasia, nonadvanced neoplasia, and AN) or binary (CRC or AN present/absent), whereas regression trees are used when the outcome or target variable is continuous (age, height, or BMI, for example). The product is an algorithm in the form of a tree with branches that explains the relationship among variables and categorizes subsequent data into specific classes or subgroups.

A generic illustration of CART output is shown in **Fig. 3**. The tree begins with the entire study population represented by a single group. This single group is known as a parent "node" because it gives rise to 2 child nodes based on the feature that provides the greatest difference with respect to the target variable. CART allows for examination of all candidate predictor variables at each level of the algorithm/tree to identify the one that results in the cleanest split or separation based on the algorithm learned by the machine. Each parent node splits into only 2 child nodes. Each of the remaining independent variables is examined to determine which one now results in the largest difference (or "best split") based on predetermined outcome variable, with each of the child nodes potentially becoming parent nodes for the 2 child nodes that result from the second independent variable. With CART, the question asked at each step of the algorithm is based on the answer to the previous question. This procedure continues for each branch/node of the tree until criteria for a predetermined

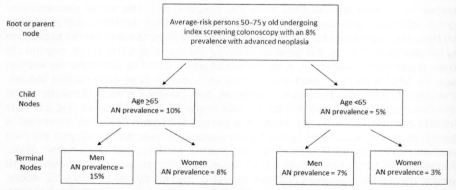

Fig. 3. CART for AN. Example of a classification tree showing variables associated with finding AN on index screening colonoscopy.

stopping rule are reached. A parameter known as the "complexity parameter" (CP) determines the number of splits in a tree by defining the minimum benefit that must be gained at each level (or split) to make that split worthwhile. The CP eliminates splits that add little or no value to the tree and, in doing so, provides a stopping rule for the tree. At this point, no further splitting occurs and each of the last nodes becomes a terminal node, representing mutually exclusive and exhaustive subgroups of the study population.

Advantages of CART include the following: (1) it is a nonparametric method of model building, which means that it requires minimal underlying assumptions; (2) it categorizes independent variables, and thus, can handle skewness without requiring transformation of variables to reduce overly influential observations; (3) it has characteristics of an automated "ground-up" learning method in that it does not require analyst input to discover cut points for continuous independent variable; and (4) it is easy for users to interpret.

For CRC risk prediction, there is at least one CART-based study worth mentioning. Shi and colleagues[26] used CART on regular health examination data for early detection of CRC, based on analysis of more than 7000 CRC cases and more than 140,000 controls without known CRC. The investigators validated the derived CART model on independent datasets, and compared its effectiveness in CRC detection with fecal immunochemical test (FIT)-based screening. The CART model included 4 variables that were dichotomized: albumin ($\geq$44 g/L vs <44 g/L), % lymphocytes ($\geq$16% vs <16%), age ($\geq$70 years vs <70 years), and hematocrit ($\geq$36% vs <36%). At a specificity of 99%, model sensitivity for CRC was 62.2%, with these test characteristics remaining fairly constant within subgroups of the validation data set having different CRC prevalence, aging rates, gender ratios, and distribution of cancer stages and locations. CART-based screening had a positive predictive value of 1.6%, which was higher than FIT (0.3%). This model and setting illustrate the potential of CART for risk stratification for CRC screening. CART-generating programs are available in both commercial statistical computing packages such as SPSS (IBM Corp, Armonk, NY), SAS (SAS Institute, Inc, Cary, NC), and STATA (Stata Corp, College Station, TX), and in open-source programs, most notably R.[27,28]

Neural Networks and Deep Learning

The basic structure of an artificial neural network is shown in **Fig. 4**, with each circle in the diagram representing a node, which some consider analogous to a neuron. A neural network is organized into 3 layers: an input layer, which consists of the independent (predictor) variables; an output layer, which generates a response to the input in the form of a dependent (predicted) variable; and a hidden layer, which connects the inner and outer layers based on intermediate values generated by the network. Hidden layers can be demystified by thinking of them as latent variables that are derived from weighted combinations of input values.[29] A neural network with many hidden layers is referred to as a deep neural network. Hidden nodes enable the modeling of complex, nonlinear relationships between predictor variables and outcome. Each input node is connected to each hidden node by connection weights, which represent the neural network counterpart of β coefficients in a regression model. These weights, like weights from other models, contain information about the strength of the relationship among input, hidden layers, and outcome.

Most neural networks "learn" through the process of backpropagation, short for "backward propagation of errors." The name is derived from how the error in a neural network system becomes minimized. Backpropagation uses the error associated with an incorrect guess to adjust its parameter estimates toward the endpoint of minimizing

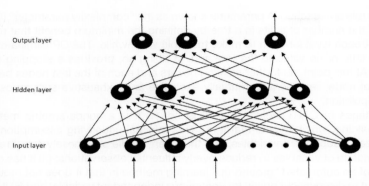

Output layer

Hidden layer

Input layer

Fig. 4. Structure of a neural network. (*From* Papik K, Molnar B, Schaefer R, Dombovari Z, Tulassay Z, Feher J. Application of neural networks in medicine-a review. Medical Science Monitor. 1998;4(3):MT538–MT546; with permission.)

error. In a multi-layer (or deep) neural network, this process occurs sequentially at each level, in which the relationship between the network's error and parameters of its last layer are optimized, then the process repeats between the last layer and second to last layer, and so forth.

A couple of examples of neural networks within the domain of CRC screening deserve mention, one involving classification of (diminutive) colorectal polyps using computer-aided diagnosis, and the other involving risk prediction for CRC using self-reportable personal health data. Both examples use artificial neural networks to accomplish these goals. Chen and colleagues[30] used images of diminutive neoplastic polyps and hyperplastic polyps to train a deep neural network, with histology used as the reference standard. The network was then tested on a separate set of images, and the results were compared with 2 expert and 4 novice endoscopists' assessments. The network identified neoplastic or hyperplastic polyps with 96.3% sensitivity and 78.1% specificity, and negative predictive value of 91.5%, the latter measure exceeding the PIVI threshold of 90%. The neural network outperformed the endoscopists, among whom both intraobserver and interobserver agreement was low. In the second example, Nartowt and colleagues[31] used data from the National Health Interview Survey to estimate CRC risk, constructing a neural network trained on 12 to 14 categories of personal health data from 1269 cases of CRC and more than 500,000 controls. Input variables included age, sex, race/ethnicity, BMI, smoking frequency, first-degree relatives with CRC, exercise frequency, and several comorbid conditions, whereas the output was a number between 0 and 1, and was treated as a risk score. When tested on an independent sample of 140 CRC cases and more than 58,000 controls, the neural network had a negative predictive value of 0.999. When compared with the US Preventive Services Task Force guidelines to stratify subjects into low-risk, intermediate-risk, and high-risk categories, the network outperformed the guidelines in subjects misclassified as low risk (from 35% to 5%) and misclassified as high risk (from 53% to 6%). These results exemplify the clinical and public health utility of neural networks for stratifying CRC risk, with the potential to improve the efficiency, effectiveness, and cost-effectiveness of screening.

Artificial Intelligence

We have already discussed some of the tools of AI. Until recently, AI conjured thoughts of robots, IBM's Watson supercomputer, smart speakers, facial recognition, and others. AI's most active area within gastroenterology, and specifically relevant to

CRC screening, has been for both polyp detection during colonoscopy[32] and real-time histologic determination.[33,34] This technology is approved for use in Europe and is under study in the United States.

In health care and other sectors, AI refers to the collection of concepts and technologies that facilitate the simulation of human intelligence processes (such as problem solving, learning, and pattern recognition) by machines, particularly computer systems. The technologies in AI's toolbox include natural language processing, artificial neural networks, data mining, and modeling methods that fit linear and nonlinear relationships. The utility of these techniques has been amplified by access to large databases and enhanced computational ability. Deep neural networks has emerged as a popular method underlying AI, as it is well suited to discovering complex nonlinear relationships; however, because many parameters are estimated, it is well suited for large samples sizes and is often outperformed by parametric logistic regression in cross-validation analysis when the underlying population data contains very few nonlinear relationships.

Although the potential of AI in medicine appears limitless, its greatest utility to date has been in the area of image analysis: discriminating between basal cell carcinoma and benign lesions, identifying retinal findings of diabetic retinopathy, and colorectal polyp recognition[32] and real-time histologic diagnosis,[33] among many others. Image analysis and other data sets that provide many observations are ideal for nonparametric methods that involve estimating many coefficients (such as neural networks) because greater numbers of observations are needed to reliably estimate models with large numbers of coefficients.

A MEDLINE search intersecting the terms "colorectal cancer screening," "risk prediction," and "artificial intelligence" yielded 12 references, 3 of which are directly relevant to this discussion. The 3 studies report on the same model, which was used to identify patients who may have had CRC based on specific factors identified from examination of routinely collected clinical data from large numbers of patients with and without CRC. Kinar and colleagues[35] used a method known as random forest modeling, which combines CART with ensemble learning by aggregating results from multiple decision trees obtained from bootstrap-derived repeat random resamples of the original data set.[16] They used a dataset of more than 600,000 Israeli patients, 3135 of whom had a CRC diagnosis, deriving the model on 80% of the sample and validating it on both the remaining 20% and an entirely separate dataset from the United Kingdom that included 5061 CRC cases and 25,613 controls. This final model was then tested completely independently on an independent dataset for external validation. The criteria by which model performance was evaluated included (1) AUROC for overall performance; (2) determination of the odds of CRC above versus below a threshold corresponding to a specificity of 99.5%; and (3) determination of the proportion of controls correctly classified as such (ie, specificity) at the model threshold corresponding to a sensitivity of 50%.

The model identified age and variables from a complete blood count (CBC) (eg, hemoglobin, mean corpuscular value, red cell distribution width, platelet count, others) obtained 3 to 6 months before the CRC diagnosis as the most discriminating features. The model's AUROC was 0.82, whereas the OR for CRC was 26 at the threshold required for a false-positive rate of 0.5% (or specificity of 99.5%). At a CRC sensitivity of 50%, model specificity was 88%. Based on these performance metrics, the investigators concluded that the model may help to detect CRC earlier in clinical practice by supplementing detection through screening. Although this review is not the forum for critical evaluation of the article, a couple of limitations are worth discussing. One is that the stage spectrum of CRCs in the Israeli and UK cohorts is not described. The model would be of greater clinical utility if most or all of the cancers detectable were of a curable stage (0, I, II). Further, the 3-month to 6-month interval between CBC and CRC diagnosis is short and may have good discrimination only because of such close proximity to the cancer diagnosis. The short interval might not allow the opportunity for intervention that favorably affects prognosis compared with the opportunity provided by a longer interval.

In the second article identified, which addressed the time interval issue, Birks and colleagues[36] tested the model using the UK's Clinical Practice Research Datalink, from which patients 40 to 89 years with full CBC data were risk stratified by the model and followed for a CRC diagnosis. In this retrospective cohort study, the investigators identified CBCs at least 18 months before the CRC diagnosis for cases and before the end date of follow-up for controls. The CBCs obtained during the 18-month to 24-month interval were considered as the primary analysis, with secondary analyses consisting of intervals of 3 to 6 months, 6 to 12 months, 12 to 18 months, and 24 to 36 months before the CRC diagnosis. For the primary analysis, which included 5141 CRC cases and 2,220,108 controls, the AUROC was 0.776 (95% confidence interval [CI] 0.771–0.781). At a specificity of 99.5% (ie, a false-positive rate of 0.5%), the positive predictive value was 8.8%. As expected, model performance improved to an AUROC of 0.84 for the 3-month to 6-month interval, validating the model developed by Kinar and colleagues.[35] Most of the model discrimination was due to age, as evidenced by an age-matched case-control analysis for which AUROC was 0.583 (CI 0.574–0.591), indicating poor discrimination of the residual factors. The investigators concluded that this model, with an 18-month to 24-month lead-time, offered an additional way to identify patients with CRC. The CRC stage distribution was not described in this study.

The third article is another evaluation of the same model using data from Kaiser Permanente's Northwest Region.[37] Hornbrook and colleagues[37] identified a random sample of 900 CRC cases and 18 controls per case (age range 40–89 years for both groups) selected from the same year of the case's diagnosis and matched on the general population's distribution of 10-year age groups and length of enrollment. Intervals of 0 to 180 days and 181 to 360 days between CBC date and CRC diagnosis were considered, with respective ORs, at 99% specificity, of 34.7 and 20.4 and an overall AUROC of 0.80. Individuals in the highest 1% of scores had a 20-fold greater CRC risk within the subsequent 12 to 18 months. The AUROC for age alone was 0.73, supporting the dominance of age in the model. Among the 605 (67%) cases for which CRC stage was available, ORs at a specificity of 99% ranged from 12.1 for in situ cancers to 40.4 for stage IV. ORs were higher for CRCs in the proximal colon, although a more advanced-stage distribution may account for this finding. These US findings are consistent with the other 2 studies, and suggest that routinely collected electronic health data may be used to supplement screening in the early identification of CRC.

Cumulatively, these articles illustrate the data mining and computational capacities and potential of current technology for identifying patterns in large, complex datasets and for deriving and testing multivariable models to identify how these patterns provide diagnostic discrimination. Given the persuasive nature of the computational capacity of AI methods, it behooves the reader/user to determine whether the underlying study methods and results are reliable and valid, what the results mean both quantitatively and clinically, and whether and to what extent the model can be applied to patients in other settings. Liu and colleagues[38] recently published a user's guide for understanding articles that use machine learning. It provides step-by-step guidance for evaluating this body of literature with a critical eye.[39]

BARRIERS TO USE OF RISK PREDICTION MODELS

Despite the proliferation of risk prediction models in medicine in general, and the several models available for prediction of current risk for AN and future CRC risk, the great majority of models are not used in clinical practice. Several factors negatively impact their use, foremost among which are (1) absence of robust validation, and (2) lack of an impact analysis. Many models have had no "external" (ie, independent) validation. A hierarchy of increasing stringent validation includes temporal, geographic, and domain validation.[40] Temporal validation tests a prediction model at a different time, but is usually done by the same investigators at the same institution and with the same population. Geographic validation varies time and place, and is carried out in a population defined by the setting and inclusion and exclusion criteria of the development study. The most rigorous test of a model, domain validation, varies time, place, setting, and patient spectrum, including demographics. The degree of validation required of a risk prediction model depends on the setting for its intended use. Most models with some degree of external validation nearly always include temporal and geographic variation, much less so, domain variation.

Impact analysis of a prediction rule requires its testing in a clinical trial, and would typically examine several outcomes, including clinical, economic, and satisfaction. Very few prediction rules in any area have had an impact analysis. For CRC risk prediction, Schroy and colleagues[41] tested a decision aid alone or with a risk assessment tool for AN in 341 asymptomatic average-risk patients, and found no differences in test concordance between patients' preference and test ordered. But this is just one study in a single setting, with the outcome of test concordance, 1 intervention (a decision aid plus a risk assessment tool), and 1 significant comparator (the decision aid itself) that likely diluted the effect of the risk assessment tool itself. We need many more impact studies that consider the setting and format for how a risk prediction model should be tested and applied.

Several other reasons contribute to the nonuse of risk prediction models, one of which is providers' understanding of these models, particularly their output. This barrier may be overcome with interface software that facilitates understanding and perhaps links to a preferred strategy or, in the case of CRC screening, to a preferred test for a particular level of risk. A related reason is provider trust of the model. To many providers, risk prediction models invoke a "black box" response, affecting their level of confidence in the model itself and uncertainty about the methodological quality of the research that belies it. An extension of this reason is provider fear of litigation. To assuage this concern, those models with consistent performance and high degrees of validity and generalizability should be supported by guideline organizations. Institutional factors also contribute to nonuse, specifically the extent of support for and integration into the workflow of prediction models. How should these tools integrate into the electronic medical record? Should they instead be available through patient portals for patients to consider before seeing a provider? The answers to these questions depend both on the prediction model being considered and the goals for its use. Related to these issues, the opportunities and challenges in moving from current guidelines to personalized CRC screening have been nicely described by Robertson and Ladabaum.[42]

AGENDA FOR RESEARCH

Despite the proliferation and promise of risk prediction models, including those for CRC screening, questions exist about whether, when, and how to use them, and whether they will improve the uptake and efficiency of screening and, most importantly, outcomes of CRC incidence, morbidity, and mortality. The most important items on the research agenda are studies assessing the extent of validation of risk prediction models, and studies assessing their impact on processes and outcomes of care. Use of large datasets may be especially helpful with validation studies, as these could be applied retrospectively if the proper factors are identifiable in those datasets. Impact analyses will require either randomized trials or quasi-randomized trials, such as before-after studies. Other research agenda items include understanding provider and patient attitudes toward risk prediction models and how these tools are best integrated into the health care system. It is likely that whether and how risk prediction models are used and which ones are used will depend on the particular health care system, requiring research at the systems level.

DISCLOSURE

The authors have nothing to disclose.

REFERENCES

1. Doyle J, Kannel W. Coronary risk factors: 10 year findings in 7446 Americans, Pooling Project. VI World Congress of Cardiology, London, England, September, 1970.
2. Truett J, Cornfield J, Kannel W. A multivariate analysis of the risk of coronary heart disease in Framingham. J Clin Epidemiol 1967;20(7):511–24.
3. MDCalc. Framingham risk score for hard coronary heart disease: estimates 10-year risk of heart attack. 2005. Updated 2019. Available at: https://www.mdcalc.com/framingham-risk-score-hard-coronary-heart-disease, Accessed December 5, 2019.
4. Blatchford O, Murray WR, Blatchford M. A risk score to predict need for treatment for uppergastrointestinal haemorrhage. Lancet 2000;356(9238):1318–21.
5. Rockall T, Logan R, Devlin H, et al. Risk assessment after acute upper gastrointestinal haemorrhage. Gut 1996;38(3):316–21.
6. Larvin M, Mcmahon M. APACHE-II score for assessment and monitoring of acute pancreatitis. Lancet 1989;334(8656):201–5.
7. Wu BU, Johannes RS, Sun X, et al. The early prediction of mortality in acute pancreatitis: a large population-based study. Gut 2008;57(12):1698–703.
8. Pugh R, Murray-Lyon I, Dawson J, et al. Transection of the oesophagus for bleeding oesophageal varices. Br J Surg 1973;60(8):646–9.
9. Said A, Williams J, Holden J, et al. Model for end stage liver disease score predicts mortality across a broad spectrum of liver disease. J Hepatol 2004;40(6):897–903.
10. Gail MH, Brinton LA, Byar DP, et al. Projecting individualized probabilities of developing breast cancer for white females who are being examined annually. J Natl cancer inst 1989;81(24):1879–86.
11. Wolf AM, Fontham ET, Church TR, et al. Colorectal cancer screening for average-risk adults: 2018 guideline update from the American Cancer Society. CA Cancer J Clin 2018;68(4):250–81.
12. Johnston S, Wilson K, Varker H, et al. Real-world direct health care costs for metastatic colorectal cancer patients treated with cetuximab or bevacizumab-containing regimens in first-line or first-line through second-line therapy. Clin Colorectal Cancer 2017;16(4):386–96.e1.
13. Subramanian S, Tangka FK, Hoover S, et al. Costs of colorectal cancer screening provision in CDC's Colorectal Cancer Control Program: comparisons of colonoscopy and FOBT/FIT based screening. Eval Program Plann 2017;62:73–80.

14. Fletcher RH. Personalized screening for colorectal cancer. Med Care 2008; 46(9):S5–9.
15. Dekker E, Tanis PJ, Vleugels JLA, Kasi PM, Wallace MB. Colorectal Cancer. Lancet 2019;394(10207):1467–80.
16. Hastie T, Tibshirani R, Friedman J. The elements of statistical learning: data mining, inference, and prediction. 2nd ed. New York: Springer; 2009.
17. Cheng X, Khomtchouk B, Matloff N, et al. Polynomial regression as an alternative to neural nets. arXiv:1806.06850v3 [cs.LG] 2019;1–26.
18. Sullivan LM, Massaro JM, D'Agostino RB Sr. Presentation of multivariate data for clinical use: the Framingham Study risk score functions. Stat Med 2004;23(10): 1631–60.
19. Imperiale TF, Monahan PO, Stump TE, et al. Derivation and validation of a scoring system to stratify risk for advanced colorectal neoplasia in asymptomatic adults: a cross-sectional study. Ann Intern Med 2015;163(5):339–46.
20. Usher-Smith JA, Walter FM, Emery JD, et al. Risk prediction models for colorectal cancer: a systematic review. Cancer Prev Res (Phila) 2016;9(1):13–26.
21. Ma GK, Ladabaum U. Personalizing colorectal cancer screening: a systematic review of models to predict risk of colorectal neoplasia. Clin Gastroenterol Hepatol 2014;12(10):1624–34.e1.
22. Peng L, Weigl K, Boakye D, et al. Risk scores for predicting advanced colorectal neoplasia in the average-risk population: a systematic review and meta-analysis. Am J Gastroenterol 2018;113(12):1788–800.
23. Imperiale TF, Yu M, Monahan PO, et al. Risk of advanced neoplasia using the national cancer institute's colorectal cancer risk assessment tool. J Natl Cancer Inst 2017;109(1). djw181.
24. Driver JA, Gaziano JM, Gelber RP, et al. Development of a risk score for colorectal cancer in men. Am J Med 2007;120(3):257–63.
25. Jeon J, Du M, Schoen RE, et al. Determining risk of colorectal cancer and starting age of screening based on lifestyle, environmental, and genetic factors. Gastroenterology 2018;154(8):2152–64.e19.
26. Shi Q, Gao Z, Wu P, et al. An enrichment model using regular health examination data for early detection of colorectal cancer. Chin J Cancer Res 2019;31(4): 686–98.
27. Kuhn L, Page K, Ward J, et al. The process and utility of classification and regression tree methodology in nursing research. J Adv Nurs 2014;70(6):1276–86.
28. Venables W, Smith D, R Development Core Team. An introduction to R. Vienna (Austria): R Foundation for Statistical Computing; 2010.
29. Papik K, Molnar B, Schaefer R, et al. Application of neural networks in medicine-a review. Med Sci Monit 1998;4(3):MT538–46.
30. Chen PJ, Lin MC, Lai MJ, et al. Accurate classification of diminutive colorectal polyps using computer-aided analysis. Gastroenterology 2018;154(3):568–75.
31. Nartowt BJ, Hart GR, Roffman DA, et al. Scoring colorectal cancer risk with an artificial neural network based on self-reportable personal health data. PLoS One 2019;14(8):e0221421.
32. Misawa M, Kudo SE, Mori Y, et al. Artificial intelligence-assisted polyp detection for colonoscopy: initial experience. Gastroenterology 2018;154(8):2027–9.e3.
33. Byrne MF, Chapados N, Soudan F, et al. Real-time differentiation of adenomatous and hyperplastic diminutive colorectal polyps during analysis of unaltered videos of standard colonoscopy using a deep learning model. Gut 2019;68(1):94–100.

34. Urban G, Tripathi P, Alkayali T, et al. Deep learning localizes and identifies polyps in real time with 96% accuracy in screening colonoscopy. Gastroenterology 2018; 155(4):1069–78.e8.

35. Kinar Y, Kalkstein N, Akiva P, et al. Development and validation of a predictive model for detection of colorectal cancer in primary care by analysis of complete blood counts: a binational retrospective study. J Am Med Inform Assoc 2016; 23(5):879–90.

36. Birks J, Bankhead C, Holt TA, et al. Evaluation of a prediction model for colorectal cancer: retrospective analysis of 2.5 million patient records. Cancer Med 2017; 6(10):2453–60.

37. Hornbrook MC, Goshen R, Choman E, et al. Early colorectal cancer detected by machine learning model using gender, age, and complete blood count data. Dig Dis Sci 2017;62(10):2719–27.

38. Liu Y, Chen PC, Krause J, et al. How to read articles that use machine learning: users' guides to the medical literature. JAMA 2019;322(18):1806–16.

39. Doshi-Velez F, Perlis RH. Evaluating machine learning articles. JAMA 2019; 322(18):1777–9.

40. Toll DB, Janssen KJ, Vergouwe Y, et al. Validation, updating and impact of clinical prediction rules: a review. J Clin Epidemiol 2008;61(11):1085–94.

41. Schroy PC 3rd, Duhovic E, Chen CA, et al. Risk stratification and shared decision making for colorectal cancer screening: a randomized controlled trial. Med Decis Making 2016;36(4):526–35.

42. Robertson DJ, Ladabaum U. Opportunities and challenges in moving from current guidelines to personalized colorectal cancer screening. Gastroenterology 2019;156(4):904–17.

Colorectal Cancer in Persons Under Age 50

Seeking Causes and Solutions

Swati G. Patel, MD MS[a],*, Clement Richard Boland, MD[b]

KEYWORDS

- Colorectal cancer • Lynch syndrome • Adenoma • Colonoscopy

KEY POINTS

- Incidence and mortality associated with colorectal cancer (CRC) is increasing in patients younger than 50 years. By the year 2030, 10% of all colon cancers and 22% of all rectal cancers will be diagnosed in patients under the age of 50.
- Approximately 16% of CRCs in patients younger than 50 years are associated with a germline genetic predisposition to cancer; another 20% to 25% of cases are associated with family history of CRC, and the remaining cases are sporadic.
- CRCs diagnosed in patients under the age of 50 are more likely to occur in the left colon, especially the rectum. They may have a distinct pathogenesis.
- Immediate ways to address this trend include continued efforts to collect and act on cancer family history, improve recognition of hereditary cancer syndromes, and immediate evaluation of colorectal symptoms in young patients.
- Lowering the screening age is another way to address this trend; however, more research is needed to determine the optimal age to start screening and the best modalities. Further work is needed to determine whether screening approaches based on risk factors can help screen the patients who will benefit from it the most.

INTRODUCTION

Over the last several decades, the overall incidence and mortality associated with colorectal cancer (CRC) has decreased in the United States. Reasons for this decline include increasing uptake of colorectal screening and colonoscopic polypectomy in those over the age of 50,[1] as well as changing risk factors (decreased smoking and increased use of hormone replacement therapy and aspirin).[2]

[a] Division of Gastroenterology & Hepatology, Rocky Mountain Regional Veterans Affairs Medical Center, Aurora, CO, USA; [b] University of California San Diego School of Medicine, 9500 Gilman Drive, 2-065 East Campus Office Building, La Jolla, CA 92093-0956, USA
* Corresponding author. 12631 East 17th Avenue, MS B-158, Aurora, CO 80045.
E-mail address: Swati.Patel@cuanschutz.edu
Twitter: @swatigp (S.G.P.)

Gastrointest Endoscopy Clin N Am 30 (2020) 441–455
https://doi.org/10.1016/j.giec.2020.03.001
1052-5157/20/Published by Elsevier Inc.
giendo.theclinics.com

Contrary to this general trend, the incidence and mortality associated with CRC are increasing in patients under age 50.[3] This article reviews the epidemiology, clinicopathological features, and proposed etiologies for these changing trends. It also presents practical approaches and opportunities to curbing these trends.

DEFINITIONS

The term early onset CRC (EOCRC) includes a heterogeneous population of patients. Most studies have defined EOCRC as CRC occurring in patients younger than 40 to 55 years of age, and have not sorted out patients at increased risk because of presence of family history or hereditary cancer syndromes. Although a specific cut-off age does not necessarily separate biologically or pathophysiologically different disease entities, 50 is an intuitive cut-off based on most currently accepted recommendations to start screening in the general population.[4–6] For the purposes of this article, EOCRC will refer to those diagnosed with CRC younger than 50 years, unless otherwise specified. This article will focus on sporadic EOCRCs. More detailed reviews of hereditary colorectal cancer syndromes can be found elsewhere.[7–10]

EPIDEMIOLOGY
Incidence

In the United States, CRC is the second most common cancer and the third leading cause of cancer-related death in individuals younger than 50 years of age.[11] Eleven percent of all CRCs diagnosed in men occur in patients younger than 50 years of age (10% for women).[12] The median age of diagnosis for those younger than age 50 is 44, with 75.2% of all CRCs occurring between the ages of 40 and 49.[13] CRC incidence has been steadily increasing in younger patients for the last several decades, with the sharpest rise seen in incidence of rectal cancer (**Fig. 1**). By the year 2030, 10% of all colon cancers and 22% of all rectal cancers in the United States are expected to be diagnosed in patients younger than 50 years of age.[14]

EOCRCs affect men and women, but with a slight male predominance. Bhandari and colleagues[11] reported age-specific incidence rates per 100,000 population for ages 30 to 34 (men 4.9 cases vs women 4.2 cases), ages 35 to 39 (men 9.9 cases

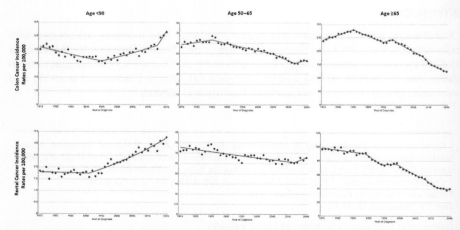

Fig. 1. Age-adjusted SEER incidence rates of colon and rectal cancer from 1975 to 2016 by age. Data plotted by accessing SEER*Explorer (https://seer.cancer.gov/explorer/index.html).

vs women 7.6 cases), ages 40 to 44 (men 16.4 cases vs women 15.3 cases), and ages 45 to 49 (men 30.8 cases vs women 25.9 cases).

The rise in EOCRC persists across racial and ethnic groups in the United States; however, the rates of change vary. Between the year 2000 and 2013, EOCRC incidence increased 2.5% in American Indian/Alaskan Natives, 2.3% in non-Hispanic whites, 1.0% in non-Hispanic blacks, and 0.2% in Asian/Pacific Islanders.[12] In an analysis of SEER (Surveillance, Epidemiology, and End Results) data, Murphy and colleagues[15] reported that from 1992 to 1996 to 2010 to 2014, CRC incidence increased from 7.5 to 11.0 cases per 100,000 population in white individuals and from 11.7 to 12.7 cases per 100,000 population in black individuals. The increase in rectal cancer was larger in whites (from 2.7 to 4.5 cases per 100,000 population) than in blacks (from 3.4 to 4.0 cases per 100,000 population).

Mortality

CRC-associated mortality in the United States in those age 20 to 54 declined from 6.3 cases per 100,000 population in 1970 to 3.9 cases per 100,000 population in 2004.[16] However, more recently there has been a 13% increase from 2000 to 2014 (4.3 cases per 100,000 population).[16] The recent increase in mortality is limited to whites, where there has been a 1.4% increase per year from 2004 to 2014 (3.6 cases per 100,000 population to 4.1 cases per 100,000 population). Among blacks, mortality declined by 0.4% to 1.1% annually, but blacks still had a higher absolute mortality rate than whites in 2014 (6.1 deaths per 100,000 population).[16] Blacks with EOCRC have an increased risk of cancer-related death (relative risk [RR] 1.35, 95% confidence interval [CI] 1.26–1.45) with a 5-year survival of 54.9% compared with 68.1% among non-Hispanic whites.[17] The racial disparities are likely multifactorial, stemming from a combination of socioeconomic, access to care, dietary, environmental, and biologic factors.[18]

Regional Variations

There are significantly different rates of EOCRC by state with higher incidence seen in the Mississippi Delta Region and Appalachia (14 cases per 100,000 population) compared with western states (9.5 cases per 100,000 population).[19] Although the western states have a lower absolute incidence, these states have seen the sharpest increase in incidence. Data from the American Association of Central Cancer Registries, which include 47 US states and the District of Columbia, showed that of the 10 states with the highest average annual percent change in incidence, 6 were located in the western United States. Comparing 1995 to 1996 with 2014 to 2015, Washington State's EOCRC incidence increased from 6.7 to 11.5 cases per 100,000 population. Over the same period, EOCRC incidence in Colorado increased from 6.0 to 9.5 cases per 100,000 population.[20]

Internationally, there is significant variability in EOCRC incidence (12.9 cases per 100,000 population in Korea vs 3.5 cases per 100,000 population in India). Of 42 countries included in a recent analysis, EOCRC incidence has been increasing in 19 countries across North America, Europe, Asia, and Australia. In 9 of these countries, EOCRC has been increasing as later-age onset CRC is stable or has been decreasing.[21]

Birth Cohort Effect

Siegel and colleagues[3] used age period cohort modeling to determine the influence of period effects (generally occur because of changes in clinical practice) versus birth cohort effects (caused by generation-specific changes in risk factors) in the rising incidence of EOCRC. SEER incidence data from 1974 to 2013 were analyzed by age group. Incidence in the 20 to 29, 30 to 39, and 40 to 49 age groups declined from the mid-1970s to the mid-1980s. The incidence started rising for those 20 to 39 starting in the mid-1980s and then in the mid-1990s for those age 40 to 54. In contrast, incidence in older individuals increased from the mid-1970s to the mid-1980s and then declined starting in the 1990s.

Interestingly, the incidence curve for those age 50 to 54 is similar to the older age groups in the 1970s to 1980s, but then reflects the younger age group after the mid-1990s. Siegel and colleagues conclude that the younger birth cohorts are carrying the elevated risk with them as they age and that this supports a strong cohort effect in the data. Wolf and colleagues[22] illustrate this cohort effect (**Fig. 2**).

CLINICAL AND PATHOLOGIC FEATURES

Most CRCs in young patients are identified because of signs and symptoms rather than incidentally or through screening (**Table 1**). In a series of over 1000 EOCRCs,

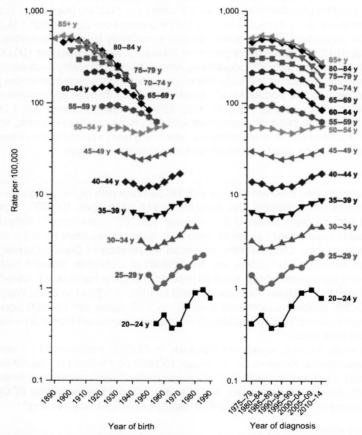

Fig. 2. Trends in colorectal cancer incidence rates by (A) age and year of birth, and by (B) age and year of diagnosis, United States, 1975 to 2014. (Data source: Surveillance, Epidemiology, and End Results (SEER) program, SEER 9 registries, delayed adjusted rates, 1975-2014, National Cancer Institute. From Wolf AMD, Fontham ETH, Church TR, et al. Colorectal cancer screening for average-risk adults: 2018 guideline update from the American Cancer Society. CA Cancer J Clin 2018;68:250-281; with permission.)

Table 1
Clinical and pathologic features of colorectal cancer diagnosed in patients under and over the age of 50

Clinical and Pathologic Features		EOCRC (<Age 50)	Later Onset CRC (≥Age 50)
Presenting with symptoms (%)		86.4[23]–94.0[81]	33.9–51.5[32]
Incidental or screen detected (%)		5.2[24]	14.6[24]
Duration of symptoms (days)		243[24]	154[24]
Time to diagnosis (days)		152–217[24,82]	29.5–87[24,82]
Family history of CRC (%)		13.8–33.5[24,32,33]	8.3–19.3[24,32,33]
Location (%)	Right colon	16.2–35.2[23,24,26,27,32,33,81]	28.5–51.5[24,32,33]
	Left colon	29.1–41.2[23,24,26,27,81]	33.6–48.5[24,33]
	Rectal	25.4–49.1[23,24,26,27,32,81]	31.3–34.9[24,32]
Histology (%)	Mucinous	10.0–14.5[26–28]	4.7–10.8[28]
	Signet ring	2.0–13.0[26,27,29]	0.9–4.0[13,83]
	Poor or no differentiation	7.2–27.9[26–28]	3.2–18.0[13,28]
Stage (%)	Early	11.0–47.0[23,26,27,33,81]	37.5–69.7[24,33,81]
	Late	61.2–89.0[23,24,26,27,32,33,81]	30.3–62.5[24,32,33,81]

he most common presenting symptom was rectal bleeding (50.8%), followed by ɪbdominal pain (32.5%) and change in bowel habits (18.0%).[23] When compared to symptomatic older patients with CRC, Chen and colleagues reported that young pa-ients are more likely to present with symptoms of hematochezia (28.8% vs 23.2%) ɪnd abdominal pain (41.2% vs 27.2%).

EOCRC patients experience symptoms for longer (243 vs 154 days) and have a ɪonger delay to diagnosis (152 vs 87 days), compared with older patients (see Table 1).[24]

Younger patients tend to more commonly present with left-sided cancers. Patients diagnosed with CRC over the age of 50 are more likely to have right-sided cancers ꜰ31.1% vs 20.0%, P<.001), and younger patients are more likely to have rectal cancer ꜰ31.2% vs 22.4%, P<.001) (see Table 1).[25]

CRCs in the young also appear to have more aggressive histopathology than those n older patients. Overall, mucinous and signet ring histologies were seen in 10.0% to ⲓ4.5%[26–29] and 2.0 to 13.0%[26,27,29] of EOCRCs, respectively, with up to 27.9% of ɪancers being poorly differentiated or undifferentiated.[24] Comparative data from the ꜰlational Cancer Database showed that young-onset CRC was modestly, but signifi-ɪantly, more likely to have a mucinous and/or signet-ring histology compared with ꝋlder-onset CRCs (12.6% vs 10.8%, P<.001) and poor or no differentiation (20.4% ꜰs 18%; P<.001).[13]

CRC in the young tends to present at a more advanced stage (see Table 1). Abdel-ɪattar and colleagues[25] reported RR of 1.37 (1.33-1.41) and 1.58 (1.53-1.63) for ꜰounger patients to present with regional or distant metastasis, respectively, ɪompared with older patients. Chen and colleagues[24] found that the difference in ꜱtage at presentation between EOCRC and later-onset CRCs could not be explained ꜱimply by a longer time between the onset of symptoms and diagnosis.

Despite seemingly later stage and more aggressive histology at presentation, ⲈOCRC patients appear to have equivalent, if not improved stage-specific outcomes. n 1 large report of SEER data, the stage-adjusted, cancer-specific survival was better n younger patients compared with those diagnosed over the age of 50 (local: 95.1% ꜰs 91.9%; regional: 76% vs 70.3%; distant: 21.3% vs 14.1%).[25]

It is important to note that the literature on EOCRC clinical and pathologic features is drawn from retrospective series that have not consistently separated sporadic cancers from those occurring in patients with hereditary cancer syndromes. Two recent studies characterized cohorts of EOCRC patients with multigene panel testing. Although these are small cohorts (450 and 430 patients, each), Pearlman and colleagues[30] reported that left-sided cancers (including rectal) comprised a larger proportion of sporadic EOCRCs compared with hereditary EOCRCs (74.9% vs 58.3%). Similarly, Stoffel and colleagues[31] reported that 72.6% of sporadic EOCRCs were left sided versus 38.0% of hereditary EOCRCs.

CAUSES OF EARLY ONSET COLORECTAL CANCER
Hereditary Cancer Syndromes

Early age of cancer onset is a hallmark of hereditary cancer syndromes, so it is not surprising that there is a larger hereditary contribution to CRC in the young. Pearlman and colleagues[30] prospectively performed comprehensive multi-gene panel germline genetic testing on 450 patients diagnosed with CRC under the age of 50 and found that 14% had at least 1 first-degree relative with CRC in the absence of an identifiable germline mutation, and 16% carried a pathogenic mutation. Ten percent were found to have a high-penetrance gene mutation (ie, Lynch syndrome genes, biallelic MutYH, APC, BRCA1/2, CDKN2A), and 6% had a moderate penetrance gene mutation (ATM, PALB2, monoallelic MutYH, CHEK2, APC-I1307 K). In a retrospective series of EOCRC patients referred to a genetics clinic, Stoffel and colleagues[31] found that 25% of patients carried a germline mutation associated with hereditary cancer syndromes. **Fig. 3** summarizes germline spectrum based on age of CRC diagnosis.

Familial Colorectal Cancer

Up to 33.5% of patients diagnosed with EOCRC have a family history of CRC[24,32,33] (see **Table 1**). Chen and colleagues[34] reported that EOCRC patients are more likely to have a family history of CRC than older patients (24.9% vs 16.8%). When definitively excluding patients with germline hereditary syndromes, 14.0%[30] to 16.3%[31] of patients with EOCRC still have a family history of CRC.

Based on these risks, the US Multi-Society Task Force (MSTF) on Colorectal Cancer[5] and the National Comprehensive Cancer Network (NCCN)[4] recommend that individuals with an FDR with CRC diagnosed younger than 60 years of age, or more than 1 FDR with CRC (any age), should undergo screening colonoscopy starting at age 40 or 10 years earlier than the earliest cancer in the family and repeat screening

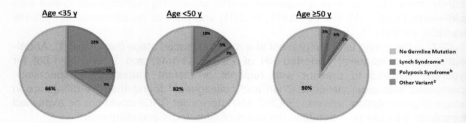

Fig. 3. Germline genetic spectrum of colorectal cancer by age. [a] *MLH1, MSH2, MSH6, PMS2.* [b] *APC, MUTYH, SMAD4, BMPR1A, PTEN, POLE.* [c] *BRCA1, BRCA2, TP53, PALB2, CDKN2A, CHEK2, ATM, NBN, BARD1, BRIP1.* (*Adapted from* Stoffel EM, Murphy CC. Epidemiology and mechanisms of the increasing incidence of colon and rectal cancers in young adults. Gastroenterology 2019; with permission.)

every 5 years. Those with an FDR diagnosed with CRC over the age of 60 should begin screening at age 40 with any of several acceptable screening strategies (annual high-sensitivity fecal occult blood test, multi-target FIT/DNA, flexible sigmoidoscopy, computed tomography [CT] colonography, colonoscopy) but can proceed at average-risk intervals.[5]

Despite this increased risk, adherence to screening recommendations is low. Lowery and colleagues[35] summarized 17 original studies where adherence to start age and appropriate interval ranged between 31% and 47%. A meta-analysis of these 17 studies determined that only 40% (range 26%–54%) of individuals with an FDR with CRC had undergone colonoscopy, and only 31% (range 12%–51%) had undergone colonoscopy at 5-year intervals.[36]

Familial Adenomas

Colorectal adenomas are known precursors to adenocarcinoma. An advanced adenoma is defined as an adenoma of at least 1 cm, the presence of villous architecture, or with high-grade dysplasia. A family history of advanced adenomas increases risk of CRC. An individual with 1 or more FDR with any advanced adenoma has a twofold increased risk of developing CRC.[37,38] Tuohy and colleagues[37] reported an odds ratio of 1.68 (95% CI 1.29-2.18) of developing CRC for those with an FDR with an advanced adenoma at any age. FDRs with an advanced adenoma at age younger than 60 years had a 1.54 (1.06-2.24) increased odds of developing CRC, and FDRs of those diagnosed with an advanced adenoma at age 60 or older had a 2.04 (1.35-3.08) increased odds of CRC. Cottet and colleagues[39] similarly reported a 2.27 (1.09-5.09) increased odds of developing CRC or a large adenoma in those with an FDR with a large adenoma.

Based on this increased risk, the MSTF and NCCN recommend that those with an FDR with an advanced adenoma at any age should undergo CRC screening at age 40 with average risk intervals. Those who have an FDR diagnosed with an advanced adenoma younger than 60 years of age should start CRC screening with colonoscopy at age 40 or 10 years earlier than the earliest advanced adenoma in the family and then every 5 years or earlier depending on the colonoscopic findings.

Although the data are sparse, there is a similar deficiency in patient knowledge of familial CRC risk associated with advanced adenomas. In a survey conducted by Schroy and colleagues,[40] only 33% of those found to have adenomas were aware that their family members may be at increased risk of developing CRC. Only 56% of patients who were aware of this increased risk indicated that they received this information from their physician.

Sporadic Early Onset Colorectal Cancer

Although precise estimates are lacking on what proportion of EOCRCs is associated with hereditary syndromes or family history of CRC or advanced adenomas, current data suggest that most EOCRCs are sporadic. Pearlman and colleagues[30] reported that 86% of their EOCRC cohort without a germline mutation had no family history of CRC (although this did not include a family history of adenomas).

POTENTIAL ETIOLOGIES FOR THE RISE IN EARLY ONSET COLORECTAL CANCER
Unrecognized Hereditary or Familial Risk

Although hereditary syndromes contribute to 16% to 25%[30,31] of all EOCRCs and they are grossly under-recognized,[41,42] there is no reason to suspect that the incidence of hereditary syndromes is increasing or that penetrance is changing. Thus, although there is much work to be done to improve recognition of hereditary syndromes, they likely have not contributed to the rise in EOCRC that has been observed over the past several decades. Similarly, although there are gross deficiencies in acquisition and follow-up of accurate cancer family history,[35,43] there are no data to suggest that this deficiency is worsening such that it would contribute to the rise in EOCRC.

Increasing Utilization of Colonoscopy and Earlier Diagnosis

Some authors have speculated that the increase in the incidence of CRC in the young is partly because of detection bias. Using commercial insurance claims and encounters data, Murphy and colleagues[44] found an overall increase in colonoscopy utilization in the 18- to 49-year-old age group from 15.2 colonoscopies per 1000 population in 2001 to 19.7 colonoscopies per 1000 population in 2009, a period when CRC incidence was increasing in the young, with the highest colonoscopy utilization in those aged 40 to 49. However, the colonoscopy rate went back down to 16 coloscopies per 1000 population in 2014, and no comparable decrease in CRC incidence has been seen in the most recent reports.

Despite this time-trend correlation, it seems unlikely that the rising incidence of EOCRC is explained by earlier diagnosis alone for several reasons. The largest increase in incidence is seen in the youngest age group (see **Fig. 2**), which is the least likely age group to undergo colonoscopy. Second, the rise in incidence started in the 1970s in the youngest age group, well before the era of widespread colonoscopy availability. Third, EOCRCs present at later stages than those in older individuals. Finally, the recent rise in EOCRC mortality rates also is consistent with increasing disease burden as opposed to detection bias.

Lifestyle, Environmental, and Metabolic Risk Factors

Established risk factors for CRC in all age groups include diabetes/metabolic syndrome,[45] obesity,[46] smoking,[47] moderate alcohol consumption,[48–50] red meats, and processed meats.[51] Protective factors include regular physical activity,[52,53] nonsteroidal anti-inflammatory drug (NSAID) use (particularly aspirin),[54,55] and diets high in fiber.[51]

Although there has been a steady rise in sedentary lifestyles, diabetes mellitus, and obesity in the United States, and these risk factors are particularly increasing in the young,[56] there is limited literature on risk factors specific to EOCRC. Liu and colleagues reported data from the Nurses' Health Study II showing a 1.93 (95% CI 1.15–3.25) adjusted RR for EOCRC in those with a body mass index of at least 30. Nguyen and colleagues[57] recently reported that those who were sedentary for more than 14 hours per week had an adjusted RR of 1.68 (95% CI 1.09–2.63) for EOCRC. The risk was more pronounced for rectal cancers (RR 2.62, 95% CI 1.15–6.00). When comparing 329 cases of CRC diagnosed younger than 45 years of age with controls, Rosato and colleagues[58] found that consumption of at least 14 alcoholic drinks per week (1.56, 95% CI 1.12-2.16) and the highest tertile of processed meat consumption (1.56, 95% CI 1.11-2.20) were risk factors. Vegetable consumption was protective (RR 0.40, 95% CI 0.28–0.56). Jung and colleagues[59] reported that chronic smoking (30-39-year-olds: 4.41, 95% CI 1.80-10.80; 40-49-year-olds: 1.64 95% CI 1.14-2.37), hepatic steatosis (30–39-year-olds: 1.71, 95% CI 1.10-2.68), and elevated triglyceride levels (30–39-year-olds: 2.00, 95% CI 1.26-3.16) were risk factors for advanced colonic neoplasia. In contrast, Gausman and colleagues[60] did not identify obesity, smoking, or diabetes as independent risk factors in the EOCRC population, suggesting that traditional risk factors may not completely explain the rise in EOCRC. All of these studies evaluated the presence of risk factors at the time of CRC diagnosis.

There are multiple additional risk factors currently under consideration as possible drivers of EOCRC. Alterations in gut microbiota can induce changes in mutational patterns, gene expression, metabolism, and local and systemic immune responses.[61] Thus, risk factors such as antibiotic use (particularly in childhood), antibiotics in the food chain, mode of birth delivery, breast feeding or periodontal disease, and unrecognized dietary toxins may be contributing.[19] Regional variations in disease burden raise the possibility of water supply or ambient exposures, although evidence for these risk factors is limited.[62] Ongoing epidemiologic research is needed to better characterize these risk factors.

APPROACHES TO ADDRESSING DISEASE BURDEN OF EARLY ONSET COLORECTAL CANCER

Improving Identification of High-Risk Populations

Family history of colorectal cancer and adenomas

At least 30% of the population likely has an FDR with CRC or an advanced adenoma. Based on data demonstrating that a first-degree relative with a large or histologically advanced adenoma or CRC increases the lifetime risk of CRC by up to fourfold,[63–66] the national guidelines are in consensus that these individuals should initiate CRC screening at age 40.[4,5,67] Unfortunately, adherence to this recommendation in the 40- to 49-year-old group is low. Tsai and colleagues[68] analyzed the National Health Interview data from 2005 and 2010 and found that overall CRC screening rates had increased by two- to threefold between 2005 and 2010 and that FDRs of patients with CRC had a slightly higher rate of colonoscopy screening than those without a family history (70% vs 68%). However, the rate of colonoscopy in those aged 40 to 49 with an FDR with CRC remained low (15% in 2005%; 41% in 2010). Screening rates for those with an FDR and an advanced adenoma are undoubtedly even lower. Improving identification of and screening in this population are immediate steps to addressing the rising CRC rates in the young.

There is a multitude of cited barriers at the provider, patient, and systems level. There is inadequate family history collection and documentation, inadequate knowledge of associated risk, and insufficient action on family history information. Fletcher and colleagues[43] reported that only 39% of patients younger than 50 years of age were asked about family history of CRC. CRC family history was only documented in 59% of patient charts, but only half of these records included relative's age of CRC diagnosis. Of those who had a strong family history of CRC, only 46% were aware that they needed to start CRC screening earlier than age 50. Not surprisingly, only 45% of these patients had undergone appropriate screening.

Universal tumor screening for Lynch syndrome

Numerous multidisciplinary professional societies endorse screening all colorectal tumors for Lynch syndrome with either immunohistochemistry for loss of mismatch repair protein expression and/or microsatellite instability testing,[42,69–71] Despite this recommendation, many health care institutions face challenges to incorporating universal tumor testing of CRC patients to screen for Lynch syndrome. Even at National Cancer Institute-designated Comprehensive Cancer Centers, only 71% reported that they routinely perform MSI/IHC testing on CRCs to screen for Lynch syndrome, whereas only 48% and 14%, respectively, perform Lynch syndrome tumor screening at American College of Surgeons–accredited Community Hospital Comprehensive Cancer Programs and Community Hospital Cancer Programs.[72] There is a need for continued efforts to overcome current challenges, including securing resources for a large-scale screening program to ensure patients are appropriately navigated through the system, ensuring access to genetics expertise for interpretation and action on tumor testing and dispelling misconceptions about cost and potential delays in care.

Avoiding Delay in Diagnosis

Another immediate opportunity to address EOCRC is to diagnose CRC as early as possible in symptomatic patients. Bleeding, abdominal pain, anemia, and change in bowel habits are the most commonly reported symptoms of CRC. Because these symptoms are often cause by benign etiologies in young patients (eg, hemorrhoids or irritable bowel), there may be a low index of suspicion among clinicians for CRC in people younger than 50 years of age. This can unfortunately lead to significant delays in the diagnosis (see **Table 1**). Although this delay in care is likely multifactorial, including patient-related delay in seeking care or difficulty accessing care, it is important to acknowledge delays in care from dismissal of symptoms by health care providers. Scant hematochezia is often dismissed as a benign anorectal source such as hemorrhoids. The presence of hemorrhoids does not exclude more proximal pathology, and bleeding hemorrhoids can obscure subtle symptoms suggestive of a more proximal source.[73] In 1 series of 145 patients presenting with rectal bleeding, primary care providers predicted an anal source (hemorrhoids or fissure) in 63 patients based on their history and physical examination. Of these 63 patients, 11 (17.5%) had a more proximal rectal or colonic source on lower endoscopy.[74] Based on these data showing how unreliable clinical history and physical examination can be and the observation that up to 15% of CRCs occur under the age of 50, the American Society for Gastrointestinal Endoscopy (ASGE) recommends endoscopic evaluation for all patients presenting with bleeding symptoms.[75]

Changing the Screening Age

In response to the rising burden of CRC in young patients, the American Cancer Society published a qualified recommendation to start screening in all average-risk patients at age 45 instead of 50.[22] The MSTF, the NCCN, and the US Preventative Services Task Force have maintained a recommendation to start screening at age 50. There are still many unanswered questions about how best to approach screening for average-risk individuals younger than 50 years of age,[76,77] although a recent analysis suggests that this strategy can be cost-effective, with a cost of $7700 or $33,900 per quality-adjusted life year for fecal immunochemical testing or colonoscopy screening for this age group, respectively.[78] Many advocate for risk-specific screening. The challenge with risk-specific screening is that the specific risk factors for EOCRC are not elucidated; thus it is not surprising that available risk models have relatively weak discriminatory power.[79] Furthermore, many of the existing models have not been specifically applied to the EOCRC population. Emerging models that include incorporation of clinical risk factors and genetic variants may provide more precise risk assessment,[80] however are far from immediate clinical application.

SUMMARY

An increase in the incidence of EOCRC in the United States has been well-documented, as has an increase in CRC-associated mortality in this group. A major concern is that this trend will continue to increase and become a serious health burden in people under 50. Increasing EOCRC has also been seen in several non-US populations. The underlying cause of this problem is unknown. Germline mutations in genes known to cause familial cancer syndromes are responsible for a minority of these cases (16%–25%). This incidence underscores the need to test all EOCRC patients for germline mutations, but this does not explain most of the problem. Young patients with lower abdominal symptoms or rectal bleeding should be fully evaluated for the possibility of CRC. Family histories need to be taken and recorded in a more systematic fashion, perhaps using online tools outside of the medical provider's office. Methods should be developed to record the presence of advanced adenomas, and this information needs to be shared with first-degree relatives along with appropriate screening recommendations. Research should be directed at determining the biological basis of this problem, which may require an analysis of mutational signatures in these tumors and possibly tracing those patterns back to changes in the microbiome or the presence of unexpected mutagens in the diet or changes in the fecal metabolome. Finally, the medical community needs to determine the optimal age to begin surveillance for CRC and the most efficient and cost-effective means to do this.

DISCLOSURE

S.G. Patel: no conflicts of interest. C.R. Boland: honoraria from Ambry Genetics.

REFERENCES

1. Edwards BK, Noone AM, Mariotto AB, et al. Annual report to the nation on the status of cancer, 1975-2010, featuring prevalence of comorbidity and impact on survival among persons with lung, colorectal, breast, or prostate cancer. Cancer 2014;120:1290–314.
2. Brenner H, Chen C. The colorectal cancer epidemic: challenges and opportunities for primary, secondary and tertiary prevention. Br J Cancer 2018;119: 785–92.
3. Siegel RL, Fedewa SA, Anderson WF, et al. Colorectal cancer incidence patterns in the United States, 1974-2013. J Natl Cancer Inst 2017;109:djw322.
4. Benson AB, Venook AP, Al-Hawary MM, et al. NCCN Guidelines Insights: Colon Cancer, Version 2.2018. *J Natl Compr Canc Netw.* 2018;16(4):359–369.
5. Rex DK, Boland CR, Dominitz JA, et al. Colorectal cancer screening: recommendations for physicians and patients from the U.S. Multi-Society Task Force on Colorectal Cancer. Gastroenterology 2017;153:307–23.
6. Force USPST, Bibbins-Domingo K, Grossman DC, Curry SJ, et al. Screening for colorectal cancer: US preventive services task force recommendation statement. JAMA 2016;315:2564–75.
7. Ballester V, Rashtak S, Boardman L. Clinical and molecular features of young-onset colorectal cancer. World J Gastroenterol 2016;22:1736–44.
8. Patel SG, Ahnen DJ. Familial colon cancer syndromes: an update of a rapidly evolving field. Curr Gastroenterol Rep 2012;14:428–38.
9. Stoffel EM, Mangu PB, Limburg PJ, et al. Hereditary colorectal cancer syndromes: American Society of Clinical Oncology clinical practice guideline endorsement of the familial risk-colorectal cancer: European Society for Medical Oncology clinical practice guidelines. J Oncol Pract 2015;11:e437–41.
10. Syngal S, Brand RE, Church JM, et al. ACG clinical guideline: genetic testing and management of hereditary gastrointestinal cancer syndromes. Am J Gastroenterol 2015;110:223–62.
11. Bhandari A, Woodhouse M, Gupta S. Colorectal cancer is a leading cause of cancer incidence and mortality among adults younger than 50 years in the USA: a

SEER-based analysis with comparison to other young-onset cancers. J Investig Med 2017;65:311–5.

12. Siegel RL, Miller KD, Fedewa SA, et al. Colorectal cancer statistics, 2017. CA Cancer J Clin 2017;67:177–93.

13. You YN, Xing Y, Feig BW, et al. Young-onset colorectal cancer: is it time to pay attention? Arch Intern Med 2012;172:287–9.

14. Bailey CE, Hu CY, You YN, et al. Increasing disparities in the age-related incidences of colon and rectal cancers in the United States, 1975-2010. JAMA Surg 2015;150:17–22.

15. Murphy CC, Wallace K, Sandler RS, et al. Racial disparities in incidence of young-onset colorectal cancer and patient survival. Gastroenterology 2019;156: 958–65.

16. Siegel RL, Miller KD, Jemal A. Colorectal cancer mortality rates in adults aged 20 to 54 years in the United States, 1970-2014. JAMA 2017;318:572–4.

17. Holowatyj AN, Ruterbusch JJ, Rozek LS, et al. Racial/ethnic disparities in survival among patients with young-onset colorectal cancer. J Clin Oncol 2016;34: 2148–56.

18. Ashktorab H, Kupfer SS, Brim H, et al. Racial disparity in gastrointestinal cancer risk. Gastroenterology 2017;153:910–23.

19. Stoffel EM, Murphy CC. Epidemiology and mechanisms of the increasing incidence of colon and rectal cancers in young adults. Gastroenterology 2020; 158(2):341–53.

20. Siegel RL, Medhanie GA, Fedewa SA, et al. State variation in early-onset colorectal cancer in the United States, 1995-2015. J Natl Cancer Inst 2019;111: 1104–6.

21. Siegel RL, Torre LA, Soerjomataram I, et al. Global patterns and trends in colorectal cancer incidence in young adults. Gut 2019;68(12):2179–85.

22. Wolf AMD, Fontham ETH, Church TR, et al. Colorectal cancer screening for average-risk adults: 2018 guideline update from the American Cancer Society. CA Cancer J Clin 2018;68:250–81.

23. Dozois EJ, Boardman LA, Suwanthanma W, et al. Young-onset colorectal cancer in patients with no known genetic predisposition: can we increase early recognition and improve outcome? Medicine (Baltimore) 2008;87:259–63.

24. Chen FW, Sundaram V, Chew TA, et al. Advanced-stage colorectal cancer in persons younger than 50 years not associated with longer duration of symptoms or time to diagnosis. Clin Gastroenterol Hepatol 2017;15:728–37.e3.

25. Abdelsattar ZM, Wong SL, Regenbogen SE, et al. Colorectal cancer outcomes and treatment patterns in patients too young for average-risk screening. Cancer 2016;122:929–34.

26. Teng A, Lee DY, Cai J, et al. Patterns and outcomes of colorectal cancer in adolescents and young adults. J Surg Res 2016;205:19–27.

27. Georgiou A, Khakoo S, Edwards P, et al. Outcomes of patients with early onset colorectal cancer treated in a UK Specialist Cancer Center. Cancers (Basel) 2019;11 [pii:E1558].

28. Liang JT, Huang KC, Cheng AL, et al. Clinicopathological and molecular biological features of colorectal cancer in patients less than 40 years of age. Br J Surg 2003;90:205–14.

29. Chang DT, Pai RK, Rybicki LA, et al. Clinicopathologic and molecular features of sporadic early-onset colorectal adenocarcinoma: an adenocarcinoma with frequent signet ring cell differentiation, rectal and sigmoid involvement, and adverse morphologic features. Mod Pathol 2012;25:1128–39.

30. Pearlman R, Frankel WL, Swanson B, et al. Prevalence and spectrum of germline cancer susceptibility gene mutations among patients with early-onset colorectal cancer. JAMA Oncol 2017;3:464–71.

31. Stoffel EM, Koeppe E, Everett J, et al. Germline genetic features of young individuals with colorectal cancer. Gastroenterology 2018;154:897–905.e1.

32. Rho YS, Gilabert M, Polom K, et al. Comparing clinical characteristics and outcomes of young-onset and late-onset colorectal cancer: an international collaborative study. Clin Colorectal Cancer 2017;16(4):334–42.

33. Strum WB, Boland CR. Clinical and genetic characteristics of colorectal cancer in persons under 50 years of age: a review. Dig Dis Sci 2019;64(11):3059–65.

34. Chen FW, Sundaram V, Chew TA, et al. Low prevalence of criteria for early screening in young-onset colorectal cancer. Am J Prev Med 2017;53:933–4.

35. Lowery JT, Ahnen DJ, Schroy PC 3rd, et al. Understanding the contribution of family history to colorectal cancer risk and its clinical implications: a state-of-the-science review. Cancer 2016;122:2633–45.

36. Ait Ouakrim D, Lockett T, Boussioutas A, et al. Screening participation for people at increased risk of colorectal cancer due to family history: a systematic review and meta-analysis. Fam Cancer 2013;12:459–72.

37. Tuohy TM, Rowe KG, Mineau GP, et al. Risk of colorectal cancer and adenomas in the families of patients with adenomas: a population-based study in Utah. Cancer 2014;120:35–42.

38. Winawer SJ, Zauber AG, Gerdes H, et al. Risk of colorectal cancer in the families of patients with adenomatous polyps. National Polyp Study Workgroup. N Engl J Med 1996;334:82–7.

39. Cottet V, Pariente A, Nalet B, et al. Colonoscopic screening of first-degree relatives of patients with large adenomas: increased risk of colorectal tumors. Gastroenterology 2007;133:1086–92.

40. Schroy PC 3rd, Lal SK, Wilson S, et al. Deficiencies in knowledge and familial risk communication among colorectal adenoma patients. J Clin Gastroenterol 2005; 39:298–302.

41. Hampel H, de la Chapelle A. The search for unaffected individuals with Lynch syndrome: do the ends justify the means? Cancer Prev Res (Phila) 2011;4:1–5.

42. Giardiello FM, Allen JI, Axilbund JE, et al. Guidelines on genetic evaluation and management of Lynch syndrome: a consensus statement by the U.S. Multi-Society Task Force on Colorectal Cancer. Gastrointest Endosc 2014;80:197–220.

43. Fletcher RH, Lobb R, Bauer MR, et al. Screening patients with a family history of colorectal cancer. J Gen Intern Med 2007;22:508–13.

44. Murphy CC, Lund JL, Sandler RS. Young-onset colorectal cancer: earlier diagnoses or increasing disease burden? Gastroenterology 2017;152:1809–12.e3.

45. Yuhara H, Steinmaus C, Cohen SE, et al. Is diabetes mellitus an independent risk factor for colon cancer and rectal cancer? Am J Gastroenterol 2011;106:1911–21 [quiz: 1922].

46. Pan SY, DesMeules M. Energy intake, physical activity, energy balance, and cancer: epidemiologic evidence. Methods Mol Biol 2009;472:191–215.

47. Botteri E, Iodice S, Bagnardi V, et al. Smoking and colorectal cancer: a meta-analysis. JAMA 2008;300:2765–78.

48. Fedirko V, Tramacere I, Bagnardi V, et al. Alcohol drinking and colorectal cancer risk: an overall and dose-response meta-analysis of published studies. Ann Oncol 2011;22:1958–72.

49. Cho E, Smith-Warner SA, Ritz J, et al. Alcohol intake and colorectal cancer: a pooled analysis of 8 cohort studies. Ann Intern Med 2004;140:603–13.

50. Mizoue T, Inoue M, Wakai K, et al. Alcohol drinking and colorectal cancer in Japanese: a pooled analysis of results from five cohort studies. Am J Epidemiol 2008; 167:1397–406.

51. Song M, Garrett WS, Chan AT. Nutrients, foods, and colorectal cancer prevention. Gastroenterology 2015;148:1244–60.e16.

52. Zheng J, Zhao M, Li J, et al. Obesity-associated digestive cancers: a review of mechanisms and interventions. Tumour Biol 2017;39. 1010428317695020.

53. Wolin KY, Yan Y, Colditz GA, et al. Physical activity and colon cancer prevention: a meta-analysis. Br J Cancer 2009;100:611–6.

54. Algra AM, Rothwell PM. Effects of regular aspirin on long-term cancer incidence and metastasis: a systematic comparison of evidence from observational studies versus randomised trials. Lancet Oncol 2012;13:518–27.

55. Arber N, Eagle CJ, Spicak J, et al. Celecoxib for the prevention of colorectal adenomatous polyps. N Engl J Med 2006;355:885–95.

56. Bhupathiraju SN, Hu FB. Epidemiology of obesity and diabetes and their cardio-vascular complications. Circ Res 2016;118:1723–35.

57. Nguyen LH, Liu PH, Zheng X, et al. Sedentary behaviors, TV viewing time, and risk of young-onset colorectal cancer. JNCI Cancer Spectr 2018;2:pky073.

58. Rosato V, Bosetti C, Levi F, et al. Risk factors for young-onset colorectal cancer. Cancer Causes Control 2013;24:335–41.

59. Jung YS, Ryu S, Chang Y, et al. Risk factors for colorectal neoplasia in persons aged 30 to 39 years and 40 to 49 years. Gastrointest Endosc 2015;81:637–45.e7.

60. Gausman V, Dornblaser D, Anand S, et al. Risk factors associated with early-onset colorectal cancer. Clin Gastroenterol Hepatol 2019. [Epub ahead of print].

61. Song M, Chan AT. Environmental factors, gut microbiota, and colorectal cancer prevention. Clin Gastroenterol Hepatol 2019;17:275–89.

62. Dwyer AJ, Murphy CC, Boland CR, et al. A summary of the fight colorectal cancer working meeting: exploring risk factors and etiology of sporadic early-age onset colorectal cancer. Gastroenterology 2019;157:280–8.

63. Lynch KL, Ahnen DJ, Byers T, et al. First-degree relatives of patients with advanced colorectal adenomas have an increased prevalence of colorectal cancer. Clin Gastroenterol Hepatol 2003;1:96–102.

64. Lieberman DA, Prindiville S, Weiss DG, et al. Risk factors for advanced colonic neoplasia and hyperplastic polyps in asymptomatic individuals. JAMA 2003; 290:2959–67.

65. Fuchs CS, Giovannucci EL, Colditz GA, et al. A prospective study of family history and the risk of colorectal cancer. N Engl J Med 1994;331:1669–74.

66. Butterworth AS, Higgins JP, Pharoah P. Relative and absolute risk of colorectal cancer for individuals with a family history: a meta-analysis. Eur J Cancer 2006;42:216–27.

67. U.S. Preventive Services Task Force. Screening for colorectal cancer: U.S. Preventive Services Task Force recommendation statement. Ann Intern Med 2008; 149:627–37.

68. Tsai MH, Xirasagar S, Li YJ, et al. Colonoscopy screening among US adults aged 40 or older with a family history of colorectal cancer. Prev Chronic Dis 2015; 12:E80.

69. Evaluation of Genomic Applications in Practice and Prevention (EGAPP) Working Group. Recommendations from the EGAPP Working Group: genetic testing strategies in newly diagnosed individuals with colorectal cancer aimed at reducing morbidity and mortality from Lynch syndrome in relatives. Genet Med 2009;11: 35–41.

70. Gupta S, Provenzale D, Llor X, et al. NCCN Guidelines Insights: Genetic/Familial High-Risk Assessment: Colorectal, Version 2.2019. J Natl Compr Canc Netw 2019;17(9):1032–41.
71. Sepulveda AR, Hamilton SR, Allegra CJ, et al. Molecular biomarkers for the evaluation of colorectal cancer. Am J Clin Pathol 2017;147(3):221–60.
72. Beamer LC, Grant ML, Espenschied CR, et al. Reflex immunohistochemistry and microsatellite instability testing of colorectal tumors for Lynch syndrome among US cancer programs and follow-up of abnormal results. J Clin Oncol 2012;30: 1058–63.
73. Bat L, Pines A, Rabau M, et al. Colonoscopic findings in patients with hemorrhoids, rectal bleeding and normal rectoscopy. Isr J Med Sci 1985;21:139–41.
74. Goulston KJ, Cook I, Dent OF. How important is rectal bleeding in the diagnosis of bowel cancer and polyps? Lancet 1986;2:261–5.
75. ASGE Standards of Practice Committee, Pasha SF, Shergill A, Acosta RD, et al. The role of endoscopy in the patient with lower GI bleeding. Gastrointest Endosc 2014;79:875–85.
76. Liang PS, Allison J, Ladabaum U, et al. Potential intended and unintended consequences of recommending initiation of colorectal cancer screening at age 45 years. Gastroenterology 2018;155:950–4.
77. Imperiale TF, Kahi CJ, Rex DK. Lowering the starting age for colorectal cancer screening to 45 years: who will come...and should they? Clin Gastroenterol Hepatol 2018;16:1541–4.
78. Ladabaum U, Mannalithara A, Meester RGS, et al. Cost-effectiveness and national effects of initiating colorectal cancer screening for average-risk persons at age 45 years instead of 50 years. Gastroenterology 2019;157(1):137–48.
79. Ma GK, Ladabaum U. Personalizing colorectal cancer screening: a systematic review of models to predict risk of colorectal neoplasia. Clin Gastroenterol Hepatol 2014;12:1624–16234.e1.
80. McGeoch L, Saunders CL, Griffin SJ, et al. Risk prediction models for colorectal cancer incorporating common genetic variants: a systematic review. Cancer Epidemiol Biomarkers Prev 2019;28:1580–93.
81. Myers EA, Feingold DL, Forde KA, et al. Colorectal cancer in patients under 50 years of age: a retrospective analysis of two institutions' experience. World J Gastroenterol 2013;19:5651–7.
82. Scott RB, Rangel LE, Osler TM, et al. Rectal cancer in patients under the age of 50 years: the delayed diagnosis. Am J Surg 2016;211:1014–8.
83. Wang R, Wang MJ, Ping J. Clinicopathological features and survival outcomes of colorectal cancer in young versus elderly: a population-based cohort study of seer 9 registries data (1988-2011). Medicine (Baltimore) 2015;94:e1402.

Colorectal Cancer Screening for the Serrated Pathway

Joseph C. Anderson, MD, MHCDS[a,b,c,*], Amitabh Srivastava, MD[d]

KEYWORDS

- Serrated polyps • Colorectal cancer • Hyperplastic polyps • Sessile serrated polyps
- Traditional serrated adenomas • Resection and surveillance

KEY POINTS

- There are 3 subtypes of serrated polyps—hyperplastic polyps, sessile serrated adenomas/polyps and traditional serrated adenomas—all with saw tooth appearance histologically.
- Distinguishing hyperplastic polyps from sessile serrated adenomas/polyp is challenging owing to varying minimum thresholds for making a diagnosis of sessile serrated adenomas/polyp and poor observer reproducibility for specific criteria.
- Traditional serrated adenomas are cytologically dysplastic lesions and sessile serrated adenomas/polyps develop cytologic dysplasia as they progress to colorectal cancer.
- Hyperplastic polyps regarded as benign but hyperplastic polyps 1 cm or more have increase long-term colorectal cancer risk.
- Flat and indistinct borders can make serrated polyps difficult to detect and resect. Close surveillance is recommended for sessile serrated adenomas/polyps, sessile serrated adenomas/polyp with dysplasia, hyperplastic polyps 10 mm or larger, and traditional serrated adenomas.

INTRODUCTION

Although hyperplastic polyps (HPs) were once believed to have a benign course with little clinical significance, they are now recognized as part of a broader group of lesions known as serrated polyps.[1–4] The associated pathway may be responsible for 20% to 30% of all colorectal cancers (CRCs).[2] Serrated polyps share characteristic colonic crypts serrations and are classified into 3 main subgroups—HPs, sessile serrated

The contents of this work do not represent the views of the Department of Veterans Affairs or the United States Government.

[a] Department of Veterans Affairs Medical Center, White River Junction, VT, USA; [b] The Geisel School of Medicine at Dartmouth, 1 Rope Ferry Road, Hanover, NH 03755, USA; [c] Division of Gastroenterology and Hepatology, University of Connecticut School of Medicine, Farmington, CT 06030, USA; [d] Brigham and Women's Hospital, 75 Francis Street, Boston, MA 02115, USA
* Corresponding author. The Geisel School of Medicine at Dartmouth, 1 Rope Ferry Road, Hanover, NH 03755.
E-mail address: joseph.anderson@dartmouth.edu

Gastrointest Endoscopy Clin N Am 30 (2020) 457–478
https://doi.org/10.1016/j.giec.2020.02.007
1052-5157/20/© 2020 Elsevier Inc. All rights reserved.

adenomas/polyps (referred to as SSPs in this article), and traditional serrated adenomas (TSAs). In addition, in this article, serrated polyps refers to the whole classification and not to SSPs in particular. This article discusses the significance of serrated polyps, histologic, and endoscopic appearance and challenges that exist in managing patients with these polyps, including detection, resection, and surveillance.

Classification and Histology

All serrated polyps share a characteristic saw tooth or serrated appearance of the colonic epithelial crypts (**Table 1**).[1] In a typical HP, the crypts are relatively straight, extending to the muscularis mucosa without significant distortion. In addition, the basal half of the crypt seems to be mucin depleted and regenerative, whereas serrations seems to be prominent in the upper half (**Fig. 1**A). Although HPs can be further divided into microvesicular HPs, goblet cell–rich HPs, and mucin-poor HPs, this distinction is not clinically significant. In contrast with HPs, SSPs are characterized by architectural disarray at the crypt bases (**Fig. 1**B) with crypt dilatation, boot- or anchor-shaped or horizontal crypts, and a mucin-rich appearance at the crypt base, with goblet cells and at times with pyloric-gland type mucin.

However, distinguishing HP from SSP can be challenging owing to varying minimum thresholds for making a diagnosis of SSP, as well as lack of observer reproducibility in determination of specific criteria used for making this diagnosis[2,5] (**Fig. 1**C). Moreover, prolapse-type changes in left-sided HPs can mimic the architectural changes of SSP. The major difficulty centers around distinguishing SSPs from microvesicular HPs.[6] Although changes in even a single crypt have recently been proposed to be sufficient for making a diagnosis of SSP, this finding is not evidence based and, despite this low threshold, consensus continues to elude pathologists in a significant number of cases[7,8] Most experts therefore agree that, given these problems in diagnosis, large (≥1 cm) serrated polyps should be treated in a similar fashion, regardless of a histologic diagnosis of HP or SSP.[1,6]

The final category of serrated polyps is a TSA that also harbors serrated crypts similar to HPs and SSP, but these polyps are cytologically dysplastic with nuclear hyperchromasia and stratification, and also display a characteristic cytoplasmic eosinophilia and ectopic crypt budding[9] (**Fig. 1**D). The distinction of TSA from SSPs and HPs is quite reproducible, but there are some issues that endoscopists need to

	Frequency	Morphology	Location	Appearance	Malignant Progression?
Table 1 Clinical features of common serrated polyps					
HPs	>90% of all serrated polyps	Typically flat or Paris IIa	Typically distal but can be proximal	Pale	No
Sessile serrated polyps	<10% of all serrated polyps	Typically flat or Paris IIa but can be sessile or Is	Typically proximal but can be distal	Pale/yellow/ mucous cap	Yes
TSA	<1% of all serrated polyps	Typically protruding or sessile (Is) or pedunculated (Ip)	Typically distal	Erythematous	Yes

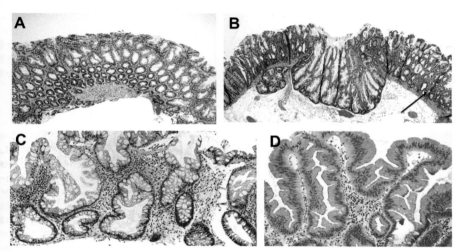

Fig. 1. (*A*) Typical HPs show a relatively mucin depleted basal zone with retained normal crypt architecture. Serrations are prominent in the upper half of the crypts. This zonation is easily discernible in well-oriented polyps at low power evaluation. (*B*) In contrast, SSP, in its most characteristic form, shows basal crypt dilatation with abundant mucin and serrations extending to the base of the crypts. HP-like areas are often present within these lesions, as seen in the right third of this image (*arrow*). (*C*) The base of the crypts are not mucin depleted and show some dilatation in this diminutive serrated polyp in the rectum. Whether this is enough to label a lesion as an SSP continues to be an issue that leads to observer variability in diagnosis. A lesion with exactly similar morphology is more likely to be diagnosed as an SSP by pathologists when located in the right colon and as an HP in the left colon. (*D*) TSAs show prominent crypt serrations similar to other serrated polyps but are characterized by intense cytoplasmic eosinophilia and cytologic dysplasia that manifests as pencillate, hyperchromatic nuclei with stratification, oriented perpendicular to the basement membrane. H&E; ×100 for A and B, ×200 for C and D.

be aware of when managing individuals with TSAs. A significant proportion of TSAs arise in a background of an HP or SSP (**Fig. 2**A). Not surprisingly, the former situation is more common in the left and the latter in the right colon. When TSA-like changes occur in an SSP, some pathologists may simply diagnose these lesions as a TSA while others may label the same lesions as SSP with dysplasia (SSP-D). The finding of a background of HP features in some TSAs is also evidence that HPs are also the earliest precursors in the serrated pathway that can rarely progress to lesions capable of giving rise to CRC. As they progress to CRC, TSAs show high-grade nuclear atypia or conventional adenoma-like changes that make distinction from typical tubular, tubulovillous, or villous adenoma quite challenging (**Fig. 2**B). This finding may explain why a significant proportion of CRC share molecular features found in TSAs despite the latter constituting only 2% to 4% of all colorectal polyps. Thus, although TSAs may have reproducible features to distinguish them from HPs and SSPs, there are instances where the distinction between a TSA with high-grade changes described elsewhere in this article from a conventional adenoma can be quite challenging.

Risk Factors

Smoking is the most important risk factor for clinically significant serrated polyps (CSSP),[10–20] especially SSPs that are large and proximal.[21] In fact, smoking has

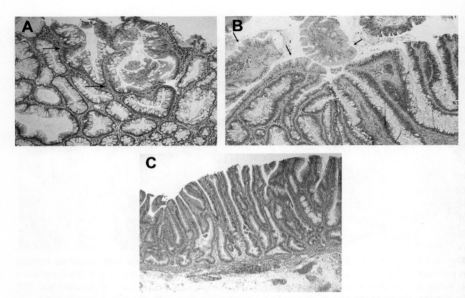

Fig. 2. (*A*) Early TSA involving just 2 crypts (*arrows*). The morphologic features in this focus are similar to the TSA illustrated in **Fig. 1D**, but the changes are occurring in a background of a rectosigmoid HP. Similar alterations can also occur in a background of SSP and are more common in right colon polyps. (*B*) When TSAs progress to cancer, they often acquire morphologic changes that resemble conventional adenomas. This large, descending colon TSA (upper left image; *arrows*) was associated with an invasive adenocarcinoma (not shown) and the crypts in the right half are indistinguishable from a conventional adenoma. Such foci are often associated with a mutant pattern of staining on a p53 immunostain suggestive of an advanced TSA. (*C*) Large, flat adenomas in the right colon also show the basal architectural disarray that is currently used in serrated polyps to distinguish HP from SSP. This endoscopic submucosal dissection from a large tubular adenoma in the right colon shows basal crypt dilatation, branching, and boot- and anchor-shaped crypts.

been linked with serrated lesions as small (<2 mm) aberrant crypt foci, precursors to serrated polyps.[22] In addition to a higher body mass index,[23] smoking is one of a few risk factors that they share with conventional adenomas.[24–27] One recent study used data from more than 20,000 asymptomatic individuals in the New Hampshire Colonoscopy Registry (NHCR) having their first screening colonoscopy to compare risk factors in 3 groups, those with CSSP only, those with conventional high-risk adenomas (HRA) only and those with CSSP and HRA to those with normal colonoscopies.[14] They observed that, although older age and male sex were risk factors for those with HRA, these factors were not associated with the risk for having only CSSP. Of note, they observed that the risk associated with smoking was significantly higher for those with both CSSP and HRA than those with HRA alone, underscoring the risk that smoking has for serrated polyps. The interesting finding regarding the null association between older age and serrated polyps has some clinical implications, which are discussed elsewhere in this article.

Carcinogenesis and Attendant Molecular Mutations

As mentioned elsewhere in this article, TSAs are cytologically dysplastic lesions and SSPs develop cytologic dysplasia (SSP-D) when they progress toward cancer.

Although TSA and SSP are widely accepted as precursors of CRC, prevailing opinion still regards HP as benign lesions with no malignant potential. The presence of a background of HP in a TSAs, as discussed elsewhere in this article, suggests that HP are best considered as the earliest precursor in the serrated pathway, albeit with a very low risk of malignant transformation. Similarly, given the difficulty in distinguishing HP from SSP, and the overlapping gene expression profiles between the 2 lesions,[28] it is conceivable that SSPs, which are currently regarded as a distinct microscopic subtype of serrated polyps, may eventually turn out to be a lateral spreading type of HP with a predilection for the right colon. Interestingly, flat adenomas in the right colon also show similar basal architectural disarray, a feature that is currently used to diagnose SSPs (**Fig. 2C**). Individuals with large serrated polyps ($\geq$1 cm) , including HPs, have been shown to have an increased long-term risk for CRC.[29–31] Thus, polyps diagnosed as HPs that are 1 cm and larger in size are also important polyps requiring close surveillance owing to this long-term CRC risk. These data also suggest that larger size rather than specific histology may be important in stratification of risk. One caveat to this assumption, however, is that 1 study did show a greater long-term risk of CRC in adults with TSAs, although there were too few cases to stratify by size.[7] However, this study included high-risk individuals, such as those with inflammatory bowel disease, and may not be generalizable to the average screening population. In addition to size, the number of serrated polyps may also be a reproducible risk factor for predicting subsequent CRC, similar to conventional adenomas. A recent study on patients with multiple serrated polyps who fell short of current criteria for the serrated polyposis syndrome (SPS) showed increased CRC risk in these individuals as well as in their first-degree relatives.[32]

In addition to size and histology, there are other potential risks for the development of CRC in adults with the serrated polyps. One significant factor is the increased risk for synchronous advanced conventional adenomas in patients with these lesions.[31,33–36] It is interesting to note that, even in patients with SPS, the best predictor of carcinoma in a large series was not histology or polyp number, but the presence of concurrent conventional adenomas.[37] This finding is consistent with those in a prospective study that observed that patients with both SSPs and advanced adenomas have the highest risk for metachronous advanced adenomas and thus may benefit from close surveillance.[38]

With respect to mutations in the serrated pathway, HP and SSP share a similar mutational profile with *BRAF* being the most commonly mutated gene in both polyps and *KRAS* in a minor subset. Mutations in *BRAF* are tightly linked to the CpG island methylator phenotype and there are progressively increasing degrees of methylation in SSP compared with HP, and in SSPs in older patients when compared with SSP in a younger age group.[6,39–41] Methylation of *MLH1* is associated with the development of cytologic dysplasia[42,43] and loss of staining for the MLH1 protein on immunohistochemistry. Some SSP-D show serrated-type dysplasia reminiscent of TSAs, whereas others show conventional adenomatous-type dysplasia.[44] Rarely, the dysplastic changes can be quite subtle and difficult to recognize (**Fig. 3**). Loss of MLH1 is seldom detected in TSA-like SSP-D, but is much more common in SSP-D with conventional adenomatous-type dysplasia.[44–46]

The time course for SSP transformation into CRC seems to be similar to that for advanced adenomas and may not be a rapid as suggested by older data.[30,47] A recent case series analyzed the mean age of individuals with SSPs with and without cancer and suggested a lag time of 17 years between patients with SSPs and those with SSPs with cancer.[48] Interestingly, the average age for SSPs with cancers and SSP-D were similar, suggesting that the progression to cancer is rapid in those with SSP-D.

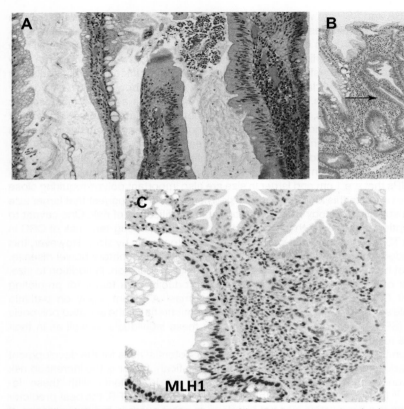

Fig. 3. (A) Dysplastic change in SSP can resemble TSAs or conventional adenomas. In this example, the crypt on the left from the precursor SSP shows small basal nuclei, whereas the one on the right shows cytoplasmic eosinophilia and pencillate nuclei similar to typical TSAs. (B, C) Abrupt transition into cytologic dysplasia in SSP (*arrow*) shows mucin depletion and nuclear enlargement. The type of dysplasia can be difficult to categorize: in this example the crypts still retain some serration but the cytoplasmic changes typical of a TSA are absent. Loss of MLH1 in dysplastic foci is clinically more important (C) than the specific morphologic type of dysplasia.

However, this observation may be a nomenclature issue as well, because SSP-D with loss of MLH1 are genetically similar to high microsatellite instability cancers and may represent intramucosal adenocarcinomas.[49] The long transformation time from SSP to SSP-D seems to support the observation that, although older age is not a risk for SSPs, older people may be at a higher risk for having SSPs with cancer than younger adults.[40,41,50] This hypothesis is also supported by the progressively increasing levels of methylation in SSPs with age.[6,39–41]

Endoscopic Appearance

Each of the serrated polyps may exhibit unique characteristics, including shape, color, and anatomic location, potentially impacting their detection. TSAs, the least common of all serrated polyps, are typically distal and erythematous with a protruding morphology, features that allow for fairly easy detection. The most common of all serrated polyps are HPs, which are flat, pale, and typically located in the distal colon.

SSPs, which tend to be proximally located, have distinctive features, including a flat morphology and indistinct borders. These polyps often have a mucous cap, which allows for easy detection.[51,52] Other features such as a cloudy surface and dome shape are demonstrated in **Fig. 4**.[53] Characteristic features of the 3 commonly observed serrated polyps are shown in **Table 1**.

The unique endoscopic appearances of serrated polyps, particularly the crypts, have allowed for real time endoscopic diagnosis of these lesions. This aspect has been important in the development of the criteria used for optical diagnosis of colorectal polyps, which can be used in strategies designed to reduce pathologic interpretation such as resect and discard.[54–56] One set of criteria, known as the Narrow Band Imaging (NBI) International Colorectal Endoscopic classification can distinguish adenomas from HPs. The Narrow Band Imaging International Colorectal Endoscopic criteria use endoscopic clues such as surface pattern and NBI imaging appearances of adenoma such as brown color to aid in differentiating adenomas from HPs.[57] Unfortunately, the Narrow Band Imaging International Colorectal Endoscopic criteria may be limited for optical diagnosis of SSPs.[58] To address this gap, the Workgroup on Serrated Polyps and Polyposis criteria were developed to help distinguish SSPs.[59] The Workgroup on Serrated Polyps and Polyposis criteria (**Fig. 5**) are predictive of an SSP if there are 2 of the following features present;

- Irregular surface,
- Indiscrete edges,
- A cloudlike appearance, and
- Large open pits.

Endoscopic Detection

Because SSPs have a potential for malignant transformation and they can be flat with indistinct borders, making them difficult to detect endoscopically, there is great concern among endoscopists for missing these lesions. This concern is supported by data demonstrating a wide variation in detection of serrated polyps, especially those that are clinically significant such as SSPS, TSAs, and large proximal HPs.[60–67] This observed variation has led some experts to question whether a serrated polyp detection rate is needed to ensure adequate detection by all endoscopits.[10] One

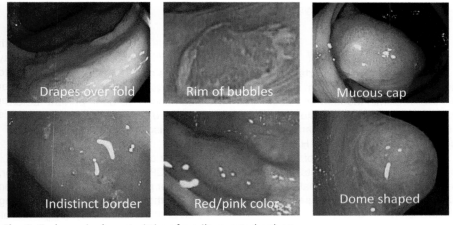

Fig. 4. Endoscopic characteristics of sessile serrated polyps.

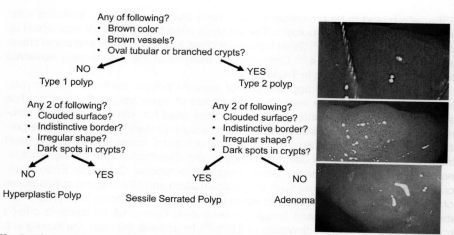

Any of following?
- Brown color
- Brown vessels?
- Oval tubular or branched crypts?

NO   YES

Type 1 polyp   Type 2 polyp

Any 2 of following?
- Clouded surface?
- Indistinctive border?
- Irregular shape?
- Dark spots in crypts?

Any 2 of following?
- Clouded surface?
- Indistinctive border?
- Irregular shape?
- Dark spots in crypts?

NO   YES   YES   NO

Hyperplastic Polyp   Sessile Serrated Polyp   Adenoma

Fig. 5. Algorithm demonstrating use of Workgroup on Serrated Polyps and Polyposis criteria to diagnose SSPs.

of the issues in developing a serrated detection is the choice of outcome for polyp detection. Although some studies have examined proximal serrated polyp detection,[60–62] others have chosen to examine only SSP detection.[63] Although SSPs are lesions that can develop into cancer, the inclusion of only these serrated polyps in a detection rate is problematic for a few reasons. The first is that this rate may be more dependent on the pathologists' interpretations of the resected serrated polyps rather than the ability of the endoscopists to detect and resect these polyps. This concept was demonstrated in a recent study that showed wide variation across centers for SSP detection, suggesting that factors outside of endoscopists' abilities may influence these rates.[65]

To address the concern regarding pathologist interpretation of serrated polyps, some investigators have examined other rates such proximal serrated detection rates.[60–62] One alternative that has also been examined is using detection rates for CSSP:

- SSP (with or without dysplasia) of any size
- TSAs of any size
- Any HP 1 cm or larger
- Any proximal HP larger than 5 mm

This rate combines important histology such as SSPs and TSAs with other factors such as HPs that are 5 mm or greater and located proximal to sigmoid or splenic flexure. Proximal location and larger size have been shown to be important factors in predicting an SSP histology in lesions that were previously diagnosed as HPs.[68,69] Thus, this rate can account for potential misdiagnosed SSPs that have been incorrectly labeled as HPs.

In addition to the choice of lesion to measure, another concern is how to develop a benchmark for endoscopists. Investigators in the NHCR used adenoma detection rates to determine an optimal serrated detection rate for proximal and CSSP.[60] Specifically, they examined the serrated detection rates for those endoscopists achieving an adenoma detection rate of 25% or higher. Based on their result, they suggested a detection rate of 7% for CSSP.

One important observation in this NHCR study was that the rates for both proximal and CSSP correlated with each other as well as with the overall adenoma detection rate. Although this finding is reassuring, there are some implications. If the proximal serrated detection rates correlate with CSSP detection rates, presumably endoscopists could use the former, which would not require size estimation or differentiation of SSPs from HPs. However, given the correlation between adenoma detection rate and serrated polyp detection rate, it raises the issue of whether a separate serrated polyp detection rate benchmark is needed. In their analysis, however, the authors observed that even among those endoscopists with adequate adenoma detection rates, a significant proportion (25%) of the endoscopists failed to meet the serrated polyp detection rate benchmark of 7%. The authors conclude that this finding demonstrates the need to measure 1 serrated polyp detection rate at least once in an endoscopists practice to assess their serrated detecting ability.

A logical question is how can endoscopists increase their serrated polyp detection rates. The first step for practices seeking to maximize serrated polyp detection would be to ensure that all of their patients are split dosing their bowel preparations.[70] A recent meta-analysis and systematic review of 28 trials examining split dose preparation found that SSP detection had a greater benefit when using split dose as compared with conventional adenoma and advanced adenoma detection.[71] A study by Clark and Laine[72] observed that SSP detection was maximized in those patients who had high-quality bowel preparation. Although intermediate quality may be adequate for conventional adenomas, the authors recommended that high-quality preparation may be required for SSP detection.

Another simple measure that endoscopists can take is to increase their withdrawal time. One study from the Netherlands suggested that the variation in proximal serrated detection rates may be due to variations in withdrawal time.[73] One analysis that examined data from nearly 8000 patients in the NHCR observed that detection of CSSPs reached the highest level in those endoscopists who had withdrawal times of 8 to 9 minutes. These data suggest that a withdrawal time of 8 to 9 minutes may be needed to ensure an adequate SSP detection.

Technology or Techniques to Increase Detection

One technique that has been used in an attempt to increase detection of polyps is chromoendoscopy or specifically chromo-colonoscopy.[74] Although studies have shown an increase is serrated polyp detection, there are limitations, which include longer withdrawal time and increased burden on endoscopy centers owing to time and resources as well attendant issues with dye use.[75–77] Therefore, the use of dye-assisted colonoscopy may not be practical. Another technique, total underwater colonoscopy, was shown to not increase detection and is potentially burdensome in a busy endoscopy unit.[78]

Among the new technologies that are widely used, high definition is likely the most effective new technology. NBI uses blue light to enhance visualization of the mucosal structures in part by highlighting superficial microcapillaries. This technology has been available for more than 10 years.[79] and has been available clinically since 2005. One randomized controlled trial observed an increased detection of proximal serrated polyps in individuals with the use of NBI as compared with white light endoscopy.[80] One recent meta analysis demonstrated a slight benefit in the detection of non adenomatous polyps as compared with white light endoscopy when bowel preparation is optimal.[81] This slight increase may not offset the length of time that using NBI may add to an examination. Therefore, although NBI is widely available it is unlikely to impact practice with respect to increasing serrated polyp detection. Full-spectrum endoscopy allows the field of view to expand from 170° to 330°. One study that randomized patients to full-spectrum endoscopy versus standard forward viewing colonoscopy observed that there was no difference in sessile serrated polyp detection.[82] These data suggest that this technology may not increase serrated polyp detection.

Attachments to the tip of the colonoscope have also been studied to examine the impact on serrated polyp detection.[83–86] One randomized controlled trial of more than 500 patients observed that a ring-fitted cap did not yield an increase detection of SSP.[86] With regard to other cuff devices, which are designed to flatten folds to maximize mucosal inspection, 1 study of more than 1000 procedures observed that there was no increase in the detection of serrated lesions using a cuff.[85] A meta-analysis that examined attachments as well as electronic chromoendoscopic technology like NBI observed that only NBI increased serrated polyp detection.[87] Finally, 1 study randomized more than 1000 patients to standard high-definition colonoscopy, high definition with a cuff, high definition with a ring, or full-spectrum endoscopy.[88] They observed no clinically significant differences for sessile serrated polyp detection among the 4 groups. Thus, it seems that there is no consensus regarding the use of new technology in terms of detecting serrated polyps and endoscopists should use those techniques or devices that assist them in their practice.

Detection of Serrated Polyps by Other Screening Tests

Owing to the flat nature of serrated polyps, colonoscopy seems to be the best screening test for the detection of serrated polyps. A randomized controlled trial comparing computed tomography colonoscopy with colonoscopy observed that colonoscopy was superior to computed tomography colonoscopy for detecting SSPs, especially flat and proximal SSPs.[89] Computed tomography colonoscopy relies on protrusion of lesions into the lumen for these lesions to be seen on the images. Thus, flat lesions may be missed by this technology. Because air is needed to inflate the bowel, SSPs that are proximal may further flatten, making their detection more challenging.

With regard to stool testing, the fecal immunochemical test seems to have a significantly lower sensitivity for serrated polyps as compared with conventional adenomas.[90–92] Fecal immunochemical testing detects hemoglobin in stool and data suggest that serrated polyps are less likely to bleed than conventional neoplasia.[93,94] Factors that predict higher fecal hemoglobin levels are distal location as compared with proximal location and protruding versus flat morphology.[94] Given the flat and proximal nature of many important serrated polyps, such as SSPs, it is not surprising that fecal immunochemical testing is not sensitive for these polyps. One study, for example, observed a high detection rate for adenomas (45%) and advanced adenomas (29%) in their sample,[91] but an unacceptably low rate for SSAs (1.8%). However, whereas serrated polyps may not bleed like conventional adenomas, these lesions do shed cellular debris that contain DNA mutations. Thus, using a multitargeted stool DNA test, which has markers for DNA methylation (NDRG4 and BMP3), may be a superior choice to fecal immunochemical testing for serrated lesions.[95]

Resection

Given the indistinct borders of the serrated polyps, especially SSPs, there is understandable concern by endoscopists about the adequacy of resection of these lesions in practice. One analysis, conducted in the Incomplete polyp resection during colonoscopy-results of the complete adenoma resection (CARE) study, examined the adequacy of resection by biopsies of the edges of resected polyps.[96] They observed that serrated lesions had a nearly 4-fold increase (relative risk, 3.7) for incomplete resection as conventional adenomas. The CARE study also found that larger size was a predictor of inadequate resection for all polyps, regardless of histology. For serrated polyps 10 to 20 mm, almost one-half (47.6%) were incompletely resected. This study underscored the need for careful resection of serrated polyps, especially those large than 10 mm.

One method that has been shown to be an effective strategy for resection of serrated polyps larger than 10 mm is endoscopic mucosal resection (EMR).[97] As shown in **Fig. 6**, this is an easy method that can be used with an injectable fluid as well as commonly used snares. By using a dye such as methylene blue or indigo carmine, the indistinct edges of serrated polyps can be made easier to delineate. One study by Rao and colleagues[98] showed, in a sample of 199 patients with 251 SSPs larger than 10 mm, that the recurrence rate was only 3.6% in a mean follow-up time of 17.8 months. Another study by Pellise and colleagues[99] prospectively the resection of SSPs and conventional adenomas 20 mm or larger using a standardized dye-based conventional EMR technique. They observed that the recurrence of SSPs was less than conventional lesions for those polyps sized 20 to 25 mm. Finally, a study by Rex and colleagues[100] observed that, among lesions greater than 20 mm, the rate for incomplete resection when using EMR was similar for SSPs and conventional adenomas. These studies support the idea that EMR should be used when resecting lesions suspected of being SSPs.

Serrated Polyposis Syndrome

SPS, which was formerly known as hyperplastic polyposis syndrome, carries an increased risk for CRC in affected individuals as well as their relatives.[32,101–103] The previous World Health Organization criteria for SPS[104] were:

- Criterion 1: 20 serrated polyps found in the colon,
- Criterion 2: at least 5 serrated polyps proximal to the sigmoid colon with 2 greater than 10 mm in diameter, or
- Criterion 3: serrated polyps found proximal to the sigmoid colon in an individual with a first-degree relative with SPS

These criteria have changed in the recent WHO publication[105]:

- Criterion 1: at least 5 serrated polyps proximal to the rectum all 5 mm or larger, with at least 2 that are 10 mm or larger.
- Criterion 2: more than 20 serrated polyps of any size but distributed throughout the large bowel, with at least 5 proximal to the rectum.

Important issues that endoscopists need to keep in mind include the observation that many SPS may be underdiagnosed in practice.[106] It is also important to remember that the diagnosis is based on a cumulative incidence of serrated polyps.

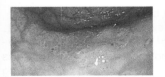 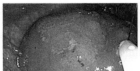 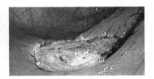

Fig. 6. EMR enables complete resection of large serrated polyps (this one presumed to be SSP) partly through the better delineation of polyp borders with dye. In this case the dye is methylene blue.

With respect to surveillance in individuals with SPS, the US Multi-Society Task Force on CRC recommend annual surveillance for those with SPS.[107] A recent study from the Netherlands and Spain suggested that 2-year intervals may be similar to annual surveillance with regard to metachronous risk of advanced neoplasia including CRC.[108] An expert panel recommended that annual colonoscopy should be performed with the goal of clearing all serrated polyps in the proximal, or at least all serrated polyps 5 mm or greater in size if there are numerous diminutive lesions. A recent study from Indiana observed that it might take 2 to 3 colonoscopies for the polyp burden to be under control.[109] This clearing of serrated polyps in the colon typically took 1 to 2 years. After clearing, patients returned after 24 months with CRC detected or requirement for surgery. These data support 2-year surveillance for those individuals with SPS in whom the polyp burden is controlled.

Surveillance

One challenging aspect in the management of serrated polyps is the follow-up in individuals who have these lesions resected on index colonoscopies. The main obstacle is that until recently there have been few data published.[38,110–113] Although many individuals may be diagnosed with serrated polyps, many of these are small HPs and are not clinically relevant. Conversely, SSPs and TSAs are much less common, but are important lesions that require follow-up. The high frequency of synchronous conventional adenomas, especially HRA, in individuals with serrated polyps can also create a challenge for investigators.[31,33–36] Specifically, it is not possible to determine if the risk for metachronous HRA arises from the serrated lesions or from the synchronous HRA. Therefore, these data cannot be used to determine risk for those individuals with only SSPs, TSAs, or significant HPs.

When examining the metachronous risk for serrated polyps, another consideration is the selection of an appropriate outcome for assessing the future risk of index serrated polyps. Although the risk for CRC is the most important, it is not a practical outcome for studies because it is relatively rare and can take years to develop. Therefore, researchers use a surrogate risk of metachronous (future) polyps. HRA, including adenomas 1 cm or larger, adenomas with villous elements or high-grade dysplasia, 3 or more adenomas, or adenocarcinoma (CRC), are used for studies examining conventional adenomas. However, prior research from a time period before the recognition of SSP suggests that individuals with HPs are at risk for future HPs and not conventional adenomas.[114,115] These data would suggest that conventional HRAs would not be an appropriate outcome for examining metachronous risk for individuals with serrated polyps.

An outcome that has been used by a few studies is the metachronous risk for large (≥1 cm) serrated polyps. This outcome makes sense for a few reasons. The first is that the size makes it less likely that a large serrated polyp detected on surveillance represents a missed lesion. In addition, including all serrated polyps as opposed to SSPs makes the pathologic interpretation, which can be difficult, less important. Finally, individuals with large serrated polyps have been shown to have increased risk for CRC in long-term studies.[29,30] Recently, a few studies have demonstrated that patients with SSPs, TSAs, or large HPs at the index examination are at increased risk for metachronous large (≥1 cm) serrated polyps.[38,111,113,116] Conversely, these studies observed that individuals with these serrated polyps were not at increased risk for conventional HRA.

The largest analysis to date has been conducted using data from the NHCR.[38] This population database had sufficient power to stratify patients by index serrated polyps and conventional adenomas. The investigators observed that, when the serrated polyps were stratified by size, those that were 1 cm or larger were associated with an increased risk for metachronous large (≥1 cm) serrated polyps. When stratified by histology, those with SSP or TSA were also associated with an increased risk. Serrated polyps less than 1 cm and HPs were not associated with an increased metachronous risk. Given the association between large HPs and long-term CRC risk in larger studies,[29,30] these data suggest that SSPs, TSAs and large serrated polyps should have closer surveillance than other serrated polyps. Conversely, serrated polyps were not associated with an increased risk for conventional HRA. Given the size of the database, the data are also the best estimate to date of the minimal risk that adults with only index serrated polyps have for metachronous conventional adenomas. Finally, a novel observation in this study is that those individuals with both SSPs or TSAs and conventional HRAs had a statistically higher risk for metachronous HRA than those with HRA alone. These data suggest that there may be 3 distinct biologic categories when assessing risk.

- Individuals with serrated polyps only,
- Individuals with only HRA, and
- Individuals with synchronous HRA and serrated polyps.

The main question for endoscopists is what appropriate intervals should be recommended for individuals with serrated polyps. Although there have been a few guidelines that addressed intervals, the recommendations have been based on little evidence. In 2012, there were 2 sets of guidelines that were published, those from an expert panel[2] and those from the US Multi-Society Task Force on Colorectal Cancer.[107] The US Multi-Society Task Force made recommendations for serrated lesions that were explicitly diagnosed as SSP or TSAs. The recommendations varied depending on size (<1 vs ≥1 cm), histology (SSP), or the presence of dysplasia in SSPs. SSPs less than 1 cm with no dysplasia had a recommended interval of 5 years, whereas TSAs, SSPs 1 cm or larger, or with dysplasia had 3-year follow-up intervals. Other potentially significant lesions such as HPs greater than 1 cm were not addressed in these guidelines, largely owing to a lack of evidence. The expert panel took a more ambitious approach by providing recommendations for HPs that are proximal and 5 mm or larger. Although this approach was helpful for endoscopists, especially for large HPs, the recommendations were based on little available data. Part of the rationale for recommending close intervals for larger HPs is correctly based on the assumption that some large and/or proximal HPs may be misclassified SSPs.[68,69,117] The European Society of Gastrointestinal Endoscopy postpolypectomy colonoscopy surveillance guidelines divide serrated polyps into high-risk groups depending on size or presence of dysplasia, but do not provide specific intervals for follow-up aside from those patients with SPS.[118] The British Society of Gastroenterology recommends a 3 year follow-up for SSPs 10 mm or larger or with dysplasia.[119] They recommend no follow-up for any HP or SSPs less than 10 mm with no dysplasia. A recent guideline from British Society of Gastroenterology/Association of Coloproctology of Great Britain and Ireland/Public Health England classify any serrated polyp 10 mm or larger or containing any grade of dysplasia as high risk, requiring repeat colonoscopy in 3 years.[120]

A new set of recommendations was published recently by the US Multi-Society Task Force on CRC.[121] One major change is that these guidelines recommended close intervals of 3 to 5 years for those individuals with only large (≥1 cm) HPs. These recommendations were based on the association of these lesions with future large serrated polyps. Other changes included providing specific recommendations for individuals with small SSPs, treating them like low-risk adenomas. For example, 1 to 2

Table 2
Take home points for serrated polyps

Section	Take Home Points
Classification and histology	Three subtypes of serrated polyps; HPs, SSPs and TSAs All have saw tooth appearance histologically HPs have straight crypts with serration at luminal surface SSPs have architectural disarray at the crypt bases with crypt dilatation, boot or anchor shaped or horizontal crypts Distinguishing HP from SSP is challenging owing to varying minimum thresholds for making a diagnosis of SSP No observer reproducibility for specific criteria used to diagnose SSP TSAs easy to distinguish from HPs/SSPs, However, distinction of TSA with high-grade changes vs a conventional adenoma can be challenging
Risk factors	Smoking is the most important risk factor Unlike conventional adenomas, older age and male sex are not risk factors
Carcinogenesis	TSAs are cytologically dysplastic lesions SSPs develop cytologic dysplasia (SSP-D) as they progress to CRC SSP to CRC transformation likely has similar time course as conventional adenomas TSA and SSP are widely accepted as precursors of CRC HP regarded as benign but HPs $\geq$1 cm have an increased long-term CRC risk Size may be as important as histology for CRC risk Strong association with synchronous advanced conventional adenomas provides additional CRC risk for those with serrated polyps
Molecular mutations	BRAF most common oncogene for HPs and SSPs BRAF is tightly linked to the CpG island methylator phenotype Degree of methylation increases with malignant progression of SSPs Methylation of MLH1 is linked with cytologic dysplasia
Endoscopic appearance	TSAs are distal and erythematous with a protruding morphology HPs are flat, pale and typically located in the distal colon SSPs are typically proximal with flat morphology SSPs can have mucous cap, indistinct edges, dome shape, cloudy surface, large open O pit patterns and irregular surface
Endoscopic detection	Detection of serrated polyps can vary across endoscopists SSPs rates can vary owing to variation in pathologic interpretation One measurement of serrated polyp detection may be prudent Increased serrated polyp detection can be achieved with longer withdrawal time and split dose bowel preparation
Endoscopic Resection	Data suggest high rate of incomplete resection for large serrated polyps Use of EMR may achieve high rates of complete resection

(continued on next page)

Table 2 (continued)	
Section	**Take Home Points**
SPS	Carries an increased CRC risk in affected individuals as well as relatives
	New SPS criteria from the World Health Organization
	Criterion 1: ≥5 serrated polyps proximal to rectum ≥5 mm, with 2 ≥ 10 mm.
	Criterion 2: >20 serrated polyps (any size) with ≥5 proximal to rectum.
	SPS is based on cumulative polyps across subsequent colonoscopies
	SPS is likely underdiagnosed in practice
	Yearly colonoscopy clearing all proximal serrated polyps or at least all serrated polyps ≥5 mm
Surveillance	Close surveillance (3–5 y) for SSPs (≥10 mm), SSP-D, HPs ≥10 mm and TSAs
	More data are needed for proximal HPs 6–9 mm

small (<10 mm) SSPs would have a follow-up colonoscopy at 5 to 10 years after the index examination. These new guidelines will hopefully provide endoscopists with intervals that will ensure adequate CRC protection in patients with serrated polyps.

SUMMARY

Serrated polyps are a heterogeneous group of lesions that require careful attention by the endoscopist with respect to detection, resection and follow-up (**Table 2**). Recognition of the endoscopic appearance of these lesions will likely allow the endoscopist to detect serrated polyps present in their patients' colons. In addition, careful attention to bowel preparation in the form of split dose preparation as well a longer withdrawal time will ensure optimal detection. Good communication with the pathologist is important in the diagnosis. However, it is important to realize that distinction among serrated polyps is not always feasible. In light of this observation, large HPs may be treated as SSP equivalent and thus require close follow-up similar to SSPs.

DISCLOSURE

The authors have no conflicts of interest to declare.

REFERENCES

1. Farris AB, Misdraji J, Srivastava A, et al. Sessile serrated adenoma: challenging discrimination from other serrated colonic polyps. Am J Surg Pathol 2008; 32:30–5.
2. Rex DK, Ahnen DJ, Baron JA, et al. Serrated lesions of the colorectum: review and recommendations from an expert panel. Am J Gastroenterol 2012;107: 1315–29 [quiz: 1314, 1330].
3. Lindholm CR, Anderson JC, Srivastava A. The dark side of the colon: current issues surrounding the significance, prevalence, detection, diagnosis and management of serrated polyps. Curr Opin Gastroenterol 2019;35:34–41.
4. Tadros M, Anderson JC. Serrated polyps: clinical implications and future directions. Curr Gastroenterol Rep 2013;15:342.

5. East JE, Vieth M, Rex DK. Serrated lesions in colorectal cancer screening: detection, resection, pathology and surveillance. Gut 2015;64:991–1000.
6. Pai RK, Bettington M, Srivastava A, et al. An update on the morphology and molecular pathology of serrated colorectal polyps and associated carcinomas. Mod Pathol 2019;32:1390–415.
7. Erichsen R, Baron JA, Hamilton-Dutoit SJ, et al. Increased risk of colorectal cancer development among patients with serrated polyps. Gastroenterology 2016; 150:895–902.e5.
8. Kolb JM, Morales SJ, Rouse NA, et al. Does better specimen orientation and a simplified grading system promote more reliable histologic interpretation of serrated colon polyps in the community practice setting? results of a nationwide study. J Clin Gastroenterol 2016;50:233–8.
9. Anderson JC, Srivastava A. Traditional serrated adenomas: what the endoscopist should know. Gastrointest Endosc 2019;90:647–50.
10. Anderson JC. Detection of serrated polyps: how do endoscopists rate? Endoscopy 2018;50:950–2.
11. Anderson JC, Rangasamy P, Rustagi T, et al. Risk factors for sessile serrated adenomas. J Clin Gastroenterol 2011;45:694–9.
12. He X, Wu K, Ogino S, et al. Association between risk factors for colorectal cancer and risk of serrated polyps and conventional adenomas. Gastroenterology 2018;155:355–73.e18.
13. Figueiredo JC, Crockett SD, Snover DC, et al. Smoking-associated risks of conventional adenomas and serrated polyps in the colorectum. Cancer Causes Control 2015;26:377–86.
14. Anderson JC, Calderwood AH, Christensen BC, et al. Smoking and other risk factors in individuals with synchronous conventional high-risk adenomas and clinically significant serrated polyps. Am J Gastroenterol 2018;113:1828–35.
15. Burnett-Hartman AN, Passarelli MN, Adams SV, et al. Differences in epidemiologic risk factors for colorectal adenomas and serrated polyps by lesion severity and anatomical site. Am J Epidemiol 2013;177:625–37.
16. Crockett SD, Snover DC, Ahnen DJ, et al. Sessile serrated adenomas: an evidence-based guide to management. Clin Gastroenterol Hepatol 2015;13: 11–26.e1.
17. Anderson JC, Weiss JE, Robinson CM, et al. Adenoma detection rates for screening colonoscopies in smokers and obese adults: data from the New Hampshire Colonoscopy Registry. J Clin Gastroenterol 2017;51:e95–100.
18. Anderson JC, Alpern ZA. Smoking and the increased risk for serrated polyps: implications for screening and surveillance. J Clin Gastroenterol 2019;53: 319–21.
19. Bailie L, Loughrey MB, Coleman HG. Lifestyle risk factors for serrated colorectal polyps: a systematic review and meta-analysis. Gastroenterology 2017;152: 92–104.
20. Bouwens MW, Winkens B, Rondagh EJ, et al. Simple clinical risk score identifies patients with serrated polyps in routine practice. Cancer Prev Res (Phila) 2013; 6:855–63.
21. Rustagi T, Rangasamy P, Myers M, et al. Sessile serrated adenomas in the proximal colon are likely to be flat, large and occur in smokers. World J Gastroenterol 2013;19:5271–7.
22. Anderson JC, Pleau DC, Rajan TV, et al. Increased frequency of serrated aberrant crypt foci among smokers. Am J Gastroenterol 2010;105:1648–54.

23. Anderson JC, Messina CR, Dakhllalah F, et al. Body mass index: a marker for significant colorectal neoplasia in a screening population. J Clin Gastroenterol 2007;41:285–90.

24. Anderson JC, Attam R, Alpern Z, et al. Prevalence of colorectal neoplasia in smokers. Am J Gastroenterol 2003;98:2777–83.

25. Anderson JC, Latreille M, Messina C, et al. Smokers as a high-risk group: data from a screening population. J Clin Gastroenterol 2009;43:747–52.

26. Anderson JC, Messina C. Smoking and risk for colorectal cancer. Arch Intern Med 2006;166:1669–70 [author reply: 1671].

27. Anderson JC, Moezardalan K, Messina CR, et al. Smoking and the association of advanced colorectal neoplasia in an asymptomatic average risk population: analysis of exposure and anatomical location in men and women. Dig Dis Sci 2011;56:3616–23.

28. Gonzalo DH, Lai KK, Shadrach B, et al. Gene expression profiling of serrated polyps identifies annexin A10 as a marker of a sessile serrated adenoma/polyp. J Pathol 2013;230:420–9.

29. He X, Hang D, Wu K, et al. Long-term risk of colorectal cancer after removal of conventional adenomas and serrated polyps. Gastroenterology 2019. https://doi.org/10.1053/j.gastro.2019.06.039.

30. Holme O, Bretthauer M, Eide TJ, et al. Long-term risk of colorectal cancer in individuals with serrated polyps. Gut 2015;64:929–36.

31. Hiraoka S, Kato J, Fujiki S, et al. The presence of large serrated polyps increases risk for colorectal cancer. Gastroenterology 2010;139:1503–10, 1510.e1-3.

32. Egoavil C, Juarez M, Guarinos C, et al. Increased risk of colorectal cancer in patients with multiple serrated polyps and their first-degree relatives. Gastroenterology 2017;153:106–12.e2.

33. Li D, Jin C, McCulloch C, et al. Association of large serrated polyps with synchronous advanced colorectal neoplasia. Am J Gastroenterol 2009;104:695–702.

34. Gao Q, Tsoi KK, Hirai HW, et al. Serrated polyps and the risk of synchronous colorectal advanced neoplasia: a systematic review and meta-analysis. Am J Gastroenterol 2015;110:501–9 [quiz: 510].

35. Ng SC, Ching JY, Chan VC, et al. Association between serrated polyps and the risk of synchronous advanced colorectal neoplasia in average-risk individuals. Aliment Pharmacol Ther 2015;41:108–15.

36. Buda A, De Bona M, Dotti I, et al. Prevalence of different subtypes of serrated polyps and risk of synchronous advanced colorectal neoplasia in average-risk population undergoing first-time colonoscopy. Clin Transl Gastroenterol 2012;3:e6.

37. Rosty C, Buchanan DD, Walsh MD, et al. Phenotype and polyp landscape in serrated polyposis syndrome: a series of 100 patients from genetics clinics. Am J Surg Pathol 2012;36:876–82.

38. Anderson JC, Butterly LF, Robinson CM, et al. Risk of metachronous high-risk adenomas and large serrated polyps in individuals with serrated polyps on index colonoscopy: data from the New Hampshire Colonoscopy Registry. Gastroenterology 2018;154:117–27.e2.

39. Fernando WC, Miranda MS, Worthley DL, et al. The CIMP phenotype in BRAF mutant serrated polyps from a prospective colonoscopy patient cohort. Gastroenterol Res Pract 2014;2014:374926.

40. Liu C, Bettington ML, Walker NI, et al. CpG island methylation in sessile serrated adenomas increases with age, indicating lower risk of malignancy in young patients. Gastroenterology 2018;155:1362–5.e2.

41. Bettington M, Brown I, Rosty C, et al. Sessile serrated adenomas in young patients may have limited risk of malignant progression. J Clin Gastroenterol 2019 53(3):e113–6.

42. Goldstein NS. Small colonic microsatellite unstable adenocarcinomas and high-grade epithelial dysplasias in sessile serrated adenoma polypectomy specimens: a study of eight cases. Am J Clin Pathol 2006;125:132–45.

43. Sheridan TB, Fenton H, Lewin MR, et al. Sessile serrated adenomas with low- and high-grade dysplasia and early carcinomas: an immunohistochemical study of serrated lesions "caught in the act. Am J Clin Pathol 2006;126:564–71

44. Cenaj O, Gibson J, Odze RD. Clinicopathologic and outcome study of sessile serrated adenomas/polyps with serrated versus intestinal dysplasia. Mod Patho 2018;31:633–42.

45. Liu C, Walker NI, Leggett BA, et al. Sessile serrated adenomas with dysplasia morphological patterns and correlations with MLH1 immunohistochemistry. Mod Pathol 2017;30:1728–38.

46. Yozu M, Kem M, Cenaj O, et al. Loss of expression of MLH1 in non-dysplastic crypts is a harbinger of neoplastic progression in sessile serrated adenomas, polyps. Histopathology 2019;75:376–84.

47. Lu FI, van Niekerk de W, Owen D, et al. Longitudinal outcome study of sessile serrated adenomas of the colorectum: an increased risk for subsequent right-sided colorectal carcinoma. Am J Surg Pathol 2010;34:927–34.

48. Bettington M, Walker N, Rosty C, et al. Clinicopathological and molecular features of sessile serrated adenomas with dysplasia or carcinoma. Gut 2017;66. 97–106.

49. Cenaj O, Yozu M, Baltay M, et al. Molecular correlates of dysplasia subtypes in sessile serrated polyps and their relationship to invasive adenocarcinoma 108th Annual Meeting of the United-States-and-Canadian-Academy-of-Pathology (USCAP) - Unlocking Your Ingenuity. Volume Modern Pathology Volume 32. National Harbor, MD, March 16–21, 2019.

50. Anderson JC, Levine JB. Age and CRC risk in the serrated pathway. J Clin Gastroenterol 2018;52:465–7.

51. Anderson JC, Pollack BJ. Predicting of hyperplastic histology by endoscopic features. Gastrointest Endosc 2000;52:149–50.

52. Rex DK, Rahmani EY. New endoscopic finding associated with hyperplastic polyps. Gastrointest Endosc 1999;50:704–6.

53. Tadepalli US, Feihel D, Miller KM, et al. A morphologic analysis of sessile serrated polyps observed during routine colonoscopy (with video). Gastrointest Endosc 2011;74:1360–8.

54. Hassan C, Pickhardt PJ, Rex DK. A resect and discard strategy would improve cost-effectiveness of colorectal cancer screening. Clin Gastroenterol Hepatol 2010;8:865–9, 869.e1-3.

55. Rex DK, Patel NJ, Vemulapalli KC. A survey of patient acceptance of resect and discard for diminutive polyps. Gastrointest Endosc 2015;82:376–80.e1.

56. Soudagar AS, Nguyen M, Bhatia A, et al. Are gastroenterologists willing to implement the "predict, resect, and discard" management strategy for diminutive colorectal polyps? Results from a national survey. J Clin Gastroenterol 2016;50:e45–9.

57. Hewett DG, Kaltenbach T, Sano Y, et al. Validation of a simple classification system for endoscopic diagnosis of small colorectal polyps using narrow-band imaging. Gastroenterology 2012;143:599–607.e1.

58. Kumar S, Fioritto A, Mitani A, et al. Optical biopsy of sessile serrated adenomas: do these lesions resemble hyperplastic polyps under narrow-band imaging? Gastrointest Endosc 2013;78:902–9.

59. JE IJ, Bastiaansen BA, van Leerdam ME, et al. Development and validation of the WASP classification system for optical diagnosis of adenomas, hyperplastic polyps and sessile serrated adenomas/polyps. Gut 2016;65:963–70.

60. Anderson JC, Butterly LF, Weiss JE, et al. Providing data for serrated polyp detection rate benchmarks: an analysis of the New Hampshire Colonoscopy Registry. Gastrointest Endosc 2017;85:1188–94.

61. Kahi CJ, Hewett DG, Norton DL, et al. Prevalence and variable detection of proximal colon serrated polyps during screening colonoscopy. Clin Gastroenterol Hepatol 2011;9:42–6.

62. Kahi CJ, Li X, Eckert GJ, et al. High colonoscopic prevalence of proximal colon serrated polyps in average-risk men and women. Gastrointest Endosc 2012;75: 515–20.

63. Crockett SD, Gourevitch RA, Morris M, et al. Endoscopist factors that influence serrated polyp detection: a multicenter study. Endoscopy 2018;50(10):984–92.

64. JE IJ, van Doorn SC, van der Brug YM, et al. The proximal serrated polyp detection rate is an easy-to-measure proxy for the detection rate of clinically relevant serrated polyps. Gastrointest Endosc 2015;82:870–7.

65. Payne SR, Church TR, Wandell M, et al. Endoscopic detection of proximal serrated lesions and pathologic identification of sessile serrated adenomas/polyps vary on the basis of center. Clin Gastroenterol Hepatol 2014;12(7): 1119–26.

66. Schramm C, Janhsen K, Hofer JH, et al. Detection of clinically relevant serrated polyps during screening colonoscopy: results from seven cooperating centers within the German colorectal screening program. Endoscopy 2018;50(10): 993–1000.

67. Mandaliya R, Baig K, Barnhill M, et al. Significant variation in the detection rates of proximal serrated polyps among academic gastroenterologists, community gastroenterologists, and colorectal surgeons in a single tertiary care center. Dig Dis Sci 2019;64:2614–21.

68. Anderson JC, Lisovsky M, Greene MA, et al. Factors associated with classification of hyperplastic polyps as sessile serrated adenomas/polyps on morphologic review. J Clin Gastroenterol 2018;52:524–9.

69. Singh H, Bay D, Ip S, et al. Pathological reassessment of hyperplastic colon polyps in a city-wide pathology practice: implications for polyp surveillance recommendations. Gastrointest Endosc 2012;76:1003–8.

70. Johnson DA, Barkun AN, Cohen LB, et al. Optimizing adequacy of bowel cleansing for colonoscopy: recommendations from the U.S. multi-society task force on colorectal cancer. Gastrointest Endosc 2014;80:543–62.

71. Zawaly K, Rumbolt C, Abou-Setta AM, et al. The efficacy of split-dose bowel preparations for polyp detection: a systematic review and meta-analysis. Am J Gastroenterol 2019;114:884–92.

72. Clark BT, Laine L. High-quality bowel preparation is required for detection of sessile serrated polyps. Clin Gastroenterol Hepatol 2016;14:1155–62.

73. de Wijkerslooth TR, Stoop EM, Bossuyt PM, et al. Differences in proximal serrated polyp detection among endoscopists are associated with variability in withdrawal time. Gastrointest Endosc 2013;77:617–23.

74. Kahi CJ, Anderson JC, Waxman I, et al. High-definition chromocolonoscopy vs. high-definition white light colonoscopy for average-risk colorectal cancer screening. Am J Gastroenterol 2010;105:1301–7.

75. Buchner A. Chromoendoscopy for detection of proximal serrated lesions in routine screening colonoscopy. Lancet Gastroenterol Hepatol 2019;4:329–31.

76. Hurt C, Ramaraj R, Farr A, et al. Feasibility and economic assessment of chromocolonoscopy for detection of proximal serrated neoplasia within a population-based colorectal cancer screening programme (CONSCOP): an open-label, randomised controlled non-inferiority trial. Lancet Gastroenterol Hepatol 2019; 4:364–75.

77. Pohl J, Schneider A, Vogell H, et al. Pancolonic chromoendoscopy with indigo carmine versus standard colonoscopy for detection of neoplastic lesions: a randomised two-centre trial. Gut 2011;60:485–90.

78. Anderson JC, Kahi CJ, Sullivan A, et al. Comparing adenoma and polyp miss rates for total underwater colonoscopy versus standard CO2: a randomized controlled trial using a tandem colonoscopy approach. Gastrointest Endosc 2019;89:591–8.

79. East JE, Vleugels JL, Roelandt P, et al. Advanced endoscopic imaging: European Society of Gastrointestinal Endoscopy (ESGE) technology review. Endoscopy 2016;48:1029–45.

80. Rex DK, Clodfelter R, Rahmani F, et al. Narrow-band imaging versus white light for the detection of proximal colon serrated lesions: a randomized, controlled trial. Gastrointest Endosc 2016;83:166–71.

81. Atkinson NSS, Ket S, Bassett P, et al. Narrow-band imaging for detection of neoplasia at colonoscopy: a meta-analysis of data from individual patients in randomized controlled trials. Gastroenterology 2019;157:462–71.

82. Hassan C, Senore C, Radaelli F, et al. Full-spectrum (FUSE) versus standard forward-viewing colonoscopy in an organised colorectal cancer screening programme. Gut 2017;66:1949–55.

83. Ngu WS, Bevan R, Tsiamoulos ZP, et al. Improved adenoma detection with endocuff vision: the ADENOMA randomised controlled trial. Gut 2019;68:280–8.

84. Subramanian V, Mannath J, Hawkey CJ, et al. High definition colonoscopy vs. standard video endoscopy for the detection of colonic polyps: a meta-analysis. Endoscopy 2011;43:499–505.

85. van Doorn SC, van der Vlugt M, Depla A, et al. Adenoma detection with Endocuff colonoscopy versus conventional colonoscopy: a multicentre randomised controlled trial. Gut 2017;66:438–45.

86. Rex DK, Kessler WR, Sagi SV, et al. Impact of a ring-fitted cap on insertion time and adenoma detection: a randomized controlled trial. Gastrointest Endosc 2020;91(1):115–20.

87. Aziz M, Desai M, Hassan S, et al. Improving serrated adenoma detection rate in the colon by electronic chromoendoscopy and distal attachment: systematic review and meta-analysis. Gastrointest Endosc 2019;90:721–31.e1.

88. Rex DK, Repici A, Gross SA, et al. High-definition colonoscopy versus Endocuff versus EndoRings versus full-spectrum endoscopy for adenoma detection at colonoscopy: a multicenter randomized trial. Gastrointest Endosc 2018;88: 335–44.e2.

89. JE IJ, Tutein Nolthenius CJ, Kuipers EJ, et al. CT-colonography vs. colonoscopy for detection of high-risk sessile serrated polyps. Am J Gastroenterol 2016;111: 516–22.

90. Chang LC, Shun CT, Hsu WF, et al. Fecal immunochemical test detects sessile serrated adenomas and polyps with a low level of sensitivity. Clin Gastroenterol Hepatol 2017;15(6):872–9.e1.

91. Zorzi M, Senore C, Da Re F, et al. Detection rate and predictive factors of sessile serrated polyps in an organised colorectal cancer screening programme with immunochemical faecal occult blood test: the EQuIPE study (Evaluating Quality Indicators of the Performance of Endoscopy). Gut 2017;66(7):1233–40.

92. Anderson JC, Robertson DJ. Serrated polyp detection by the fecal immuno-chemical test: an imperfect FIT. Clin Gastroenterol Hepatol 2017;15:880–2.

93. Digby J, Fraser CG, Carey FA, et al. Faecal haemoglobin concentration is related to severity of colorectal neoplasia. J Clin Pathol 2013;66:415–9.

94. van Doorn SC, Stegeman I, Stroobants AK, et al. Fecal immunochemical testing results and characteristics of colonic lesions. Endoscopy 2015;47:1011–7.

95. Imperiale TF, Ransohoff DF, Itzkowitz SH, et al. Multitarget stool DNA testing for colorectal-cancer screening. N Engl J Med 2014;370:1287–97.

96. Pohl H, Srivastava A, Bensen SP, et al. Incomplete polyp resection during colonoscopy-results of the complete adenoma resection (CARE) study. Gastro-enterology 2013;144:74–80.e1.

97. Gupta V, East JE. Optimal endoscopic treatment and surveillance of serrated polyps. Gut Liver 2019. https://doi.org/10.5009/gnl19202.

98. Rao AK, Soetikno R, Raju GS, et al. Large sessile serrated polyps can be safely and effectively removed by endoscopic mucosal resection. Clin Gastroenterol Hepatol 2016;14:568–74.

99. Pellise M, Burgess NG, Tutticci N, et al. Endoscopic mucosal resection for large serrated lesions in comparison with adenomas: a prospective multicentre study of 2000 lesions. Gut 2017;66:644–53.

100. Rex KD, Vemulapalli KC, Rex DK. Recurrence rates after EMR of large sessile serrated polyps. Gastrointest Endosc 2015;82:538–41.

101. Boparai KS, Mathus-Vliegen EM, Koornstra JJ, et al. Increased colorectal can-cer risk during follow-up in patients with hyperplastic polyposis syndrome: a multicentre cohort study. Gut 2010;59:1094–100.

102. Boparai KS, Reitsma JB, Lemmens V, et al. Increased colorectal cancer risk in first-degree relatives of patients with hyperplastic polyposis syndrome. Gut 2010;59:1222–5.

103. Edelstein DL, Axilbund JE, Hylind LM, et al. Serrated polyposis: rapid and relentless development of colorectal neoplasia. Gut 2013;62:404–8.

104. Snover DC, Ahnen DJ, Burt RW, et al. Serrated polyps of the colon and rectum and serrated polyposis. In: Bosman FT, Carneiro F, Hruban RH, et al, editors. WHO classification of tumors of the digestive system. 4th edition. Lyon (France): International Agency for Research on Cancer; 2010. p. 160–5.

105. Rosty C, Brosens LA, Dekker E, et al. Serrated polyposis. In: WHO classification of tumours of the digestive system, 5th edition, p. 163–9. Lyon (France): Interna-tional Agency for Research on Cancer.

106. Vemulapalli KC, Rex DK. Failure to recognize serrated polyposis syndrome in a cohort with large sessile colorectal polyps. Gastrointest Endosc 2012;75: 1206–10.

107. Lieberman DA, Rex DK, Winawer SJ, et al. Guidelines for colonoscopy surveillance after screening and polypectomy: a consensus update by the US Multi-Society Task Force on Colorectal Cancer. Gastroenterology 2012;143:844–57.

108. Bleijenberg AG, JE IJ, van Herwaarden YJ, et al. Personalised surveillance for serrated polyposis syndrome: results from a prospective 5-year international cohort study. Gut 2020;69:112–21.

109. MacPhail ME, Thygesen SB, Patel N, et al. Endoscopic control of polyp burden and expansion of surveillance intervals in serrated polyposis syndrome. Gastrointest Endosc 2019;90:96–100.

110. Melson J, Ma K, Arshad S, et al. Presence of small sessile serrated polyps increases rate of advanced neoplasia upon surveillance compared with isolated low-risk tubular adenomas. Gastrointest Endosc 2016;84:307–14.

111. Macaron C, Vu HT, Lopez R, et al. Risk of metachronous polyps in individuals with serrated polyps. Dis Colon Rectum 2015;58:762–8.

112. Pereyra L, Zamora R, Gomez EJ, et al. Risk of metachronous advanced neoplastic lesions in patients with sporadic sessile serrated adenomas undergoing colonoscopic surveillance. Am J Gastroenterol 2016;111:871–8.

113. Burnett-Hartman AN, Chubak J, Hua X, et al. The association between colorectal sessile serrated adenomas/polyps and subsequent advanced colorectal neoplasia. Cancer Causes Control 2019;30:979–87.

114. Bensen SP, Cole BF, Mott LA, et al. Colorectal hyperplastic polyps and risk of recurrence of adenomas and hyperplastic polyps. Polyps Prevention Study. Lancet 1999;354:1873–4.

115. Laiyemo AO, Murphy G, Sansbury LB, et al. Hyperplastic polyps and the risk of adenoma recurrence in the polyp prevention trial. Clin Gastroenterol Hepatol 2009;7:192–7.

116. Symonds E, Anwar S, Young G, et al. Sessile serrated polyps with synchronous conventional adenomas increase risk of future advanced neoplasia. Dig Dis Sci 2019;64:1680–5.

117. Schramm C, Kaiser M, Drebber U, et al. Factors associated with reclassification of hyperplastic polyps after pathological reassessment from screening and surveillance colonoscopies. Int J Colorectal Dis 2016;31(2):319–25.

118. Hassan C, Quintero E, Dumonceau JM, et al. Post-polypectomy colonoscopy surveillance: European Society of Gastrointestinal Endoscopy (ESGE) guideline. Endoscopy 2013;45:842–51.

119. East JE, Atkin WS, Bateman AC, et al. British Society of Gastroenterology position statement on serrated polyps in the colon and rectum. Gut 2017;66:1181–96.

120. Rutter MD, East J, Rees CJ, et al. British Society of Gastroenterology/Association of Coloproctology of Great Britain and Ireland/Public Health England post-polypectomy and post-colorectal cancer resection surveillance guidelines. Gut 2020;69(2):201–23.

121. Gupta S, Lieberman D, Anderson JC, et al. Recommendations for follow-up after colonoscopy and polypectomy: a consensus update by the US Multisociety Task Force on Colorectal Cancer. Gastroenterology 2020;91(3):463–85.e5.

Cost-Effectiveness of Current Colorectal Cancer Screening Tests

Uri Ladabaum, MD, MS

KEYWORDS

- Colorectal cancer • Screening • Cost-effectiveness • Cost-utility
- Health economics • Quality-adjusted life-year • Colonoscopy
- Fecal immunochemical test

KEY POINTS

- Cost-effectiveness analysis is used to compare strategies based on the cost per quality-adjusted life-year (QALY) gained.
- Thresholds of one to three times a country's gross domestic product per capita are often accepted as cost-effective, and in the United States, $100,000–$150,000/QALY gained is generally considered acceptable.
- Multiple cost-effectiveness analyses of colorectal cancer (CRC) screening performed around the world under a wide range of assumptions suggest that all CRC screening modalities are highly cost-effective (eg, cost/QALY gained well lower than $100,000 in the United States).
- At present, the established strategies of fecal immunochemical testing and colonoscopy are generally considered more cost-effective than the emerging strategies of computed tomography colonography, multitarget stool DNA, and methylated Septin9 based on current costs and performance characteristics, and assuming comparable participation rates.
- Cost-effectiveness analysis can inform decisions in ongoing debates, including the preferred age to begin average-risk CRC screening, and the implementation of CRC screening tailored to predicted CRC risk.

CONCEPTUAL FRAMEWORK

To appreciate what it means to say that colorectal cancer (CRC) screening is cost-effective, or that a given CRC screening strategy is more cost-effective than another one, it is valuable to understand how cost-effectiveness estimates are derived, and how cost-effectiveness or willingness-to-pay thresholds are determined. This includes

Division of Gastroenterology and Hepatology, Department of Medicine, Stanford University School of Medicine, 430 Broadway Street, Pavilion C, 3rd Floor C-326, Redwood City, CA 94063-6341, USA
E-mail address: uri.ladabaum@stanford.edu

Gastrointest Endoscopy Clin N Am 30 (2020) 479–497
https://doi.org/10.1016/j.giec.2020.02.005
1052-5157/20/© 2020 Elsevier Inc. All rights reserved.

being familiar with the overarching conceptual framework of cost-effectiveness analysis, and key methodological details (**Box 1**).

The purpose of cost-effectiveness analysis is to compare the relative value of different interventions, taking into account their effectiveness and cost.[1] President Obama once famously said when discussing health care reform: "If there's a blue pill and a red pill, and the blue pill is half the price of the red pill and works just as well, why not pay half price for the thing that's going to make you well?"[2] One does not need a complex analysis to conclude that the blue pill is the preferred choice in this scenario. But what if the blue pill is half the price of the red pill, but the red pill extends life by 9 more months than the blue pill? Or what if both the blue and red pills are costly, and their benefits are modest? As the Second Panel on Cost-Effectiveness in Health and Medicine wrote in its recommendation statement: "Cost-effectiveness analysis provides a framework for comparing the relative value of different interventions, along with information that can help decision makers sort through alternatives and decide which ones best serve their programmatic and financial needs."[1] This framing includes the important point that cost-effectiveness analysis cannot provide absolute answers; decisions depend on values, and on a society's willingness to pay for specific outcomes.

In general, it is preferable to measure something directly than to estimate it. But to arrive at cost-effectiveness estimates that account for a long time horizon, including a lifetime, estimation is required. It is not practical to design a clinical trial comparing several programs of CRC screening that are implemented from ages 50 to 80 years, with full ascertainment of all relevant clinical outcomes and all costs, including costs of screening, complications, and CRC care, with follow-up of all participants until death. It is possible, however, to construct a decision analytical model that uses the best available inputs to simulate such a trial. Over the last several decades, a rich

---

Box 1
Conceptual framework for cost-effectiveness analysis

A tool to examine benefit and cost trade-offs between alternative interventions or no intervention

Often uses model-based extrapolation to long time horizons, including a lifetime

May take the perspective of a specific payer, the health sector, or society (considering all indirect costs)

Outcome can be narrow and disease-specific (eg, cost per advanced adenoma detected), but this is difficult to interpret, and cannot be easily compared with other outcomes

Ideally, an incremental cost-effectiveness ratio reflecting cost per quality-adjusted life-year (QALY) gained is calculated, allowing for comparisons across disease states

Cannot determine what decision should be taken; it can only help inform decision makers

The cost-effectiveness threshold, or willingness to pay, varies depending on the population, but its determination is less rigorous than one might imagine

A commonly quoted cost-effectiveness threshold of 1 to 3 times gross domestic product per capita is attributed to the World Health Organization

In the United States, it is common to use a cost-effectiveness threshold of $100,000–$150,000/QALY gained

Cost-effectiveness thresholds <$1000/QALY gained have been estimated for resource-poor countries

iterature has evolved using such modeling methods to tackle a broad range of questions related to the cost-effectiveness of CRC screening, and it has been suggested that screening programs consider modeling as an important component of evaluation.[3]

Some studies do directly measure outcomes and costs related to CRC screening, but it is challenging to interpret the results when there is no established benchmark regarding the incremental cost required to achieve a change in the specific outcome under study. For instance, in a study of the yield of colonoscopy in 80-year-old persons with prior colorectal adenomas, how would one interpret the "cost per advanced adenoma detected"? Or in a study of mailed outreach to improve participation with screening, how would one interpret the "cost per additional patient participating in one round of fecal-based screening"? One is left wanting to know the long-term consequences: the cost per CRC death averted, and ultimately the cost per life-year gained. Many interventions do not prolong life expectancy but can improve the quality of life. In those cases, and in cases that do prolong life and improve its quality, it is desirable to estimate the cost per quality-adjusted life-year (QALY) gained.

When comparing strategy 1 with strategy 2, this incremental cost-effectiveness ratio (ICER) is defined as:

$$\frac{Cost_1 - Cost_2}{Effectiveness_1 - Effectiveness_2}$$

To achieve the incremental effectiveness that strategy 1 delivers versus strategy 2 (Effectiveness$_1$ – Effectiveness$_2$), one needs to spend the incremental difference between the costs of strategy 1 and strategy 2 (Cost$_1$ – Cost$_2$). This yields a cost/life-year gained or a cost/QALY gained. The advantage of using cost/life-year gained or cost/QALY gained as the measure of cost-effectiveness is that there is some degree of consensus on what a given society is willing to pay to gain a life-year or a QALY. This allows for comparisons across a broad range of interventions and diseases. In theory, in the context of an explicit process to allocate a fixed budget, it could help decide among funding cancer screening, addiction treatment, or prenatal care programs.

It is standard methodology to discount future costs and future clinical measures, such as life-years or QALYs, commonly by 3% annually. Therefore, the estimates for discounted life-years gained or discounted QALYs gained must be interpreted with caution. Over a long time horizon, these are substantially lower than the estimated gains in undiscounted life-years or QALYs.

WHAT IS A "COST-EFFECTIVE" INTERVENTION?

Although subject to judgment, the traditional threshold in the United States of $50,000/QALY gained has increased over time to $100,000 to $150,000/QALY gained.[4,5] This is consistent with the threshold attributed to the World Health Organization that defined as cost-effective those interventions that have a cost-effectiveness ratio of one to three times a country's gross domestic product (GDP) per capita.[4–6]

It should be recognized that although there may be some degree of consensus on what cost-effectiveness thresholds should be used in decision analyses in a given country, these thresholds have traditionally not been rigorously derived.[7] This is remarkable when one considers that much care and effort can go into estimating the cost/QALY gained of a certain intervention, only to then be compared with a threshold that stands on less firm ground than what is desirable, and that has less rigorous underpinnings than what is commonly believed.

The frequently used thresholds attributed to the World Health Organization stem from the work of its' Commission on Macroeconomics and Health, which cites research on the value per statistical life, and relies on the underlying concept that it is reasonable for the willingness to pay for a life-year to exceed the GDP per capita because the value of living includes more than the effects on earnings or economic productivity.[7] Cost-effectiveness thresholds are "demand-side," reflecting a population's willingness to pay for a given outcome, or "supply-side," reflecting the opportunity cost of an intervention, that is, what could have been funded instead.[7] The Commission on Macroeconomics and Health considered demand-based values in developing its thresholds.[7]

The exact threshold may vary depending on the setting and the available resources. Thresholds that are tied to the GDP per capita recognize that societies differ in their ability to pay for a given health outcome, although from a humanistic viewpoint, the value of a life is the same regardless of where a person lives. A recent article on the growing use of an ICER threshold to guide drug pricing in the United States referenced work by the economics consulting firm Bernstein Research that reported cost/QALY gained thresholds of $150,000 to $200,000 for Belgium and Norway; $75,000 to $100,000 for Canada, the Netherlands, and Japan; $50,000 to $75,000 for Australia, Ireland, and Sweden; $25,000 to $50,000 for the United Kingdom, Portugal, the Czech Republic, Brazil, Hungary, and South Korea; and less than $25,000 for Poland and Thailand.[8] The lack of universal agreement on an acceptable threshold, however, is illustrated by a recent analysis from the Netherlands that used the Dutch GDP per capita (€36,602) as the threshold for an acceptable ICER in terms of life-years gained, as opposed to two to three times this value.[9]

Furthermore, cost-effectiveness thresholds based on opportunity costs, as opposed to a one to three ratio versus the GDP per capita, were recently estimated as $3 to $166 for Malawi, $44 to $518 for Cambodia, $422 to $1967 for El Salvador, $4485 to $8018 for Kazakhstan, $25,292 to $31,915 for Canada, and $24,283 to $40,112 (46%–75% of GDP) for the United States.[10] A systematic review of studies eliciting willingness-to-pay per QALY identified only 14 studies for inclusion, which covered a broad range of conditions, such as viral infection, knee osteoarthritis, paralysis, blindness, allergy, prostatitis, serious illness, or a chronic health state.[11] In these studies, which were performed in Asia, America, or Europe, the ratio between willingness to pay and GDP per capita varied widely from 0.05 to 5.40, and the mean ratio was higher for interventions that extend life (2.03) compared with those that improve quality of life (0.59).[11]

It is useful to keep all of these considerations in mind when evaluating estimates of the cost-effectiveness of CRC screening from around the world, and when placing results for the United States in a global context.

EFFECTIVENESS FIRST, COST-EFFECTIVENESS SECOND

Before one can discuss the cost-effectiveness of an intervention, one has to consider its effectiveness. The potential effectiveness of an intervention is estimated with decision analytical models when there are no empirical data supporting a clinical benefit. But the argument is much more powerful if effectiveness has been demonstrated in clinical studies, and modeling is then used to extrapolate to a longer time horizon and to generalize beyond what is achieved in a typical clinical study.

In CRC screening, robust evidence has accumulated that screening decreases CRC incidence and CRC-related mortality. In randomized controlled trials, guaiac-based fecal occult blood testing (gFOBT) decreased CRC incidence and mortality,[12–15] as did one-time flexible sigmoidoscopy.[16–19] The evidence supporting the effectiveness of fecal immunochemical testing (FIT) and colonoscopy in CRC screening is observational up to now, and by extension from the trials of gFOBT and sigmoidoscopy. Prospective trials of FIT and colonoscopy are ongoing.

Given the required large study sample sizes and long periods of follow-up, it is challenging to prove that a given screening test decreases CRC incidence and mortality. The number of patients enrolled ranged from 46,551 to 150,251 in the gFOBT trials and from 34,292 to 170,432 in the sigmoidoscopy trials, with follow-up for the initial reports of approximately 8 to 13 years and 11 to 12 years, respectively. The reduction in CRC incidence with gFOBT was only detected after longer follow-up to 18 years.[13] This challenge highlights the attractiveness of using a decision analytical model that reproduces the natural history of colorectal neoplasia, from precancerous polyp through invasive CRC through all its stages, to generate estimates of effectiveness for novel tests, and of comparative effectiveness for established and emerging tests, based on their sensitivities and specificities for precancerous colorectal lesions and CRC, and their risks.

Is it reasonable to measure the effectiveness of CRC screening in terms of life-years gained or QALYs gained? That is, is there evidence that CRC screening reduces overall mortality? Or is that a potentially tenuous assumption built into decision analytical models? Although no CRC screening trial has demonstrated a statistically significant reduction in overall mortality, the UK Flexible Sigmoidoscopy Trial, which has been the largest trial to date, reported a hazards ratio for overall mortality in the intervention versus control arm of 0.97 (95% confidence interval, 0.94–1.00; $P = .0519$). The screening trials have not been powered to detect differences in overall mortality, which is considered the ultimate "hard outcome," but one that is difficult to prove in screening studies given the sample size and length of follow-up requirements. Nonetheless, an insightful meta-analysis of the four large randomized trials of screening sigmoidoscopy that appropriately stratified the results of the Norwegian Colorectal Cancer Prevention (NORCCAP) study has reported a relative risk of all-cause mortality of 0.975 (0.959–0.992) for screening versus control.[20] Based on this, and on the clinical experience that some CRCs are prevented with screening, and that some screen-detected CRCs are treated successfully, in people who then go on to live for many years as opposed to dying in the short term from competing causes, such as cardiovascular disease, it is reasonable to accept that modeling studies project reductions in overall mortality attributable to CRC screening, even if individual screening trials are not powered to detect this.

LONG-TERM COMPARATIVE EFFECTIVENESS: MODELING

At present, there are no published intermediate-term or longer-term randomized, controlled comparisons between screening tests regarding their impact on CRC incidence or mortality. Available comparative data are derived from the first rounds of testing in randomized trials, with lesion detection as a surrogate marker, such as the results of the first round of screening of the COLONPREV study, which is comparing screening with biennial FIT versus one-time colonoscopy.[21]

Computerized decision analytical models of CRC screening have been developed to address questions that are unlikely to be answered directly by clinical trials, including long-term estimates of CRC cases and deaths prevented with screening, and life-years or QALYs gained. The best established models construct a natural history module that reflects the evolution through premalignant polyps to CRC, calibrated to epidemiologic data, and then superimpose screening tests with various test performance characteristics and testing intervals on this natural history module, accounting for potential complications. Costs are also considered when performing a cost-effectiveness analysis. Because it is impossible to directly validate some of the deep assumptions in models, including the natural history of adenomas, validation of a model's predictions against the results of observational studies, and the intermediate-term results of randomized controlled trials, increases the level of confidence in a model.

In the United States, three models that are part of the National Cancer Institute's Cancer Intervention and Surveillance Modeling Network consortium have informed the screening guidelines of the US Preventive Services Taskforce[22,23] and the American Cancer Society (ACS).[24–26] These three models are the Simulation Model of Colorectal Cancer, the Microsimulation Screening Analysis for Colorectal Cancer, and the Colorectal Cancer Simulated Population Model for Incidence and Natural History. **Table 1** shows the long-term effectiveness of screening, in terms of reductions in CRC incidence and mortality, that is projected for five current screening modalities by the three Cancer Intervention and Surveillance Modeling Network models[23,27] and a fourth model that has been validated against prospective trials of gFOBT and sigmoidoscopy,[28,29] as recently summarized.[30] Assuming optimal participation with screening over time, the estimated CRC incidence reductions with annual FIT and colonoscopy, the two most common CRC screening tests in the United States, range from 47% to 72% and from 62% to 88%, respectively. Furthermore, the estimated CRC mortality reductions with annual FIT and colonoscopy range from 72% to 81% and from 77% to 90%, respectively.

These estimates of effectiveness come first in any cost-effectiveness analysis. The ICERs that reflect relative cost-effectiveness are built on the differences in effectiveness that are predicted between strategies (the denominator in the ICER formula presented previously). In general, CRC screening models tend to predict that, among those participating consistently in screening, colonoscopy every 10 years yields the most profound reductions in CRC incidence and mortality, but that the programmatic impact of FIT-based screening with consistent participation is similar to that of colonoscopy (see **Table 1**).

Deep assumptions within the models probably account in large part for the key differences in results between models, including assumptions that determine adenoma dwell time either directly or indirectly,[31] and assumptions about the fraction of CRCs that arise from potentially identifiable, and removable, precursors. Assumptions about the potential impact of sigmoidoscopy on proximal CRC incidence or the behavior of distal versus proximal adenomas may account for differences in the models' predictions for sigmoidoscopy (see **Table 1**).

Estimates reflecting optimal participation are useful to benchmark the potential maximum effectiveness of a given strategy. As is expected and desired, the models' predictions of comparative effectiveness are affected profoundly if differential participation patterns are assumed between strategies. Such differential participation patterns can have a powerful impact on a modeling study's conclusions.

COST-EFFECTIVENESS OF ESTABLISHED COLORECTAL CANCER SCREENING TESTS

CRC screening emerges as highly cost-effective in multiple models across a wide range of assumptions. Many model-based cost-effectiveness analyses of CRC screening have been performed around the world, reflecting the regional epidemiology of CRC, the applicable medical costs in local currencies based on the details of the regional health system, and the relevant strategies in various countries and regions.

Table 1
Projected long-term comparative effectiveness of CRC screening strategies with optimal participation

	Colorectal Cancer Incidence, % Reduction Versus No Screening					Colorectal Cancer Mortality, % Reduction Versus No Screening				
	SimCRC[23,27]	MISCAN[23,27]	CRC-SPIN[23,27]	Ladabaum and Mannalithara,[28] 2016, Ladabaum et al,[29] 2019		SimCRC[23,27]	MISCAN[23,27]	CRC-SPIN[23,27]	Ladabaum and Mannalithara,[28] 2016, Ladabaum et al,[29] 2019	
Colonoscopy every 10 y, ages 50–75 y	81	62	88	70		87	79	90	77	
FIT yearly, ages 50–75 y	67	47	72	57		81	72	81	72	
MT-sDNA every 3 y, ages 50–75 y	63	43	68	52		78	68	76	67	
CT colonography every 5 y, ages 50–75 y	77	51	78	67		85	72	82	77	
Sigmoidoscopy every 5 y, ages 50–75 y	68	56	59	44		74	72	62	49	

SimCRC, MISCAN, and CRC-SPIN are part of the National Cancer Institute's Cancer Intervention and Surveillance Modeling Network consortium.
Abbreviations: CRC-SPIN, colorectal cancer simulated population model for incidence and natural history; CT, computed tomography; MISCAN, Microsimulation screening analysis for colorectal cancer; MT-sDNA, multitarget stool DNA; SimCRC, simulation model of colorectal cancer.

Because the epidemiology of CRC differs regionally, and the costs of medical interventions depend on the regional health systems, the results and conclusions of these analyses are, to some extent, setting-dependent. Some conclusions may be broadly generalizable, and others not. Here, a global perspective is provided when possible, and focused attention is devoted to studies relevant to the US setting.

It is challenging to synthesize all pertinent CRC screening studies given the multiple models, modeling approaches, and region-specific inputs. Three systematic reviews published in 2000, 2010, and 2016, together covering 1993 to 2016, provide useful summaries, and a sense of how the field has changed over time.[32–34] Not all potentially relevant studies were included in these reviews, but a tabulation of key findings in these three reviews is nonetheless highly informative (**Table 2**), as recently summarized.[30]

When first encountering the apparently small average gains in discounted life-years per person attributed to CRC screening by the models (see **Table 2**), readers used to scrutinizing data from clinical trials may wonder whether these differences are meaningful at all. The predicted gains with screening translate into several undiscounted life-weeks gained per person on average, over a lifetime. Is this clinically significant? It is important to appreciate that the average gains are not evenly distributed throughout the population. Most screening participants at average risk of CRC do not benefit from screening. How could they if lifetime risk of CRC without screening is only 5% to 6%, or slightly higher now as epidemiologic trends might suggest?[35] The gains in life expectancy with screening are actually concentrated in the small percentage of people who benefit from averted CRC death, and for these persons, the gains are actually several undiscounted life-years.[36] It is only when the population total of these gains is divided out by the entire screened population, as is standard methodology for calculating mean gains in effectiveness, that the gains might seem small on a per-person basis.

The comparison between a given strategy and no screening only tells a part of the story. All strategies may seem cost-effective versus no screening in nearly all models, but this does not mean that they are all preferred equally. The incremental comparisons between strategies may be much more informative. However, at this level, more substantial differences in results and conclusions can emerge between models. This may be caused by differences in deep model assumptions regarding natural history and specific model inputs. Small differences in assumptions can potentially change the ranking of strategies and the conclusions about which strategies emerge as cost-effective compared with each other. The uncertainty surrounding these and other conclusions is explored with probabilistic sensitivity analyses. Readers are referred to individual studies for such analyses. Although the differences in average QALYs per person between different strategies can be several digits to the right of the decimal point, these are still informative, particularly if they remain robust in sensitivity analyses.

Despite the subtleties, when the predicted gains in life-expectancy are considered in the context of the predicted incremental costs accrued to achieve these gains, several overarching points emerge regarding the cost-effectiveness of CRC screening (see **Table 2**), as recently summarized:[30]

1. Compared with no screening, all screening modalities are generally predicted to be cost-effective at the willingness-to-pay levels of the relevant country or region.[32–34]
2. As the costs of treatments for advanced CRC have increased, with proportionately modest gains in survival, the cost-effectiveness of CRC screening has improved, with some strategies becoming cost-saving in the United States.[32–34,37,38]

Table 2
Cost-effectiveness of CRC screening strategies versus no screening

	Annual gFOBT	Biennial gFOBT	Annual FIT	Biennial FIT	FS Every 5 y	Colonoscopy Every 10 y	CT Colonography Every 5 y	MT-sDNA Test Every 3 y
Systematic Review 2010–2017, 33 studies (17 Europe, 11 North America, 4 Asia, 1 Australia), 2016 $[28,34]								
LY gained	0.01–0.12	0.01–0.05	0.01–0.15	0.01–0.10	0.02–0.14	0.02–0.18	—	—
QALY gained	0.07–0.49	0.01–0.32	0.01–0.80	0.01–0.70	0.01–0.07	0.02–0.22	—	—
Cost/LY gained	CS - $4000; [$50,000]	CS - $3000; [$45,000]	CS - $9000; [$24,000]	CS - $4000; [$24,000]	CS - $7000; [$67,000]	CS - $27,000; [$52,000]	CS - $16,000	$9000– $11,000
Cost/QALY gained	CS - $15,000	CS - $6000	CS - $5000; [$33,000]	CS - $7000	CS - $8000; [$45,000]	CS - $15,000; [$40,000]	$3000–$11,000; [$59,000]	$15,000– $30,000
Review 1993–2009, 32 unique models (10 Europe, 14 North America, 5 Asia, 3 Australia), 2010 $[33]								
LY or QALY gained	0.01–0.16	0.01–0.03	—		0.01–0.11	0.02–0.18	—	—
Cost/LY or Cost/QALY gained	CS - $26,000; [$53,000]	$3000– $16,000	CS - $26,000		CS - $30,000; [$57,000]	CS - $32,000	CS - $36,000	$600– $32,000
Systematic Review for USPSTF 1993–2001, 7 studies (7 United States), 2000 $[32]								
Cost/LY gained	$6000–$18,000	—	—		$12,000–$39,000	$9000–$22,000	—	—

Notes: Ranges reported in published studies are shown; single values judged to be outliers at the high end of the range are shown separately in brackets. Costs are rounded to nearest $1000, and LYs and QALYs are rounded to nearest 0.01, and all reflect annual discounting, usually at rates 3%–5%.
Not all potentially relevant published studies were included in the systematic reviews. Some studies reported LYs, and some QALYs, so both outcomes are shown.
All currencies were converted to US dollars and updated to a given year, which differed in each review.
Columns are not directly comparable with each other because not all studies in a review contributed to every cell or explicitly compared all strategies with each other.

Abbreviations: CS, cost saving; CT, computed tomography; FS, flexible sigmoidoscopy; LY, life-year; MT-sDNA, multitarget stool DNA; USPSTF, US preventive services task force.

3. There seems to be no uniformly favored strategy when participation levels are the same across strategies, but the established strategies are generally favored over the emerging strategies of computed tomography colonography, multitarget stool DNA (MT-sDNA), and plasma methylated Septin9 (mSeptin9).[32–34]

Another review has reached similar conclusions,[39] and a systematic review that examined model structure and parameterization reported that the ICERs compared with no screening were higher in models that did not make deep assumptions about the polyp to carcinoma sequence compared with more complex models that did simulate this (eg, annual FIT $28,867 vs $5185, and colonoscopy every 10 years $17,890 vs $4299).[40]

A set of recent analyses that have used the same underlying model, with updates over time, illustrate the cost-effectiveness of current CRC screening tests compared with no screening, and compared with each other, in the United States.[28,29,41,42] The range of estimates points to the influence of underlying assumptions, such as the change in payments for screening tests and CRC care over time, screening participation, patient support costs for organized programs, and changes in the age-specific risk of CRC in the United States over time:

1. Compared with no screening, yearly FIT starting at age 50 is estimated to gain QALYs and also to be cost-saving (ie, dominant) when only the cost of the FIT test itself is considered, but to cost $14,300/QALY gained when imperfect participation over time and programmatic costs including outreach and patient support are considered.[28,29,42]
2. Compared with no screening, colonoscopy every 10 years starting at age 50 is estimated to cost $3400–$15,000/QALY gained, depending on the year of the analysis and whether Medicare payment rates are assumed for all ages or commercial payment rates are used in those younger than age 65 years.[28,42] However, when considering the birth cohort effect of CRC risk increasing over time in the United States, colonoscopy every 10 years starting at age 50 is most recently estimated to gain QALYs and also to be cost-saving (ie, dominant), compared with no screening.[29]
3. Compared with no screening, flexible sigmoidoscopy every 5 years starting at age 50 is estimated to cost $350–$13,100/QALY gained, depending on whether Medicare payment rates are assumed for all ages or commercial payments rates are used in those younger than age 65.[42]
4. Compared with no screening, MT-sDNA every 3 years starting at age 50 is estimated to cost $27,500–$29,500/QALY gained, accounting for commercial insurance and Medicare payment rates, and depending on participation levels.[28]
5. Compared with no screening, the first version of the mSeptin9 test every 2 years starting at age 50, with test performance characteristics based on the largest available prospective trial of that marker,[43] was estimated to cost $8400–$11,500/QALY gained.[41]
6. When these strategies are compared with each other assuming optimal adherence with all screening strategies, colonoscopy every 10 years is estimated to prevent more CRCs than yearly FIT, but FIT is estimated to gain slightly more QALYs when CRC stages are considered, and FIT is less costly (dominant) compared with colonoscopy[28,29,42]; FIT yearly and colonoscopy every 10 years are more effective and less costly (dominant) compared with either MT-sDNA every 3 years or mSeptin9 every 2 years[28,41]; FIT yearly is more effective and less costly (dominant) compared with sigmoidoscopy every 5 years[42]; and colonoscopy every 10 years is more effective and less costly (dominant), or cost $18,800/QALY gained compared with sigmoidoscopy every 5 years, depending on whether Medicare or commercial insurance payment rates are used for those younger than age 65.[42]

. All comparisons are affected dramatically if there are substantial differences in sustained screening participation rates over time between strategies.

CRC screening is most established in high-income countries, reflecting the availability of resources and the relative burden of disease and public health priorities, because CRC incidence is closely related to the level of development.[44] Recent analyses suggest that stool-based CRC screening may be attractive in some middle- and low-income countries, provided that abnormal tests are followed up appropriately and CRC is treated.[44,45]

The perspective of an analysis and the range of costs that are considered can affect cost-effectiveness estimates. Considering the nonmedical and indirect costs of screening, including patient and driver time costs, makes screening seem less cost-effective. However, considering the averted productivity losses associated with CRC prevention would make screening seem more cost-effective.

PAYER PERSPECTIVE: COMMERCIAL INSURANCE VERSUS MEDICARE IN THE UNITED STATES

Most US-based CRC screening cost-effectiveness analyses have used Medicare payment rates, but many Americans younger than age 65 have commercial insurance. A recent analysis accounted for commercial insurance payment rates younger than age 65,[46] and contrasted the cost-effectiveness of CRC screening from the perspectives and time-horizons of commercial insurers versus Medicare.

When commercial payment rates were considered, the lifetime costs of CRC screening were estimated to be 20% to 44% higher than when Medicare rates were assumed, but CRC screening still emerged as highly cost-effective.[42] For commercial payers with a time horizon of ages 50 to 64, FIT yearly was estimated to be cost-effective ($60,700/QALY gained), but colonoscopy every 10 years was estimated to be costly ($189,000/QALY gained). However, Medicare was projected to reap substantial clinical benefits and cost-savings from screening done at ages less than 65, even if screening was not continued. Among those previously screened, continuing FIT under Medicare was estimated to be cost-saving and continuing colonoscopy was highly cost-effective (<$30,000/QALY gained), and initiating any screening in those previously unscreened was highly effective and cost-saving. In sum, recent modeling suggests that screening at ages 50 to 64 under commercial insurance in the United States yields substantial clinical and economic benefits that accrue primarily at ages greater than or equal to 65 under Medicare.[42] This delayed benefit was also observed in another modeling study.[47]

CRC screening is just one of many interventions that are likely to show primarily a delayed benefit, including, for instance, control of hypertension, diabetes, and hypercholesterolemia. Thus, it is argued that commercial insurers should use a lifetime perspective when assessing the cost-effectiveness of covered services, including CRC screening, and not a perspective focused on short-term cost-effectiveness, which would lead to the underuse of services whose benefit is derived primarily in the distant future.

PARTICIPATION RATES AND PROGRAMMATIC COSTS: THE COST OF UPTAKE AND ADHERENCE

Uptake of CRC screening and adherence to consistent participation over time are far from perfect in any population. This is particularly the case for opportunistic screening with tests that require annual or biennial participation to achieve good programmatic results, such as FIT or gFOBT. Organized programs with outreach designed to increase participation, and navigation designed to increase completion of colonoscopy, have demonstrated substantial improvements in patient participation.[48,49] These services accrue their own costs, and can vary substantially by program[50,51] and by country.[52] Recent cost-effectiveness analyses have begun to take account of these important factors.[53,54] Limitations persist regarding the availability of data on consistent screening participation over the long term with various tests, and the variability in estimates of outreach and navigation costs. But the inclusion of these variables, and thus the recognition that at a societal level it may cost an incremental amount beyond a screening test's cost to actually achieve screening participation with that test, has added a level of sophistication to cost-effectiveness estimates.

For example, the critical impact of participation, and the costs accrued by patient support programs to improve participation, are illustrated by a recent analysis comparing FIT yearly with MT-sDNA every 3 years and colonoscopy every 10 years.[28] With optimal adherence, yearly FIT and colonoscopy every 10 years were predicted to be more effective and less costly than MT-sDNA every 3 years. The most successful organized FIT programs have achieved approximately 50% consistent and 27% intermittent participation levels over several cycles.[28] In the Centers for Disease Control and Prevention CRC screening pilot programs, patient support costs averaged $153/cycle.[55,56] Extrapolating to a lifetime horizon based on these numbers, it was estimated that the patient support program that is included in the cost of the MT-sDNA test would need to yield 68% consistent and 32% intermittent participation levels for the MT-sDNA test to be preferred. In the opportunistic setting, compared with yearly FIT screening that achieved 15% consistent and 30% intermittent participation, it was estimated that a participation rate more than 1.7-fold that of FIT would be required for MT-sDNA to be cost-effective versus FIT. A study focusing on the Medicare population reached qualitatively similar conclusions.[57]

In a recent randomized controlled trial of mailed outreach for FIT in a safety net system, prospective cost accounting of the outreach intervention was embedded, and its long-term cost-effectiveness was projected.[58] FIT screening was higher in the outreach group than in the usual care control group (57.9% vs 37.4%; $P<.001$), and outreach cost approximately $23 per patient and $112 per additional patient screened. Projecting long-term outcomes, outreach was estimated to cost $9200/QALY gained versus usual care. Essentially, paying to boost participation rates was estimated to be highly cost-effective. The costs were $24 to $29 per additional patient screened by FIT in another study in federally qualified health centers.[59]

TOTAL BUDGE IMPACT

The total budge impact of CRC screening depends on the population size, the specific screening program costs balanced against CRC treatment costs averted, and any costs of an organized population management program, and the phase of implementation (initial launch vs steady state). Program management and patient support costs are not negligible.[55,56] For example, opportunistic FIT screening is estimated to be cost-saving in the United States; in contrast, an organized FIT program is estimated to be substantially more effective and highly cost-effective, but may not be cost-saving[28] Navigation for one-time screening colonoscopy may be cost-saving, and navigation for a program of repeated colonoscopic screening is estimated to be highly cost-effective.[49,53,54] It can take years for screening programs to realize savings in averted CRC care.

CURRENT DEBATE 1: AVERAGE-RISK SCREENING STARTING AT AGE 45 YEARS IN THE UNITED STATES

A recent analysis examined the 2018 ACS recommendation[24] to begin CRC screening at age 45 years in average-risk persons.[29] This analysis concluded that screening initiation at age 45 versus 50 years is likely to be cost-effective, with costs/QALY gained of $33,900 for colonoscopy and $7700 for FIT. Because greater benefit, at lower cost, could be achieved by deploying the same resources to increase participation rates for unscreened older and higher-risk persons or improving follow-up rates after abnormal FIT, the critical questions came into focus: can the new recommendation be instituted without displacing efforts to achieve high screening participation rates in older or higher-risk persons and higher FIT follow-up rates, and is society willing to bear the incremental costs?

The national impact on disease burden, resources demand, and total budget was estimated for various scenarios. If current age-specific screening participation patterns in the United States were shifted by 5 years to younger ages based on the ACS recommendation, it was estimated that 29,400 CRC cases and 11,100 CRC deaths could be averted over the next 5 years, at an incremental cost of $10.4 billion and requiring 10.7 million additional colonoscopies. By comparison, achieving the aspirational goal of 80% screening participation beginning at age 50 years, without screening initiation at age 45 years, was estimated to avert 2.6-fold more CRC cases and 2.9-fold more CRC deaths at approximately one-third the incremental cost and with the need for 13% more additional colonoscopies, compared with shifting current age-specific participation rates to 5 years earlier. A national health system might be able to act based on these types of estimates, but it is not clear how decision-makers in the US health system will use this information. An analysis of shifting the age of screening initiation in Australia reached similar conclusions regarding cost-effectiveness.[60]

CURRENT DEBATE 2: TAILORED SCREENING BASED ON PREDICTED COLORECTAL CANCER RISK

Uniform CRC screening recommendations currently apply to the average risk population, which represents most people. Higher intensity screening is recommended for persons identified as high risk based on family history, and high-intensity screening is recommended for persons with certain hereditary cancer predisposition syndromes.[61-64] Age is used to define a younger group in whom CRC risk is low enough that screening is not yet recommended.[22,24,61] The ACS's recent recommendation that average-risk CRC screening begin at age 45 instead of 50[24] has spurred debate about whether this age-based approach is reasonable, or whether the CRC screening field should be pushed now into a new era of risk-stratification and personalized screening. Tailoring screening to predicted CRC risk could maximize the effectiveness of CRC screening while minimizing complications, and optimizing resource use,[65] but it is not clear that current CRC risk prediction tools, which have modest discriminatory ability,[65-68] are ready for implementation.

Cost-effectiveness analyses can shed light on the potential consequences of CRC screening based on predicted CRC risk, including the performance and cost requisites for risk prediction tools. A recently published clinical practice guideline made the provocative recommendation that CRC screening not be offered to persons with an estimated risk of CRC of <3% over the next 15 years.[69] However, the risk prediction tool recommended by the guidelines panel, QCancer10, had area under the curve of 0.66 and 0.70 for 5-year predictions in women and men, respectively, in a UK validation study.[68] The authors of this risk prediction validation study point out that their findings do not allow for specific recommendations regarding risk-based screening versus the current age-based criteria, and they suggest that decision-analytic studies be performed, followed by implementation studies.

One recent cost-effectiveness analysis examined uniform versus screening tailored to low-, moderate-, and high-risk tiers that were identified as CRC risk after age 50 of less than or equal to 3%, greater than 3% to less than 12%, and greater than or equal to 12%, respectively, based on threshold analyses with willingness-to-pay less than $50,000/QALY gained.[70] Tailored colonoscopy (once at 60 for low risk, every 10 years for moderate risk, and every 5 years for high risk) was compared with colonoscopy every 10 years for all. Tailored FIT/colonoscopy (annual FIT for low and moderate risk, colonoscopy every 5 years for high risk) was compared with annual FIT for all, consistent with the recommendation of the US Multisociety Task Force on CRC to follow a risk-stratified approach regarding test choice.[61]

In this analysis, assuming no CRC risk misclassification or risk-prediction tool costs, tailored screening was preferred over uniform screening. Tailored colonoscopy was minimally less effective than uniform colonoscopy, but it saved $90,200 to $889,000/QALY depending on the assumed underlying CRC risk distribution in the population, making tailored colonoscopy the preferred option based on cost-effectiveness considerations. Tailored FIT/colonoscopy yielded more QALYs/person than annual FIT at $10,600 to $60,000/QALY gained, depending on the assumed underlying CRC risk distribution in the population, making tailored FIT/colonoscopy the preferred option based on effectiveness and cost-effectiveness considerations. However, modest CRC risk misclassification rates or risk-prediction tool costs resulted in uniform screening as the preferred approach, suggesting that current risk prediction tools are probably not accurate enough to warrant their application, particularly to select people into lower intensity screening.

Similarly, a second recent cost-effectiveness analysis concluded that CRC screening based on currently available polygenic risk scores is unlikely to be cost-effective compared with uniform screening.[71] However, in this model, this conclusion was expected to change with only modest improvements in risk-score performance or modest reductions in risk tool cost.

The reasons behind the apparently different conclusions of these two analyses remain to be fully clarified. It is possible that differences in assumptions about the underlying true CRC risk distribution in the average risk population, which is not known and cannot be observed directly, and different approaches to modeling misclassification of risk (ie, when the risk predicted by the risk tool does not match the actual underlying risk for an individual) may have contributed to differences in the conclusions regarding the discriminatory ability and cost of a risk prediction tool that are required to make tailored screening cost-effective.

SUMMARY

Cost-effectiveness analysis is a tool that integrates a broad range of data to make projections that can inform public policy. Building on the demonstrated clinical effectiveness of CRC screening, a rich body of literature supports the cost-effectiveness of multiple CRC screening strategies. Although specific cost-effectiveness estimates, comparisons between strategies, and willingness to pay to achieve a given health outcome vary depending on the specific population and health system considered, the current strategies, particularly FIT and colonoscopy, seem to be highly cost-effective in a broad range of settings. As debates arise regarding specific aspects of CRC screening, including whether screening initiation age should be lowered based on changing epidemiology or whether CRC screening based on predicted risk is ready for implementation, cost-effectiveness analysis can make a valuable contribution to clarify issues, prompt research, and inform policy.

DISCLOSURE

Advisory board (UniversalDx, Lean Medical), consultant (Covidien, Motus GI, Quorum, Clinical Genomics).

REFERENCES

1. Sanders GD, Neumann PJ, Basu A, et al. Recommendations for conduct, methodological practices, and reporting of cost-effectiveness analyses: second panel on cost-effectiveness in health and medicine. JAMA 2016;316:1093–103.
2. Available at: https://www.cbsnews.com/news/obama-why-not-pay-half-price/ Accessed November 23, 2019.
3. Rabeneck L, Lansdorp-Vogelaar I. Assessment of a cancer screening program. Best Pract Res Clin Gastroenterol 2015;29:979–85.
4. Neumann PJ, Cohen JT, Weinstein MC. Updating cost-effectiveness: the curious resilience of the $50,000-per-QALY threshold. N Engl J Med 2014;371:796–7.
5. Institute for Clinical and Economic Review. Overview of the ICER value assessment framework and update for 2017-2019. 2018.
6. Reducing risks, promoting healthy life. Geneva (Switzerland): World Health Organization; 2002.
7. Robinson LA, Hammitt JK, Chang AY, et al. Understanding and improving the one and three times GDP per capita cost-effectiveness thresholds. Health Policy Plan 2017;32:141–5.
8. Roland D. Obscure model puts a price on good health—and drives down drug costs. Wall Street Journal 2019.
9. Greuter MJE, de Klerk CM, Meijer GA, et al. Screening for colorectal cancer with fecal immunochemical testing with and without postpolypectomy surveillance colonoscopy: a cost-effectiveness analysis. Ann Intern Med 2017;167:544–54.
10. Woods B, Revill P, Sculpher M, et al. Country-level cost-effectiveness thresholds: initial estimates and the need for further research. Value Health 2016;19:929–35.
11. Nimdet K, Chaiyakunapruk N, Vichansavakul K, et al. A systematic review of studies eliciting willingness-to-pay per quality-adjusted life year: does it justify CE threshold? PLoS One 2015;10:e0122760.
12. Mandel JS, Bond JH, Church TR, et al. Reducing mortality from colorectal cancer by screening for fecal occult blood. Minnesota Colon Cancer Control Study. N Engl J Med 1993;328:1365–71.
13. Mandel JS, Church TR, Bond JH, et al. The effect of fecal occult-blood screening on the incidence of colorectal cancer. N Engl J Med 2000;343:1603–7.
14. Kronborg O, Jorgensen OD, Fenger C, et al. Randomized study of biennial screening with a faecal occult blood test: results after nine screening rounds. Scand J Gastroenterol 2004;39:846–51.
15. Hardcastle JD, Chamberlain JO, Robinson MH, et al. Randomised controlled trial of faecal-occult-blood screening for colorectal cancer. Lancet 1996;348:1472–7.
16. Atkin WS, Edwards R, Kralj-Hans I, et al. Once-only flexible sigmoidoscopy screening in prevention of colorectal cancer: a multicentre randomised controlled trial. Lancet 2010;375:1624–33.

17. Segnan N, Armaroli P, Bonelli L, et al. Once-only sigmoidoscopy in colorecta cancer screening: follow-up findings of the Italian Randomized Controlled Trial SCORE. J Natl Cancer Inst 2011;103:1310–22.

18. Schoen RE, Pinsky PF, Weissfeld JL, et al. Colorectal-cancer incidence and mor tality with screening flexible sigmoidoscopy. N Engl J Med 2012;366:2345–57.

19. Holme O, Loberg M, Kalager M, et al. Effect of flexible sigmoidoscopy screening on colorectal cancer incidence and mortality: a randomized clinical trial. JAMA 2014;312:606–15.

20. Swartz AW, Eberth JM, Josey MJ, et al. Re-analysis of all-cause mortality in the U.S. preventive services task force 2016 evidence report on colorectal cancer screening. Ann Intern Med 2019;118:104–12.

21. Quintero E, Castells A, Bujanda L, et al. Colonoscopy versus fecal immunochem-ical testing in colorectal-cancer screening. N Engl J Med 2012;366:697–706.

22. Bibbins-Domingo K, Grossman DC, Curry SJ, et al. Screening for colorectal can-cer: US preventive services task force recommendation statement. JAMA 2016; 315:2564–75.

23. Knudsen AB, Zauber AG, Rutter CM, et al. Estimation of benefits, burden, and harms of colorectal cancer screening strategies: modeling study for the US pre-ventive services task force. JAMA 2016;315:2595–609.

24. Wolf AMD, Fontham ETH, Church TR, et al. Colorectal cancer screening for average-risk adults: 2018 guideline update from the American Cancer Society. CA Cancer J Clin 2018;68:250–81.

25. Meester RGS, Peterse EFP, Knudsen AB, et al. Optimizing colorectal cancer screening by race and sex: microsimulation analysis II to inform the American Cancer Society colorectal cancer screening guideline. Cancer 2018;124: 2974–85.

26. Peterse EFP, Meester RGS, Siegel RL, et al. The impact of the rising colorectal cancer incidence in young adults on the optimal age to start screening: Microsi-mulation analysis I to inform the American Cancer Society colorectal cancer screening guideline. Cancer 2018;124:2964–73.

27. Zauber A, Knudsen A, Rutter CM, et al. Evaluating the benefits and harms of colo-rectal cancer screening strategies: a collaborative modeling approach. AHRQ Publication No. 14-05203-EF-2 2015.

28. Ladabaum U, Mannalithara A. Comparative effectiveness and cost effectiveness of a multitarget stool DNA test to screen for colorectal neoplasia. Gastroenter-ology 2016;151:427–39.e6.

29. Ladabaum U, Mannalithara A, Meester RGS, et al. Cost-effectiveness and na-tional effects of initiating colorectal cancer screening for average-risk persons at age 45 years instead of 50 years. Gastroenterology 2019;157:137–48.

30. Ladabaum U, Dominitz JA, Kahi C, et al. Strategies for colorectal cancer screening. Gastroenterology 2020;158:418–32.

31. van Ballegooijen M, Rutter CM, Knudsen AB, et al. Clarifying differences in nat-ural history between models of screening: the case of colorectal cancer. Med Decis Making 2011;31:540–9.

32. Pignone M, Saha S, Hoerger T, et al. Cost-effectiveness analyses of colorectal cancer screening: a systematic review for the U.S. Preventive Services Task Force. Ann Intern Med 2002;137:96–104.

33. Lansdorp-Vogelaar I, Knudsen AB, Brenner H. Cost-effectiveness of colorectal cancer screening. Epidemiol Rev 2011;33:88–100.

34. Ran T, Cheng CY, Misselwitz B, et al. Cost-effectiveness of colorectal cancer screening strategies-a systematic review. Clin Gastroenterol Hepatol 2019; 17(10):1969–81.e15.

35. Siegel RL, Jemal A, Ward EM. Increase in incidence of colorectal cancer among young men and women in the United States. Cancer Epidemiol Biomarkers Prev 2009;18:1695–8.

36. Ladabaum U, Song K. Projected national impact of colorectal cancer screening on clinical and economic outcomes and health services demand. Gastroenterology 2005;129:1151–62.

37. Parekh M, Fendrick AM, Ladabaum U. As tests evolve and costs of cancer care rise: reappraising stool-based screening for colorectal neoplasia. Aliment Pharmacol Ther 2008;27:697–712.

38. Lansdorp-Vogelaar I, van Ballegooijen M, Zauber AG, et al. Effect of rising chemotherapy costs on the cost savings of colorectal cancer screening. J Natl Cancer Inst 2009;101:1412–22.

39. Patel SS, Kilgore ML. Cost effectiveness of colorectal cancer screening strategies. Cancer Control 2015;22:248–58.

40. Silva-Illanes N, Espinoza M. Critical analysis of Markov models used for the economic evaluation of colorectal cancer screening: a systematic review. Value Health 2018;21:858–73.

41. Ladabaum U, Allen J, Wandell M, et al. Colorectal cancer screening with blood-based biomarkers: cost-effectiveness of methylated septin 9 DNA vs. current strategies. Cancer Epidemiol Biomarkers Prev 2013;22:1567–76.

42. Ladabaum U, Mannalithara A, Brill JV, et al. Contrasting effectiveness and cost-effectiveness of colorectal cancer screening under commercial insurance vs. Medicare. Am J Gastroenterol 2018;113:1836–47.

43. Church TR, Wandell M, Lofton-Day C, et al. Prospective evaluation of methylated SEPT9 in plasma for detection of asymptomatic colorectal cancer. Gut 2014;63: 317–25.

44. Ginsberg GM, Lauer JA, Zelle S, et al. Cost effectiveness of strategies to combat breast, cervical, and colorectal cancer in sub-Saharan Africa and South East Asia: mathematical modelling study. BMJ 2012;344:e614.

45. Sullivan T, Sullivan R, Ginsburg OM. Screening for cancer: considerations for low- and middle-income countries. In: Gelband H, Jha P, Sankaranarayanan R, et al, editors. Cancer: disease control priorities, vol. 3, 3rd edition, chapter 12. Washington, DC: The International Bank for Reconstruction and Development/The World Bank (c) 2015 International Bank for Reconstruction and Development/The World Bank; 2015.

46. Ladabaum U, Levin Z, Mannalithara A, et al. Colorectal testing utilization and payments in a large cohort of commercially insured US adults. Am J Gastroenterol 2014;109:1513–25.

47. Chen C, Stock C, Hoffmeister M, et al. How long does it take until the effects of endoscopic screening on colorectal cancer mortality are fully disclosed? A Markov model study. Int J Cancer 2018;143:2718–24.

48. Dougherty MK, Brenner AT, Crockett SD, et al. Evaluation of interventions intended to increase colorectal cancer screening rates in the united states: a systematic review and meta-analysis. JAMA Intern Med 2018;178:1645–58.

49. Jandorf L, Gutierrez Y, Lopez J, et al. Use of a patient navigator to increase colorectal cancer screening in an urban neighborhood health clinic. J Urban Health 2005;82:216–24.

50. Subramanian S, Tangka FKL, Hoover S, et al. Costs of colorectal cancer screening provision in CDC's colorectal cancer control program: comparisons of colonoscopy and FOBT/FIT based screening. Eval Program Plann 2017;62: 73–80.

51. Tangka FKL, Subramanian S, Hoover S, et al. Costs of promoting cancer screening: evidence from CDC's colorectal cancer control program (CRCCP). Eval Program Plann 2017;62:67–72.

52. Subramanian S, Tangka FK, Hoover S, et al. Recommendations from the international colorectal cancer screening network on the evaluation of the cost of screening programs. J Public Health Manag Pract 2016;22:461–5.

53. Jandorf L, Stossel LM, Cooperman JL, et al. Cost analysis of a patient navigation system to increase screening colonoscopy adherence among urban minorities. Cancer 2013;119:612–20.

54. Ladabaum U, Mannalithara A, Jandorf L, et al. Cost-effectiveness of patient navigation to increase adherence with screening colonoscopy among minority individuals. Cancer 2015;121:1088–97.

55. Subramanian S, Tangka FK, Hoover S, et al. Costs of planning and implementing the CDC's colorectal cancer screening demonstration program. Cancer 2013; 119(Suppl 15):2855–62.

56. Subramanian S, Tangka FK, Hoover S, et al. Clinical and programmatic costs of implementing colorectal cancer screening: evaluation of five programs. Eval Program Plann 2011;34:147–53.

57. Naber SK, Knudsen AB, Zauber AG, et al. Cost-effectiveness of a multitarget stool DNA test for colorectal cancer screening of Medicare beneficiaries. PLoS One 2019;14:e0220234.

58. Somsouk M, Rachocki C, Mannalithara A, et al. Effectiveness and cost of organized outreach for colorectal cancer screening: a randomized controlled trial. J Natl Cancer Inst 2019. https://doi.org/10.1093/jnci/djz110.

59. Lara CL, Means KL, Morwood KD, et al. Colorectal cancer screening interventions in 2 health care systems serving disadvantaged populations: screening uptake and cost-effectiveness. Cancer 2018;124:4130–6.

60. Lew JB, St John DJB, Macrae FA, et al. Benefits, harms, and cost-effectiveness of potential age extensions to the national bowel cancer screening program in Australia. Cancer Epidemiol Biomarkers Prev 2018;27:1450–61.

61. Rex DK, Boland CR, Dominitz JA, et al. Colorectal cancer screening: recommendations for physicians and patients from the U.S. multi-society task force on colorectal cancer. Gastroenterology 2017;153:307–23.

62. Giardiello FM, Allen JI, Axilbund JE, et al. Guidelines on genetic evaluation and management of lynch syndrome: a consensus statement by the US multisociety task force on colorectal cancer. Am J Gastroenterol 2014;109:1159–79.

63. Ladabaum U, Ford JM, Martel M, et al. American Gastroenterological Association technical review on the diagnosis and management of lynch syndrome. Gastroenterology 2015;149:783–813.e20.

64. Rubenstein JH, Enns R, Heidelbaugh J, et al. American Gastroenterological Association Institute guideline on the diagnosis and management of lynch syndrome. Gastroenterology 2015;149:777–82 [quiz: e16–7].

65. Robertson DJ, Ladabaum U. Opportunities and challenges in moving from current guidelines to personalized colorectal cancer screening. Gastroenterology 2019;156:904–17.

56. Ma GK, Ladabaum U. Personalizing colorectal cancer screening: a systematic review of models to predict risk of colorectal neoplasia. Clin Gastroenterol Hepatol 2014;12:1624–34.e1.

57. Usher-Smith JA, Walter FM, Emery JD, et al. Risk prediction models for colorectal cancer: a systematic review. Cancer Prev Res (Phila) 2016;9:13–26.

58. Usher-Smith JA, Harshfield A, Saunders CL, et al. External validation of risk prediction models for incident colorectal cancer using UK Biobank. Br J Cancer 2018;118:750–9.

59. Helsingen LM, Vandvik PO, Jodal HC, et al. Colorectal cancer screening with faecal immunochemical testing, sigmoidoscopy or colonoscopy: a clinical practice guideline. BMJ 2019;367:l5515.

70. Ladabaum U, Mannalithara A, Mitani A, et al. Clinical and economic impact of tailoring screening to predicted colorectal cancer risk: a decision analytic modeling study. Cancer Epidemiol Biomarkers Prev 2020;29(2):318–28.

71. Naber SK, Kundu S, Kuntz KM, et al. Cost-effectiveness of risk-stratified colorectal cancer screening based on polygenic risk: current status and future potential. JNCI Cancer Spectr 2019;4(1):pkz086.

The National Colorectal Cancer Roundtable

Past Performance, Current and Future Goals

Richard Wender, MD[a],*, Durado Brooks, MD, MPH[b],
Katherine Sharpe, MTS[c], Mary Doroshenk, MA[d]

KEYWORDS

- Colorectal cancer • Colon cancer • Screening • American Cancer Society
- Cancer screening • 80% by 2018

KEY POINTS

- The National Colorectal Cancer Roundtable, a program of the American Cancer Society, is an organization of organizations dedicated to increasing colorectal cancer screening rates.
- The National Colorectal Cancer Roundtable has proposed an extensive library of resources and tools to help every interested sector promote uptake of colorectal cancer screening, particularly to bridge disparities.
- The National Colorectal Cancer Roundtable's 80% by 2018 campaign combined helped drive a substantial increase in colorectal cancer screening rates.
- The 80% in Every Community is a new campaign.

INTRODUCTION

The American Cancer Society (ACS) has a long history as a leader in promotion of cancer prevention and screening. In the mid-1990s, experts at ACS recognized that screening for colorectal cancer (CRC) presented one of our nation's best opportunities to reduce cancer incidence and mortality but that, as a result of low screening rates, the potential of CRC screening was not being realized. Robert Smith, PhD, of the ACS and Marion Nadel, PhD, from the Centers for Disease Control and Prevention (CDC) recognized that screening rates were unlikely to increase without a coordinated national effort to engage all relevant stakeholders to overcome barriers to screening.

[a] American Cancer Society, 250 Williams Street, Suite 4B, Atlanta, GA 30303, USA; [b] Cancer Control Interventions, American Cancer Society, 250 Williams Street, Suite 6C, Atlanta, GA 30303, USA; [c] Sharpe Consulting, LLC, 1 Sycamore Station, Decatur, GA 30030, USA; [d] Exact Sciences Corporation, 441 Charmany Dr., Madison, WI 53719, USA
* Corresponding author.
E-mail address: Richard.Wender@cancer.org
Twitter: @RichWender (R.W.)

Gastrointest Endoscopy Clin N Am 30 (2020) 499–509
https://doi.org/10.1016/j.giec.2020.02.013   giendo.theclinics.com
1052-5157/20/© 2020 Elsevier Inc. All rights reserved.

These leaders proposed that the ACS, create an "organization of organizations" to drive increasing CRC screening. In 1997, the ACS launched the National Colorectal Cancer Roundtable (NCCRT), with the sole aim of increasing the proportion of eligible US residents who are up to date with high-quality CRC screening. Today the NCCRT is composed of more than 150 member organizations, with nationally known experts, thought leaders, and decision makers on CRC screening policy and delivery serving as member representatives. The combined energy of the members of the NCCRT, working individually and collectively, has become the nation's most important catalyst to increase CRC screening rates. The purpose of this article is to present the history of the NCCRT with the specific objectives of identifying key elements that have contributed to its success and to spur additional efforts to bring organizations together to accomplish critical public health goals.

CREATION OF THE NATIONAL COLORECTAL CANCER ROUNDTABLE

The first steps taken by the ACS and CDC were the identification of leaders to serve as the initial Steering Committee of the new organization and the recruitment of Bernard Levin, MD, a gastroenterologist and leader of preventive health at MD Anderson, as its founding chair. These decisions proved crucial to the success of the NCCRT; the engagement of a respected, committed, and passionate Steering Committee added to the legitimacy of the organization, while allowing the work of the NCCRT to benefit from some of the best minds in the field. The multiyear leadership of Dr Bernard Levin, a universally respected statesman in the public health and medical professional communities, reinforced the stature of the organization and provided continuity during the formative years.

An important decision from the outset was to include member organizations from every relevant sector. The NCCRT included then, as it does today, government, nongovernmental, business, public health groups, professional organizations, patient advocacy groups, and key individual leaders, which allowed for critical thought and problem solving from a range of perspectives. It was determined that a meeting of the entire NCCRT membership would take place in the fall of each year to facilitate the sharing of information on the state of CRC screening, new scientific knowledge, and progress toward organizational goals. Although the ACS serves as the primary sponsoring organization, providing full-time staff and funding, the CDC remains a strong partner, providing funding, guidance, planning and execution.

EARLY NATIONAL COLORECTAL CANCER ROUNDTABLE INITIATIVES: 2002 TO 2005

In 2002, the NCCRT published its first strategic plan. The plan highlighted the challenges to CRC screening that existed at that time, including patient and physician barriers, insurance barriers, and the lack of incentives to motivate adherence to screening guidelines.[1] This initial strategic plan focused on the need to promote the value of screening by both patients and providers. Task groups were formed to identify initiatives to accelerate the awareness and uptake of high-quality CRC screening. The task groups focused on ways to better inform the general public about the importance of CRC screening, support for clinicians in the delivery of quality care, and the identification of public policy interventions to support CRC screening. In 2003, the NCCRT hired a full-time program manager to assist in the implementation of the steering committee vision. Early efforts in each of these areas are briefly discussed in the following sections.

The Public Awareness task group engaged a marketing group to identify ways in which the NCCRT might develop resources to support a public awareness campaign. The group recommended the creation of a universal symbol to represent CRC screening, leading to the design and adoption of the Blue Star as this universal symbol. Introduced on April 1, 2004, the Blue Star is intended to raise awareness about how to prevent CRC through screening, and to celebrate shared successes (Fig. 1).

The NCCRT Policy task group collaborated with The Lewin Group in 2003 and developed a cost model that explored how increased CRC screening among pre-Medicare eligible individuals (aged 50–64 years) could translate into Medicare savings realized through earlier detection and treatment, specifically polypectomy and treatment of early stage cancer. The study also looked at net costs to pre-Medicare payers.[2]

The Provider Awareness task group conducted a national survey of CRC screening education, prioritization, and self-perceived preparedness among resident physicians in family medicine, internal medicine, and obstetrics and gynecology training programs. Several publications resulted from the surveys, highlighting opportunities for curricular changes to enhance current perceptions about and practices for CRC screening tests.[3]

The NCCRT formed a Best Practices task group, which was charged with gathering evidence-based practices that could be broadly disseminated among the NCCRT membership and health systems nationwide. Ultimately these resources were used by public health experts from Thomas Jefferson University and the Prevent Cancer Foundation to develop a primary care guide to implementing high-quality CRC screening.[4] This toolkit was deployed through NCCRT members to medical professional societies, state health departments, advocacy organizations, and health systems, and became the template for future NCCRT toolkits and resource guides.

A wealth of additional tools and resources have been developed by the NCCRT. These evidence-based innovations and tools, designed to increase quality CRC

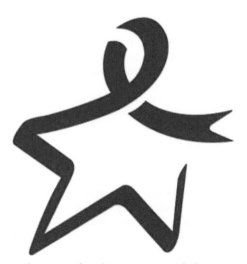

Fig. 1. Introduced on April 1, 2004, the Blue Star is intended to raise awareness about how to prevent CRC through screening, and to celebrate shared successes. (*Courtesy of* The American Cancer Society; with permission.)

screening in a range of settings and populations, are housed on the NCCRT's Resource Center (https://nccrt.org/resource-center/). In addition to resources developed by the NCCRT, members are encouraged to submit field-tested tools for inclusion as external partner resources.

BUILDING BLOCK PHASE: 2006 THROUGH 2012

Between 2006 and 2012, the NCCRT was chaired by Thomas Weber, MD, a colorectal surgeon in New York City and a passionate champion promoting CRC screening. During these years, the NCCRT continued to build momentum and expand productivity by identifying and working to address emerging issues. In 2009, state implementation of CRC screening accelerated, as the CDC Colorectal Cancer Control Program moved beyond a pilot phase to a mature program that awarded 5-year cooperative agreements to 25 states and 4 tribal organizations to both screen uninsured adults and promote screening at the population level.[5] Throughout this period, the NCCRT hosted a series of workshops with stakeholders, thought leaders, and outside experts to advance priority issues. The NCCRT worked to build goodwill among its members by not just convening members, but by actively working to deliver needed tools and resources as identified through these workshops. Task groups expanded and evolved to adapt to the changing landscape and new challenges. This work took place as CRC screening acceptance by providers grew, but struggles with incorporating CRC screening recommendations into primary care practice and moving consumers to action remained challenging.

NATIONAL COLORECTAL CANCER ROUNDTABLE SITE VISITS

In 2007, Dr Weber instituted the NCCRT Steering Committee site visit program to identify emerging trends, innovations, barriers, and solutions around CRC screening at the local level. These trips included visits to an urban federally qualified health center (FQHC) in Baltimore; visits with rural and frontier coalitions and clinics in South Carolina and the Four Corners area of Colorado; and finally a visit to the Bay area of California that included a daylong session with Kaiser Permanente of Northern California to explore their innovative integrated approach to CRC screening delivery. These visits served several purposes, namely, identifying pioneering work to share with NCCRT members, enhancing understanding of barriers and solutions to local delivery, identifying unique cultural challenges, and connecting with dynamic local leaders who subsequently became enduring contributors to the NCCRT. An unintended secondary outcome was that these visits tended to spur local excitement and action.

EVOLUTION OF THE TASK GROUPS

The work of the task groups matured and entered a period of robust productivity during this phase. Existing task groups expanded their charge and new groups were formed to address practice implementation, evidence-based education and outreach, community health centers and family history. The task groups allowed the NCCRT to pool and leverage the talents of a diverse membership base to produce publications, programs and tools. Ultimately, the task groups helped to strengthen the collective energy behind any given priority. Signature achievements that emerged from the NCCRT task groups are described.

The Professional Education Task Group expanded its charge to focus on practice implementation. This Task Group produced publications on *Promoting cancer screening within the patient centered medical home*[6] and *Strategies for expanding colorectal cancer screening at community health centers,*[7] both of which laid the foundation for a long term effort by the NCCRT to increase CRC screening in the FQHC setting, including the *Links of Care* pilot program, which aimed to ensure that FQHC patients had access to follow-up colonoscopy when needed. The task group also developed a physician's brochure on stool testing, designed to introduce physicians to the value of modern stool-based screening (https://nccrt.org/resource/fobt-clinicians-reference-resource/). Additionally, the Professional Education Task Group spawned the Community Health Center Task Group, chaired by Drs. James Hotz and Durado Brooks, which helped prioritize the NCCRT's focus on screening in the community health center setting.

The Quality Assurance Task Group published reports on evidence- and consensus-based standards for the performance of high-quality colonoscopy, the components of a quality screening colonoscopy referral system in primary care practice, and on the responsibilities of referring clinicians to ensure quality colonoscopy.[8,9]

The Public Awareness Task Group created a marketing kit containing tools and resources for members to use to heighten awareness about CRC screening during March (https://nccrt.org/resource/blue-star-marketing-kit/). This group also developed the Family PLZ! campaign, which provided member organizations an out-of-the box campaign to spur family conversations about CRC family history and CRC screening.

The Policy Action Task Group assessed both state and federal policy barriers to CRC screening. Notably, the task group released a joint report with the Kaiser Family Foundation entitled, *Coverage of Colonoscopies under the Affordable Care Act's Prevention Benefit,*[10] which helped lead to February 2013 guidance from the Center for Consumer Information and Insurance Oversight to clarify that health plans or issuers may not impose cost sharing with respect to a polyp removal during a colonoscopy performed as a screening procedure (https://www.cms.gov/CCIIO/Resources/Fact-Sheets-and-FAQs/aca_implementation_faqs12). This rules clarification addressed this frustrating issue among commercial insurers, although the problem persists in Medicare as of this writing.

Finally, the Evidence-Based Interventions and Outreach Task Group developed an Evaluation 101 toolkit (https://nccrt.org/resource/evaluation-toolkit/), which provided much needed guidance to organizations and communities on how to evaluate a wide variety of CRC screening interventions, reflecting a ripening appreciation in the field for the need to assess, learn and adjust screening interventions for impact.

ESTABLISHING THE FOUNDATION FOR A UNIFIED CAMPAIGN

Notably, it was during this period that the Public Awareness Task Group, chaired by Dr Paul Limburg of the Mayo Clinic and Amy Manela, an individual NCCRT member, began to explore the value of developing a unified national strategy to increase CRC screening rates. The effort was supported by a grant from the Colon Cancer Challenge Foundation (now known as the Colon Cancer Foundation). The task group determined that a united approach would (1) leverage the diverse NCCRT membership around a unified theme, (2) integrate and mature CRC Awareness Month efforts, (3) consolidate existing resources and invite new resources, and (4) strengthen the collective energy behind the priority of increasing public awareness of CRC screening through collaborative efforts.

The task group launched a comprehensive effort that included conducting member surveys and interviews and hosting strategy meetings to establish the buy in and ground rules for such a campaign from the membership. This work ultimately laid the groundwork needed to launch the NCCRT's 80% by 2018 campaign, discussed elsewhere in this article.

NATIONAL COLORECTAL CANCER ROUNDTABLE GROWTH AND EXPANSION: 2012 TO 2018

The impact and effectiveness of the NCCRT was magnified dramatically in recent years by 4 key developments: passage and implementation of the Patient Protection and Affordable Care Act (ACA); organizational restructuring of the ACS, which included creation of a new nationwide health systems staff structure; addition of a CRC screening measure to the Uniform Data System (UDS) measure set; and the creation and launch of the 80% by 2018 initiative. The impact of each of these factors is discussed.

The Patient Protection and Affordable Care Act

The ACA dramatically expanded insurance coverage and access to health care. After the ACA's first open enrollment period in the fall of 2013, the number of uninsured Americans rapidly decreased from 41 million to 27 million.[11] The ACA resulted in increased access to CRC screening through 2 mechanisms. First, the law requires that private health plans cover all evidence-based cancer screening tests that receive a rating of A or B from the US Preventive Services Task Force, including screening for CRC in adults beginning at age 50 and continuing until age 75. Furthermore, the ACA requires that the cost of preventive care is covered at 100%, and without cost sharing by nongrandfathered private and public health insurance plans.[12] Studies indicate that these factors have led to an increased use of CRC screening, particularly among socioeconomically disadvantaged groups.[13,14]

American Cancer Society Transformation

Changes in ACS leadership and structure was another critical factor that heightened the influence of the NCCRT in the national arena. In 2012, the ACS completed a 3-year nationwide reorganization that included both leadership and staff alignment, and in 2013 Richard Wender, MD, an expert on cancer screening and NCCRT Chair, was named as first Chief Cancer Control Officer of the ACS, a new position responsible for leading all ACS cancer control activities. Dr Wender elevated the importance of CRC screening within ACS, raised awareness of the NCCRT across the organization, and fostered greater engagement of ACS staff with the NCCRT. The ACS transformation process also led to the establishment of a cadre of 50 ACS health systems staff, responsible for addressing cancer control priorities in partnership with multiple sectors of the health care system (primary care, hospitals and health systems, public health and other governmental entities, including payors) at the regional and local level. Many of the new ACS health systems staff were trained in quality improvement and disseminated and assisted with the implementation of the growing suite of NCCRT tools and resources, while also bringing many new partners to the organization.

Uniform Data System Measure

A third factor that expanded the reach of the NCCRT was the inclusion of CRC screening in the UDS measure set. The UDS is a standardized reporting system used for required annual data collection and reporting for Health Resources and Service Administration grantees, including more than 1300 FQHCs, which provide primary and preventive care services to 28 million patients in every state, territory, and the District of Columbia (http://www.nachc.org/wp-content/uploads/2019/03/NACHC_Guide_Policy-Brief_web.pdf). FQHCs are located in medically underserved urban and rural areas and provide comprehensive primary care services to all individuals regardless of insurance status; they therefore care for a disproportionate share of the nation's socially and economically disadvantaged persons. FQHCs were first required to begin tracking and reporting their CRC screening rates in 2012. Based on UDS reporting, 30.2% of screen-eligible FQHC patients nationwide were up to date with CRC screening in 2012 compared with 65.1% of the general US population reported by CDC that same year.[15,16] This new measure motivated clinicians and administrators in many of the nations' FQHCs to invest energy and resources into improving screening rates in their centers. The NCCRT had a longstanding interest in improving screening rates among the medically underserved and in 2011 had initiated a community health center task group to explore ways in which the organization might assist FQHC clinicians and patients in overcoming some of the barriers to CRC screening that are commonly encountered in these settings. In 2012, the NCCRT collaborated with the ACS, CDC, Health Resources and Service Administration, the National Association of Community Health Centers, and other organizations to identify strategies to support CRC screening in FQHCs and other safety net environments. This collaboration resulted in a strategy document that has guided the FQHC-related work of ACS and NCCRT,[7] as well as the creation of a manual that combines step-by-step guidance on CRC screening improvement with evidence-based tools for practice change that are geared toward the unique needs and challenges experienced by FQHC patients and providers entitled *Steps for Increasing Colorectal Cancer Screening Rates: A Manual for Community Health Centers* (https://nccrt.org/manual-for-community-health-centers-2/).

The 80% by 2018 Initiative

The final—and most impactful—contributor to the heightened influence of the NCCRT was the establishment of a nationwide goal to regularly screen 80% of recommended adults for CRC by the end of 2018 (80% by 2018). This initiative arose in response to a challenge from then Assistant Secretary for Health, Dr Howard Koh, to the ACS, National Association of Community Health Centers, federal agencies and member organizations of the NCCRT to launch a "bold and audacious goal" to accelerate CRC screening progress. This initiative built on the member assessment, buy-in, and other foundational work led by the NCCRT Public Awareness Task Group. The 80% initiative by 2018 was designed to support and build on existing initiatives, including those of the NCCRT and the CDC's Colorectal Cancer Control Program. The NCCRT convened a series of planning meetings that resulted in the development of an 80% by 2018 strategic plan framed around 4 key objectives: (1) move consumers to action, (2) activate providers, payers, and employers to support screening, (3) increase access and remove barriers to screening, and (4) evaluate existing and new efforts and maintain momentum. Partners made a formal commitment to the initiative by signing the 80% by 2018 pledge. The initial goal established by NCCRT leadership was for 50 organizations to sign the pledge.[17]

The 80% by 2018 initiative was formally launched in March 2014 with a media event at the National Press Club in Washington, DC. The initiative attracted immediate attention around the country and stimulated a host of new scientific and public health activities. Researchers estimated that if the 80% CRC screening goal was achieved, 277,000 fewer new CRCs would be diagnosed, and 203,000 CRC deaths would be prevented by 2030.[18,19]

ACS cancer control and NCCRT leaders and experts traveled around the United States and its territories, delivering hundreds of presentations on the evidence supporting the importance and value of CRC screening, current screening recommendations, including the importance of offering different screening options, and information on the 80% by 2018 initiative. Targeted resources were developed to provide guidance on how primary care, hospitals and health systems, elected officials and other entities could contribute to this shared goal.

The 80% initiative by 2018 served as a force multiplier, building on the existing work of the NCCRT and taking advantage of the changes within ACS and the health care environment outlined elsewhere in this article. It also led to a new focus on CRC screening at the regional and local level and spawned an explosion of new activities around the country. New collaborations were forged at the national, regional, and local levels. New state-level CRC screening coalitions appeared and existing entities were re-energized. A series of CRC screening training and technical assistance opportunities for state teams were jointly developed by the National Cancer Institute, CDC, ACS, and NCCRT to enhance partnerships at the state level. State teams is composed of representatives from the state's Comprehensive Cancer Control program, Primary Care Association, the ACS, an FQHC, and others (such as a state health department representative and a physician champion) attended intensive 2-day trainings framed around the NCCRT's *Steps for Increasing Colorectal Cancer Screening Rates*. Teams drafted an action plan to increase CRC screening through enhanced partnerships in their states and were then provided virtual technical assistance over the following year as they moved to put their plan into action. Teams from 35 states and US territories received this training and assistance.

The 500 nationally deployed ACS health systems staff embraced the 80% goal and played a number of important roles, including assistance with the development of state roundtables and coalitions, engaging FQHCs, and providing practice facilitation and quality improvement support around CRC screening improvement, and enlisting many organizations to sign the 80% pledge and implement actions designed to increase screening among their constituencies.

The 80% by 2018 initiative proved to be one of the most successful endeavors of its kind; by the end of 2018, more than 1750 organizations from all 50 states, the District of Columbia, Puerto Rico, and Guam had signed the pledge (https://nccrt.org/national-map-of-pledges/). The level of engagement and accomplishment among partnering organizations was nothing short of amazing: more than 350 organizations reported CRC screening rates of 80% or higher among their patients or constituents (https://nccrt.org/hall-of-fame/); hundreds of other pledge signers reported increased CRC screening activities and increased rates in their organization. The 80% by 2018 National Achievement Awards program (awards/"title="https://nccrt.org/awards/">https://nccrt.org/awards/), launched in 2015 and held annually, showcases the exemplary work of 5 or more organizations and individuals each year, many of whom have either reached 80% in the communities they serve or made tremendous progress in increasing CRC screening rates. Their stories of success serve as an inspiration for NCCRT members and pledgees.

While the 2018 CRC screening rate for the nation fell short of the 80% nationwide target, preliminary data from BRFSS 2018 indicate a nationwide rate of 68.8% (https://www.cdc.gov/cancer/colorectal/statistics/use-screening-tests-BRFSS.htm). This improvement is significant compared with the 2012 baseline figure of 65.1%, representing approximately 9.3 million additional individuals being up to date with screening since 2012. Rates improved for all national datasets, including the National

Health Interview Survey and the Healthcare Effectiveness Data and Information Set.[20,21] UDS rates increased from 30.2% in 2012 to 44.1% nationwide by 2018. This finding is particularly striking given the barriers to screening experienced by many of those cared for in these centers. Even more impressive is the fact that 31 health centers reported screening rates of 80% or higher in 2018.[21]

The 80% by 2018 initiative changed the national conversation about CRC screening. Before this initiative the only national goal related to CRC screening was the Healthy People 2020 target of 70.5%, which was little known and seldom mentioned (https://www.healthypeople.gov/2020/topics-objectives/objective/c-16). Since the launch of this initiative, scores of researchers and academics have referred to the 80% screening rate goal in their publications and the goal has been widely touted by mainstream media. Eighty percent has become the target for any organization focused on increasing screening CRC screening rates and indeed, other preventive services, as well.

Unfortunately, not everyone is benefiting equally. In many racial and ethnic communities, low-income communities and rural communities low CRC screening rates persist. To address these disparities and build on the momentum generated by the 80% by 2018 initiative, the NCCRT has launched a new endeavor called 80% in Every Community. This initiative is specifically designed to catalyze work in the many and varied communities that confront substantial obstacles to screening.

In addition to initiatives to address racial/ethnic and geographic disparities in screening, the 80% in Every Community effort will target low screening rates in the early part of the eligible age spectrum (particularly among individuals age 50–54 years for whom the screening rate is only 50%)[22] and low colonoscopy completion rates after an initial abnormal noninvasive screen, which have been linked to increased risk of a CRC diagnosis and worse outcomes.[23] The 80% in Every Community campaign will develop strategies and tools to help systems monitor and address these issues. For information and resources on 80% in Every Community visit https://nccrt.org/80-in-every-community/.

THE NATIONAL COLORECTAL CANCER ROUNDTABLE TODAY

The NCCRT is entering its 23rd year of existence. The 80% by 2018 initiative was by no means the end of its work. Rather, this concentrated 5-year effort helped to engage new organizations, more precisely identify new challenges, and define a new campaign. More than 150 organizations are now official members (https://nccrt.org/about/roundtable-members/), with more members joining every quarter. Enthusiasm around making the campaign increasingly local is high, driven by a desire to eliminate health disparities and achieve health equity. Although the members of the NCCRT and the nation as a whole have much to celebrate, numerous challenges remain. In fact, as more and more people are up to date with screening, reaching those who have not been screened will require more intensive efforts with different interventions than the ones that worked for individuals who face fewer screening barriers. This work will require new resources, appropriate funding, innovative strategies, expanding the number and diversity of partners, engagement of all sectors, retention of the improved coverage provided by the Affordable Care Act, and the sustained will to prevent deaths from CRC. The NCCRT is committed to building on its rich history, its ties to the ACS and the Centers for Disease Control, and its network of members to stay the course in our national efforts to decrease the burden of CRC.

DISCLOSURE

No disclosures (R. Wender, D. Brooks). K. Sharpe – Has served as a consultant for Genentech for work not related to the topic of this article. K. Sharpe is a former director of the NCCRT. M. Doroshenk is employed by Exact Sciences Corporation that manufactures a colorectal cancer screening test that is not discussed in this article. She is a former director of the NCCRT.

REFERENCES

1. Levin B, Smith RA, Feldman GE, et al. Promoting early detection tests for colorectal carcinoma and adenomatous polyps: a framework for action: the strategic plan of the National Colorectal Cancer Roundtable. Cancer 2002;95(8):1618–28.
2. Available at: http://www.lewin.com/content/dam/Lewin/Resources/Site_Sections/Publications/3888.pdf. Accessed November 26, 2019.
3. Oxentenko AS1, Goel NK, Pardi DS, et al. Colorectal cancer screening education, prioritization, and self-perceived preparedness among primary care residents: data from a national survey. J Cancer Educ 2007;22(4):208–18.
4. Sarfaty M, Wender R. How to increase colorectal cancer screening rates in practice. CA Cancer J Clin 2008;57(6):31.
5. Hannon PA, Maxwell AE, Escoffery C, et al. Colorectal Cancer Control Program grantees' use of evidence-based interventions. Am J Prev Med 2013;45(5): 644–8.
6. Sarfaty M, Wender R, Smith R. Promoting cancer screening within the patient centered medical home. CA Cancer J Clin 2011;61(6):397–408.
7. Sarfaty M, Doroshenk M, Hotz J, et al. Strategies for expanding colorectal cancer screening at community health centers. CA Cancer J Clin 2013;63(4):221–31.
8. Lieberman D, Nadel M, Smith RA, et al. Standardized colonoscopy reporting and data system: report of the Quality Assurance Task Group of the National Colorectal Cancer Roundtable. Gastrointest Endosc 2007;65(6):757–66.
9. Fletcher RH, Nadel MR, Allen JI, et al. The quality of colonoscopy services–responsibilities of referring clinicians: a consensus statement of the Quality Assurance Task Group, National Colorectal Cancer Roundtable. J Gen Intern Med 2010;25(11):1230–4. Components of a quality screening colonoscopy referral system in primary care practice.
10. Pollitz K, Lucia K, Keith K, et al. Coverage of colonoscopies under the affordable care act's prevention benefit. 2012. Available at: https://www.kff.org/health-costs/report/coverage-of-colonoscopies-under-the-affordable-care/. Accessed February 02, 2020.
11. Gareld R, Majerol M, Anthony D. The uninsured: a primer—key facts about health insurance and the uninsured in the era of health reform (Kaiser Commission on Medicaid and the Uninsured, Nov. 2016). Available at: https://www.kff.org/uninsured/report/the-uninsured-and-the-aca-a-primer-key-facts-about-health-insurance-2and-the-uninsured-amidst-changes-to-the-affordable-care-act/. Accessed February 02, 2020.
12. Blumenthal D, Collins SRP. Health care coverage under the affordable care act - a progress report. N Engl J Med 2014;37(13):275–81.
13. Hamman MK, Kapinos KA. Affordable care act provision lowered out-of-pocket cost and increased colonoscopy rates among men in Medicare. Health Aff 2015;34(12):2069–76.

4. Fedewa SA, Goodman M, Flanders WD, et al. Elimination of cost-sharing and receipt of screening for colorectal and breast cancer. Cancer 2015;121(18): 3272–80.
5. Riehman KS, Stephens RL, Henry-Tanner J, et al. Evaluation of colorectal cancer screening in federally qualified health centers. Am J Prev Med 2018;54(2):190–6.
6. Centers for Disease Control and Prevention (CDC). Vital signs: colorectal cancer screening test use–United States, 2012. MMWR Morb Mortal Wkly Rep 2013; 62(44):881–8.
7. Wender RC, Doroshenk M, Brooks D, et al. Implementing a national public health campaign: the American Cancer Society's and National Colorectal Cancer Roundtable's 80% by 2018 initiative. Am J Gastroenterol 2018;113(12):1739–41.
8. Meester RG, Doubeni CA, Zauber AG, et al. Public health impact of achieving 80% colorectal cancer screening rates in the United States by 2018. Cancer 2015;121:2281–5.
9. Hall IJ, Tangka FKL, Sabatino SA, et al. Patterns and trends in cancer screening in the United States. Prev Chronic Dis 2018;15:E97.
20. National Commission for Quality Assurance. HEDIS measures. Available at: http://www.ncqa.org/hedis-quality-measurement/hedis-measures. Accessed November 26, 2019.
21. Health Services Research Administration. Uniform data system. Available at: https://bphc.hrsa.gov/uds/datacenter.aspx?q=t6b&year=2018&state=&fd=. Accessed October 13, 2019.
22. Joseph DA, King JB, Dowling NF, et al. Vital signs: colorectal cancer screening test use — United States, 2018. MMWR Morb Mortal Wkly Rep 2020;69:253–9.
23. Corley DA, Jensen CD, Quinn VP, et al. Association between time to colonoscopy after a positive fecal test result and risk of colorectal cancer and cancer stage at diagnosis. JAMA 2017;317(16):1631–41.

Fecal Immunochemical Test
The World's Colorectal Cancer Screening Test

Douglas J. Robertson, MD, MPH[a,b,*], Kevin Selby, MD, MAS[c]

KEYWORDS

- Fecal immunochemical test • Screening • Colorectal cancer
- Fecal occult blood test

KEY POINTS

- The fecal immunochemical test (FIT) has many advantages over older, guaiac-based fecal occult blood tests, including greater sensitivity for neoplasia and ease of use for the individuals being screened.
- Important instructions to those considering FIT include the need for regular (eg, annual) use and, if the test is positive, the need for colonoscopy.
- For programs using FIT, laboratory quality control and continuous quality monitoring are key to success.
- FIT has a 1-time sensitivity for detecting cancer of more than 70% and programmatic studies suggest that FIT use can reduce colorectal cancer mortality up to 50%.
- The future of FIT likely includes greater personalization of the test, using the quantitative FIT data, adjusting for factors like age and sex.

INTRODUCTION

Stool testing as a mechanism to screen for colorectal cancer (CRC) dates back decades and has been shown to be highly effective in CRC mortality. In the United States, recommendations to perform stool-based screening date back to approximately 1980.[1] Guidance at that time was based on few direct clinical data, but several large-scale clinical trials of fecal occult blood testing (FOBT) with guaiac-impregnated cards subsequently were performed (**Table 1**).[2–4] Effectiveness of screening FOBT in reducing CRC mortality ranged from 15% (biennial) to 33% (annual). The benefits of screening FOBT in reducing CRC mortality appear to persist for decades.[5]

The contents of this work do not represent the views of the Department of Veterans Affairs or the United States Government.
^a Department of Veterans Affairs Medical Center, White River Junction, VT, USA; ^b The Geisel School of Medicine at Dartmouth, The Dartmouth Institute, Hanover, NH, USA; ^c Center for Primary Care and Public Health (Unisanté), University of Lausanne, Rue de Bugnon 44, 1010 Lausanne, Switzerland
* Corresponding author. VA Medical Center, Section of Gastroenterology (111E), 215 North Main Street, White River Junction, VT 05009.
E-mail address: douglas.robertson@va.gov

Gastrointest Endoscopy Clin N Am 30 (2020) 511–526
https://doi.org/10.1016/j.giec.2020.02.011
1052-5157/20/Published by Elsevier Inc.

Table 1
Large randomized controlled trials of screening fecal occult blood testing in colorectal cancer mortality prevention

Location	Age (y)	N, Randomized	Follow-up	Deaths from Colorectal Cancer (N)	Colorectal Cancer Mortality Ratio (95% CI)
Minnesota, US[2]	50–80	46,551	13 y		
		Annual (N = 15,570)		82	0.67 (0.50–0.87)
		Biennial (N = 15,587)		117	0.94 (0,68–1.31)
		Control (N = 15,394)		121	1.00
Nottingham Area of UK[3]	45–74	150251	7.8 y		
		Control (N = 74,998)		420	1.00
		Biennial (N = 75,253)		360	0.85 (0.74–0.98)
Funen, Denmark[4]	45–75	61,933			
		Control (N = 30,966)		249	1.00
		Biennial (N = 30,967)	10 y	205	0.82 (0.68–0.99)

The fecal immunochemical test (FIT) builds on a rich history of stool-based testing for CRC screening. Unlike guaiac-based testing, FIT is a direct measure of human hemoglobin in stool. The development of immunoassays for fecal hemoglobin date back to the late 1970s. It is only more recently, however, the FIT has supplanted FOBT in many screening programs.

This article provides a detailed review of FIT-based CRC screening. The basic principles underlying FIT use and the FIT types available in clinical practice are reviewed. The test characteristics of FIT for detecting various preneoplastic lesions and cancer are summarized. Programmatic FIT is being utilized in some countries and those results are outlined as well. How to apply FIT screening (from patient and program perspectives) are outlined, including information on quality control for such programs. Finally, although use of FIT for CRC screening is growing rapidly, there remain many open and important questions about its use. Some of the most important areas are outlined, including current thinking about how application might be optimized to enhance program results.

PRINCIPLES OF THE FECAL IMMUNOCHEMICAL TEST, INCLUDING FECAL IMMUNOCHEMICAL TEST TYPES AND PERFORMANCE
Principles of Fecal Immunochemical Test

Historically, stool-based screening for CRC relied on guaiac-based methods for detecting blood in the stool. These tests used guaiac-impregnated cards to which stool sampled from 3 consecutive bowel movements was added. Processing the cards required the addition of hydrogen peroxide solution and, if heme was present, it would catalyze a pseudoperoxidase-type reaction and result in color change that could be interpreted by the reader. Although screening with FOBT is effective in reducing CRC mortality, the test has limitations, including that it is an indirect measure of the actual biomarker target of interest (ie, human hemoglobin) and the sensitivity of the test for hemoglobin is relatively low.[6]

Like conventional FOBT, FIT relies on examining stool for blood, but the mechanism underlying the test is quite different. FITs are directly specific for human hemoglobin, relying on antibody-antigen reactions to the globin moiety. The advantages of FIT over FOBT are many, but none more important than the fact that FIT can detect much lower concentrations of hemoglobin. FIT can detect hemoglobin at a concentration of 1/100 of guaiac-based FOBT (gFOBT).[7] Not only does the degree of sensitivity improve test performance but also it allows for the implementation of programs that require more limited stool collection (eg, only a single stool sample yearly). This directly influences adherence, and FIT-based programs have been shown to have better performance in that regard.[8]

Types of Fecal Immunochemical Test (Qualitative vs Quantitative)

There are 2 distinctly different types of FIT products: qualitative and quantitative (**Fig. 1**). Both qualitative and quantitative tests utilize antibodies specific to the globin moiety. Qualitative tests function like point-of-service pregnancy tests. The antibodies are impregnated on a card. Buffer is added to the deposited stool and, through lateral flow immunochromatographic methods, the sample is determined to be positive or

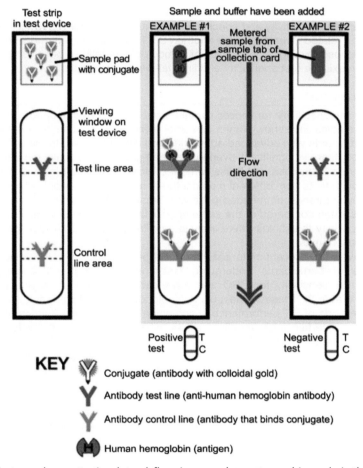

Fig. 1. Cartoon demonstrating lateral flow immunochromatographic analysis that underpins qualitative-type fecal immunochemical testing. (*From* Allison JE. Population Screening for Colorectal Cancer Means Getting FIT: The Past, Present, and Future of Colorectal Cancer Screening Using the Fecal Immunochemical Test for Hemoglobin (FIT). Gut Liver 2014; 8(2): 117-130; with permission.)

negative for blood. The amount of globin required to determine positivity is prese within the device and varies by manufacturer. With quantitative devices, stool i sampled and admixed with a buffer solution directly within the collection device The intermixing of globin (if present) and the antibodies within the buffer creat turbidity that is then read quantitatively by the analytical device.

Although qualitative and quantitative FITs are both widely available, quantitativ FITs frequently are selected for use within large programs[9–11] and clinical trials.[12–1] There are several advantages of quantitative FIT platforms relative to qualitative test (**Box 1**). Most importantly, there is some concern about the reliability of qualitative de vices across manufacturers. This has been shown in studies comparing several qua itative devices head to head and demonstrating large differences in performance.[15,1] For example, in a study of 6 different qualitative devices with German practices, th sensitivity for advanced adenoma detection ranged from 25% to 72%.[16] When quan titative FIT platforms have been compared, differences are much less.[17,18] Also, quan titative testing allows the end user (eg, the program) to determine the definition of positive test. The sensitivity and specificity of FIT are related directly to the hemoglo bin level and related inversely to one another. So, for programs with more limited ac cess to colonoscopy, higher thresholds of hemoglobin to define a positive test can b chosen to maximize test specificity and limit false-positive results.

Test Characteristics

Sensitivity and specificity for cancer, conventional and serrated neoplasia

Numerous studies have shown that mean stool hemoglobin concentrations are highe among participants with advanced adenomas and highest among those with cancer Nonetheless, there is significant overlap between groups, especially between thos with advanced adenomas and those without clinically significant lesions.[19] Further more, although tests from different manufacturers have different reported sensitivitie at the manufacturer-recommended positivity threshold, they appear to have simila sensitivities when compared at the same specificity.[20] Thus, even when considerin very low positivity thresholds, there likely is a ceiling of FIT sensitivity, especially fo advanced adenomas.

There have been 3 recent meta-analyses of FIT performance,[21–23] including primar ily studies of participants undergoing first-time screening colonoscopy. Tw compared FIT sensitivity for CRC and advanced adenomas at varying positivit thresholds (**Table 2**). These studies, using a colonoscopy gold standard, are corrob orated by reports of FIT performance in screening programs with 2 years of registr follow-up to ascertain false-negative results, which show a sensitivity for CRC c 75% and specificity of 94%.[23] FITs thus have a much better sensitivity for CRC an lower specificity than nonrehydrated Hemoccult II (Beckman Coulter Inc, Brea, CA tests, reported at 25% to 38% and 98% to 99%, respectively.[24] Furthermore, thei

---

Box 1
.**Potential advantage of quantitative versus qualitative fecal immunochemical testing**

- Automated processing
  - High throughput processing possible
  - Eliminate interobserver and interobserver variations in interpreting test positivity

- Results are numeric estimates of fecal hemoglobin concentration in stool sample
  - Less variation in performance across brands (assuming same hemoglobin cutpoint)
  - Ability to adjust definition of a positive test based on resources

Table 2
Fecal immunochemical testing performance for detecting colorectal cancer and advanced adenomas at various quantitative thresholds

Thresholds (μg Stool/g Feces)	Sensitivity for Colorectal Cancer (%)	Specificity for Colorectal Cancer (%)	Sensitivity for Advanced Adenoma (%)	Specificity for Advanced Neoplasia (%)
≤10 μg/g	78–91	90–91	31–40	90–93
<10 and ≤20 μg/g	69–82	93–95	21–30	94–96
>20 and ≤30 μg/g	71–73	95–96	18–27	95–98
>30 μg/g	66	96	19	97

Ranges represent results from 2 meta-analyses presenting data at these thresholds (data from Imperiale and colleagues,[22] 2019 and Selby and colleagues,[23] 2019) and not 95% CI.

ability to detect advanced adenomas may decrease CRC incidence, which was not seen in trials of gFOBT.

Although 1-time FIT has reasonable sensitivity for cancer and modest sensitivity for advanced neoplasia, it is poorly sensitive for serrated polyps (see Joseph C. Anderson and Amitabh Srivastava's article, "Colorectal Cancer Screening for the Serrated Pathway," in this issue, for details on serrated polyps). This was examined directly in a large study (N = 9989) comparing the FIT-DNA test (Cologuard [Exact Sciences, Madison, WI]) to conventional FIT (OC Sensor, Polymedco, Cortlandt, NY; cutoff 20 μg/g). In that study, the sensitivity for large (≥1 cm) serrated lesions was 42.4% for the FIT-DNA test but only 5.1% for FIT alone.[25]

Factors having an impact on test characteristics
Hemoglobin threshold defining a positive test The positivity threshold used to define a positive test has the most impact on FIT performance (see **Table 2**). Heterogeneity between screening populations and FIT brands have made it difficult to determine the precise trade-off of positive tests requiring colonoscopy and additional cancers or advanced adenomas, detected at varying positivity thresholds. Six months after the start of the Dutch national screening program, the positivity threshold was increased to 47 μg/g from 15 μg/g because of inadequate colonoscopy capacity, resulting in a drop in age-adjusted sensitivity from 90.5% to 82.9%, while halving the number of positive tests.[26] A large American screening program predicted that a drop in positivity threshold from 20 μg/g to 10 μg/g would increase programmatic sensitivity by only 5% (from 74.3% to 79.3%), while increasing the number of positive results per 1 cancer case detected from 52 to 85.[27] Neither of these studies, however, could calculate sensitivity for advanced adenomas. In an uninsured American population, dropping from 20 μg/g to 10 μg/g increased the detection of advanced neoplasia but again doubled the number of positive tests.[28] The meta-analyses, discussed previously, showed that positivity thresholds of less than or equal to 10 μg/g increased sensitivity for advanced adenomas by 10% compared with higher thresholds. Thus, positivity thresholds below 20 μg/g are likely to have a larger numeric effect on advanced adenoma than cancer detection and generate large numbers of positive tests, especially in programs screening annually. In summary, low thresholds to define a positive test are, in the authors' opinion, more likely to be useful

- In biennial screening
- In programs already performing primary screening colonoscopy, suggesting that there already is sufficient colonoscopy capacity (eg, United States)

- If quantitative results are available, for individuals who desire greater certainty that they do not have an advanced adenoma

With regards to the use of quantitative results, the US Food and Drug Administration has only a binary test approved the commonly used OC Sensor (Polymedco, Cortlandt, NY) test as a binary test at a threshold 20 μg/g and reporting of individual quantitative results is not allowed.

Other factors (eg, age and sex) Several recent studies have suggested that FITs have a lower sensitivity for CRC in women than in men, possibly due to lower mean stool hemoglobin concentrations or a higher incidence of harder-to-detect, right-sided lesions in women.[26,27] One article also showed decreasing sensitivity with increasing age.[27] A systematic review identified few studies stratified by sex or age, however, and no statistically significant differences were identified.[23]

APPLICATION OF FECAL IMMUNOCHEMICAL TESTING FROM PATIENT AND PROGRAM PERSPECTIVES
Patient Invitation

How best to introduce FIT as an option for screening varies based on the setting in which the test is being offered (**Table 3**). In the United States, CRC screening often is opportunistic in nature and offers to screen occur within the framework of a routine office interaction between a primary care provider and patient. Although colonoscopy is the dominant screening modality, FIT can be offered alongside colonoscopy or sequentially (ie, for those refusing colonoscopy). In such settings, both the benefits of CRC screening and options for screening can be introduced. The American Cancer Society provides guidance on how to enhance shared decision making around screening.[29] Decision aids, designed to be distributed before an office visit, and conversation cards to facilitate discussions within a visit have been developed. For those considering FIT, the advantages of this approach can be reviewed (eg, noninvasive, at-home testing). Key requirements of a FIT-based screening are emphasized, including the need for regular testing (ie, annual or biennial when negative) and completion of colonoscopy if the test is positive for blood.

In settings where FIT application is programmatic, there are different considerations related to FIT invitation. Generally, programmatic FIT utilizes large-scale outreach to populations, so determining who is eligible for such screening is an initial challenge. Administrative data often are utilized to identify individuals eligible for screening. There

Table 3	
Approaches to improving uptake of fecal immunochemical testing	
Program Type	**Practices to Consider**
Opportunistic (office-based setting)	• Development/implementation of electronic medical record–based reminder to offer screening • Offering FIT as 1 of several screening options or sequentially for those refusing an initial offered primary screening option • Use of decision aids and conversation cards can facilitate discussions about screening.
Programmatic (mailed FIT)	• Use of administrative date to identify screen eligible cohort • Preinvitation letters prior to mailing the FIT • Mailing of FIT with simplified instructions • Both mailed and telephone reminders

s an extensive literature surrounding approaches to optimize outreach, including the utility and design of invitations to participate in such programs, that is reviewed elsewhere (see Jason A. Dominitz and Theodore R. Levin's article, "What Is Organized Screening and What Is Its Value?," in this issue). In brief, evidence supports the use of

- Preinvitation letters prior to mailing the FIT
- Mailing of FIT with simplified instructions
- Both mailed and telephone reminders

Mailed FIT is associated with a 28% absolute increase[30] and 2.3-fold relative increase[31] in screen completion compared with usual care. The Dutch organized screening program has achieved a cumulative participation rate of 77% using mailed FITs.[32]

Patient Instructions

An advantage of FIT (relative to FOBT) is that patient preparation to complete FIT can be greatly simplified (**Box 2**). There is no need for an individual to modify dietary intake around the time of stool collection and to maximize adherence that should be made explicit.

The impact of drugs that increase bleeding (eg, aspirin, warfarin, and direct oral anticoagulant [DOAC]) on FIT performance is a separate consideration. A recently published meta-analysis examining the positive predictive value of FIT across 8 studies suggested that FIT accuracy was not significantly impacted by intake of aspirin/nonsteroidal anti-inflammatory drug (NSAID) use.[33] The findings of the meta-analysis also are consistent with a recently published trial that showed no increase in test sensitivity for those randomized to aspirin prior to stool collection relative to placebo.[34] Based on these data, no adjustments in NSAIDs or aspirin should be made, and this is consistent recently published US guidelines.[35]

Although current US guidelines also do not recommend adjusting warfarin prior to FIT collection, the impact of DOACs on FIT test characteristics is a more complicated issue. In the meta-analysis, discussed previously, there was no impact on FIT performance.[33] A recent report from Norway, however, came to a differing conclusion. In particular, DOACs had a significant impact on reducing the positive predictive value of FIT for cancer to 0.9% in users versus 6.8% in nonusers.[36] Programs using lower thresholds to determine the definition of a positive test would be more impacted (ie, reduced efficiency) if, for example, DOAC use was not restricted. Further data on this issue are needed.

Beyond issues of modification of dietary intake and medication at the time of completing FIT, instructions should be clear on effective sampling and rapid return of the specimen to a laboratory for processing. Sampling devices vary based on manufacturer and those should be provided to the individual completing FIT. Degradation of the hemoglobin in stool after deposit and before processing is a concern for any FIT-based program, which is an issue particularly for those relying on wet

---

Box 2
Highlights of patient instruction for those receiving fecal immunochemical testing

- No need to adjust diet.

- No need to adjust aspirin, NSAID, or conventional anticoagulation (eg, warfarin).

- Follow manufacturer guidance for sampling stool.

- Return sample QUICKLY after deposit and refrigerate overnight if the sample cannot be mailed that day.

sampling using quantitative tests with buffer. Improvement in such buffers have been made.[37] Nonetheless, participants completing FIT should be advised to mail their samples back to a laboratory on the day of collection. If not possible, then the sample should be refrigerated and mailed the following day.

Follow-up of a Positive Fecal Immunochemical Test

For those with a positive test, evaluation for colonoscopy is critical. There is evidence both from clinical and modeling studies that delays in time from FIT positivity to colonoscopy results in worse cancer outcomes.[38,39] For example, in a retrospective study from Kaiser Permanente Northern California and Kaiser Permanente Southern California, delays in follow-up greater than 10 months were associated with a significant increase in cancer and advanced-stage disease relative to those with timely follow up (8–30 days).[39] There is no consensus regarding targets for colonoscopy completion; European guidelines of 90% colonoscopy completion within 30 days may not be feasible for many patients or programs.[40]

Patient-reported barriers to completing a diagnostic colonoscopy in the setting of a positive FIT recently were reported from a safety net hospital system in Tarrant County, Texas. The most important factors cited included issues with health insurance, comorbid illness, and barriers to transportation, including lack of social support.[41] Using systematic review, Selby and colleagues[42] examined interventions to improve follow-up on positive FOBTs. The most effective patient-level intervention was navigation. At the provider level, there was some evidence that reminders to providers where follow-up action was inadequate were effective.

Programmatic Considerations, Including Quality Control and Metrics

Whether applied opportunistically or programmatically, several important decisions about how to apply FIT at the level of the provider, practice, or program need to be made. These include decisions about type of FIT (qualitative vs quantitative), number of FITs (eg, 1 vs 2), frequency of FIT (eg, annual vs biennial), and cutoff to determine a positive test. The considerations re discussed in detail elsewhere.[6,35] Generally, recommendations balance pragmatism and resource use with maximizing test sensitivity.

The challenges of setting up appropriate laboratory quality-control mechanisms for FIT-based programs recently has been reviewed[43] and include the lack of an analytical standard for FIT. The approach to quality control in the Dutch FIT program recently has been described.[44] Processing of samples at a laboratory varies depending on type of FIT used. Manufacturer guidance needs to be followed meticulously. After processing, expert guidance recommends the reporting of quantitative results in micrograms of hemoglobin per gram of feces rather than nanograms of hemoglobin per milliliter buffer.[45] Such reporting facilitates comparison of FIT performance across manufactures.

Rapid return of the completed FIT from the participant and processing of samples at a laboratory are key to avoid missed opportunities for screening. Following-up on positive tests with high-quality colonoscopy also is critical to program success. Ongoing quality improvement work is key to improving program performance in this regard.[46] The US Multi-Society Task Force on Colorectal Cancer has suggested the following quality-management standards for FIT-based programs:

- FIT completion rate greater than 60% or greater for those offered screening
- Proportion that cannot be processed by a laboratory of less than 5%
- Colonoscopy completion rate for those with a positive test greater than or equal to 80%

- Adenoma detection rate greater than 45% in men and 35% in women for those completing colonoscopy for a positive FIT

CURRENT USE OF FECAL IMMUNOCHEMICAL TESTING IN ORGANIZED SCREENING PROGRAMS AND ESTIMATES OF EFFECTIVENESS

Overview

FITs are the most commonly used screening test worldwide, especially by organized programs. For instance, in the European Union, of 23 countries or regions responding to a recent survey, 10 used FIT and 9 used gFOBTs; however, among programs using gFOBTs, at least are 4 are transitioning to FIT (in the United Kingdom and France).[47,48] In the same study, use of FIT was associated with higher overall participation than use of gFOBTs (49.5% vs 33.2%). Kaiser Permanente and the Veterans Health Administration, the 2 largest organized screening programs in the United States, both use FIT.

Fecal Immunochemical Testing Performance in Organized Screening

The meta-analyses of FIT sensitivity, discussed previously, were based primarily on first-time screenees completing a FIT prior to diagnostic colonoscopy, raising concerns regarding FIT performance in real-world settings. People who have never or have not recently been screened are more likely to have advanced CRC that may be more easily detected (known as the prevalent screening round). Furthermore, although 1-time participation with FIT clearly is greater than with colonoscopy, failure to participate in subsequent rounds could make FIT less effective over time.[49]

Several recent studies have assuaged these fears. First, FIT performs well over multiple rounds of screening, continuing to detect important numbers of advanced adenomas, maintaining a similar positive predictive value for advanced neoplasia, and with a small drop in the number of positive tests. For example, over 4 rounds of annual screening at Kaiser Permanente, the positive predictive value for an adenoma was 51.4% in the first round and between 47.4% and 48.5% in subsequent rounds.[50] FIT participation was between 78% and 89% among those who had previously participated, and in total 7% crossed over to colonoscopy because of a positive FIT.[50] In an Italian program using the OC-Hemodia test (Eiken Chemical, Japan) biennially, the positive predictive value of FIT for advanced neoplasia dropped by 18% from the first to the second round, and then remained stable.[51]

Impact of Fecal Immunochemical Testing on Colorectal Cancer Incidence and Mortality

There are not yet data from a randomized controlled trial to quantify the impact of FIT on CRC incidence and mortality. Modeling studies done for the US Preventive Services Task Force suggest that annual FIT between ages 50 and 75 can reduce CRC mortality, over a person's lifetime, by approximately 80% which was comparable to the benefit of screening colonoscopy.[52] Another modeling study done for the *British Medical Journal*, using a time horizon of 15 years and a baseline CRC risk of 3%, suggested that annual FIT could reduce CRC mortality by 59% and incidence by 15%. Biennial FIT would give a 50% reduction in mortality and only a 5% reduction in incidence.[53] There now is observational evidence that organized FIT programs are associated with decreases in CRC mortality (**Table 4**). For instance, an Italian study comparing regions with and without biennial FIT screening showed that an increase from 4% to 51% screening participation was associated with a 22% drop in CRC mortality after 10 years.[54] A prospective cohort study from Taiwan showed that 21% coverage with 1 to 3 rounds of biennial FIT screening led to a 10% reduction in

Table 4
Selected studies examining programmatic fecal immunochemical testing use on colorectal cancer mortality

Setting	Population Age (y)	Years of Study	Frequency Fecal Immunochemical Testing Brand	Hemoglobin Cutpoint	Design/Comparison	Impact on Colorectal Cancer Mortality
Veneto Region, Italy[54]	50–69	1995–2011	Biennial OC Sensor/FOB Gold	20 µg hemoglobin/g feces	Early adoption screen areas to late screen areas	22% lower in early screening area
Taiwan[55]	50–69	2004–2009	Annual OC Senor/HM Jackarc	20 µg hemoglobin/g feces	Early participants vs not participants	10% reduction in early participants
US (Kaiser Permanente)[11]	51–75	2000–2015	Annual OC Sensor	20 µg hemoglobin/g feces	Before and after implementation of mailed FIT program	52% reduction in CRC mortality

CRC mortality, after adjustments for self-selection bias.[55] Finally, a before-and-after study in the Kaiser Permanente population also showed a drop in CRC incidence, suggesting an important impact of advanced adenoma detection. It showed that the implementation of annual FIT screening increased the proportion of the population up to date with screening from 39% to 82% and was associated with a 26% reduction in annual CRC incidence and 52% reduction in CRC mortality.[11]

FUTURE OF FECAL IMMUNOCHEMICAL TESTING
Questions to Be Answered

Optimal number of tests for each screening round

Due to the low sensitivity of individual tests, guidelines recommended 3 gFOBTs be performed on 2 consecutive bowel movements each screening round. There has been similar interest in whether 2 FITs per screening round, with colonoscopy if either is positive, would be significantly better than 1 FIT. Results to date have been mixed. For instance, a Dutch study found that 2 FITs resulted in a higher detection rate of advanced neoplasia (4.1% vs 3.1%), without affecting participation (61% in both groups). However, 13% had a positive result instead of 8%.[56] Other similar studies have not shown an advantage in sensitivity for advanced neoplasia, and there are concerns regarding increased costs and lower adherence.[57–59] Furthermore, an update from the Dutch study found that 1-sample screening performed similarly over 4 rounds of screening.[60] Given the uncertain benefits, nearly all programs use and recommendations advocate a single FIT per screening round.

Which fecal immunochemical test is best—comparison of brands

There are more than 15 FIT brands reported in the literature. The OC FIT-CHEK quantitative test (from Eiken chemicals and distributed by Polymedco in the United States) that is analyzed using the OC Sensor platform has appeared in by far the largest number of scientific articles.[23] Direct comparison of FIT brands, both within 1 study using a library of frozen samples[20] or by meta-analysis,[22,23] have not given a clear answer. Tests appear to have similar sensitivity when compared at the same level of specificity. Several screening programs recently have performed large-scale, population-level comparisons of commonly used FIT. A study among approximately 50,000 participants in Italy showed that the HM-JACKarc (Alpha Laboratories, United Kingdom) and OC Sensor tests perform similarly at an identical threshold of 20 μg/g.[61] More than 21,000 participants in the Dutch program simultaneously completed both the OC Sensor and FOB Gold tests (Sentinel Diagnostics, Italy).[9] Although the distribution of positive tests differed (more OC Sensor positive at thresholds between 5 μg/g and 10 μg/g and more FOB Gold positive at thresholds 25–150 μg/g), test performance was nearly identical when set to the same positivity rate.[9] More participants preferred the FOB Gold, but most had no preference.[62] Thus, although the OC Sensor test has appeared in the most clinical studies, at the moment, no 1 test can be recommended over another.

Which screening test is best—comparative effectiveness of FIT to other screening modalities

Globally, there is significant interest in the performance of screening colonoscopy versus FIT, and there are 3 ongoing trials comparing those modalities. The US trial employs annual FIT but with a higher hemoglobin level defining a positive test.[12] Biennial testing with lower definitions of FIT positivity is used in the studies from Spain[13] and Sweeden.[14] Although long-term results from these trials are not expected soon, the Colonprev trial[13] did report the results of the first round of screening in that study.

Adherence to FIT was superior to colonoscopy (34.2% vs 24.6%) and, in the intention-to-screen analysis, there was no significant difference in cancer detection between the 2 groups (33 cancers FIT and 30 cancers colonoscopy).

Opportunities to Be Explored

Personalization

Generally speaking, whether applied programmatically or opportunistically, FIT is applied in a singular fashion across all members of the population. As discussed previously, the significance of a positive test varies based on factors, such as the age and sex of the individual being screened. In 1 meta-analysis, male sex was associated with a significantly lower risk of false positivity (relative rate 0.84; 95% CI, 0.74, 0.94).[63] To improve performance, it would be possible to tailor the definition of a positive test based on such factors. This would be accomplished most easily using a quantitative FIT platform, where the hemoglobin result could be combined with other factors known about the participants that could have an impact on FIT performance. Using these 3 factors (ie, quantitative result, age, and sex), Auge and colleagues[64] were able to delineate 16 risk categories that varied 11-fold in risk for advanced neoplasia when comparing the highest and lowest risk groups. More work is needed to better define factors to be used in such categorization and better understand the impact of tailoring on issues of adherence and follow-up over multiple rounds of testing.

Fecal immunochemical testing as part of a 2-step screening strategy

There are multiple options for screening but, generally speaking, they are offered exclusively from one another. Within programmatic settings, individuals are offered the program screening options. In opportunistic settings, individuals are offered a single test preferentially or given a choice of modalities and then choose which best meets their priorities. Using known information about risk factors for neoplasia, however, an alternative model could include applying a predictive model, allowing that to dictate screening options. Based on known risk factors and pretest probability for advanced lesions, higher-risk individuals could be offered a more invasive and more sensitive test like colonoscopy whereas lower-risk individuals could perform FIT. In a proof-of-principle study, 1 group applied the Asia-Pacific Colorectal Screening scoring system to 5657 individuals and triaged the group into low risk (N = 3243), medium risk (3243), and high risk (N = 1768).[65] Although all received colonoscopy in this study, outcomes were analyzed where the low-risk and medium-risk groups would get FIT first and only proceed to colonoscopy if the FIT were positive (all high-risk groups were assumed to go directly to colonoscopy). Using this approach, 95% of the prevalent cancers identified would have been detected but requiring less than half the colonoscopy if total colonoscopy was going to be applied to the entire cohort.

SUMMARY

Over the past decade, FIT largely has supplanted older gFOBT and globally is now the dominant stool-based screening platform. There exist a large amount of clinical data demonstrating FIT has a 1-time sensitivity for cancer that is better than 70% (and up to 90% if very low hemoglobin thresholds are used) while maintaining good specificity. The test clearly detects advanced adenoma less well, but programmatic data do demonstrate that FIT can reduce cancer incidence. Although FITs currently are applied uniformly across populations, the future of FIT may include personalized application that could improve performance even more.

DISCLOSURE

D.J. Robertson—Freenome, Metabolomic Technologies Inc, and Amadix. K. Selby—none to declare.

REFERENCES

1. Cancer of the colon and rectum. CA Cancer J Clin 1980;30:208–15.
2. Mandel JS, Bond JH, Church TR, et al. Reducing mortality from colorectal cancer by screening for fecal occult blood. Minnesota Colon Cancer Control Study. N Engl J Med 1993;328:1365–71.
3. Hardcastle JD, Chamberlain JO, Robinson MH, et al. Randomised controlled trial of faecal-occult-blood screening for colorectal cancer. Lancet 1996;348:1472–7.
4. Kronborg O, Fenger C, Olsen J, et al. Randomised study of screening for colorectal cancer with faecal-occult-blood test. Lancet 1996;348:1467–71.
5. Shaukat A, Mongin SJ, Geisser MS, et al. Long-term mortality after screening for colorectal cancer. N Engl J Med 2013;369:1106–14.
6. Tinmouth J, Lansdorp-Vogelaar I, Allison JE. Faecal immunochemical tests versus guaiac faecal occult blood tests: what clinicians and colorectal cancer screening programme organisers need to know. Gut 2015;64:1327–37.
7. Carroll MR, Seaman HE, Halloran SP. Tests and investigations for colorectal cancer screening. Clin Biochem 2014;47:921–39.
8. Vart G, Banzi R, Minozzi S. Comparing participation rates between immunochemical and guaiac faecal occult blood tests: a systematic review and meta-analysis. Prev Med 2012;55:87–92.
9. de Klerk CM, Wieten E, Lansdorp-Vogelaar I, et al. Performance of two faecal immunochemical tests for the detection of advanced neoplasia at different positivity thresholds: a cross-sectional study of the Dutch national colorectal cancer screening programme. Lancet Gastroenterol Hepatol 2019;4:111–8.
10. Chiang TH, Chuang SL, Chen SL, et al. Difference in performance of fecal immunochemical tests with the same hemoglobin cutoff concentration in a nationwide colorectal cancer screening program. Gastroenterology 2014;147:1317–26.
11. Levin TR, Corley DA, Jensen CD, et al. Effects of organized colorectal cancer screening on cancer incidence and mortality in a large community-based population. Gastroenterology 2018;155:1383–91.e5.
12. Dominitz JA, Robertson DJ, Ahnen DJ, et al. Colonoscopy vs. fecal immunochemical test in reducing mortality from colorectal cancer (CONFIRM): rationale for study design. Am J Gastroenterol 2017;112:1736–46.
13. Quintero E, Castells A, Bujanda L, et al. Colonoscopy versus fecal immunochemical testing in colorectal-cancer screening. N Engl J Med 2012;366:697–706.
14. Ribbing Wilen H, Blom J, Hoijer J, et al. Fecal immunochemical test in colorectal cancer screening: colonoscopy findings by different cut-off levels. J Gastroenterol Hepatol 2019;34:103–12.
15. Daly JM, Bay CP, Levy BT. Evaluation of fecal immunochemical tests for colorectal cancer screening. J Prim Care Community Health 2013;4:245–50.
16. Hundt S, Haug U, Brenner H. Comparative evaluation of immunochemical fecal occult blood tests for colorectal adenoma detection. Ann Intern Med 2009;150:162–9.
17. Santare D, Kojalo I, Liepniece-Karele I, et al. Comparison of the yield from two faecal immunochemical tests at identical cutoff concentrations - a randomized trial in Latvia. Eur J Gastroenterol Hepatol 2016;28:904–10.

18. Grobbee EJ, van der Vlugt M, van Vuuren AJ, et al. A randomised comparison of two faecal immunochemical tests in population-based colorectal cancer screening. Gut 2017;66:1975–82.
19. Fraser CG, Mathew CM, McKay K, et al. Automated immunochemical quantitation of haemoglobin in faeces collected on cards for screening for colorectal cancer. Gut 2008;57:1256–60.
20. Gies A, Cuk K, Schrotz-King P, et al. Direct comparison of diagnostic performance of 9 quantitative fecal immunochemical tests for colorectal cancer screening. Gastroenterology 2018;154:93–104.
21. Gies A, Bhardwaj M, Stock C, et al. Quantitative fecal immunochemical tests for colorectal cancer screening. Int J Cancer 2018;143:234–44.
22. Imperiale TF, Gruber RN, Stump TE, et al. Performance characteristics of fecal immunochemical tests for colorectal cancer and advanced adenomatous polyps: a systematic review and meta-analysis. Ann Intern Med 2019;170:319–29.
23. Selby K, Levine EH, Doan C, et al. Effect of sex, age, and positivity threshold on fecal immunochemical test accuracy: a systematic review and meta-analysis. Gastroenterology 2019;157(6):1494–505.
24. Whitlock EP, Lin JS, Liles E. Screening for colorectal cancer: a targeted, updated systematic review for the US preventive services task force. Ann Intern Med 2008;149:638–58.
25. Imperiale TF, Ransohoff DF, Itzkowitz SH, et al. Multitarget stool DNA testing for colorectal-cancer screening. N Engl J Med 2014;370:1287–97.
26. Toes-Zoutendijk E, Kooyker AI, Dekker E, et al. Incidence of interval colorectal cancer after negative results from first-round fecal immunochemical screening tests, by cutoff value and participant sex and age. Clin Gastroenterol Hepatol 2019 [pii:S1542-3565(19)30896-1].
27. Selby K, Jensen CD, Lee JK, et al. Influence of varying quantitative fecal immunochemical test positivity thresholds on colorectal cancer detection: a community-based cohort study. Ann Intern Med 2018;169:439–47.
28. Berry E, Miller S, Koch M, et al. Lower abnormal fecal immunochemical test cutoff values improve detection of colorectal cancer in system-level screens. Clin Gastroenterol Hepatol 2019;18(3):647–53.
29. Volk RJ, Leal VB, Jacobs LE, et al. From guideline to practice: new shared decision-making tools for colorectal cancer screening from the American Cancer Society. CA Cancer J Clin 2018;68:246–9.
30. Issaka RB, Avila P, Whitaker E, et al. Population health interventions to improve colorectal cancer screening by fecal immunochemical tests: a systematic review. Prev Med 2019;118:113–21.
31. Dougherty MK, Brenner AT, Crockett SD, et al. Evaluation of interventions intended to increase colorectal cancer screening rates in the United States: a systematic review and meta-analysis. JAMA Intern Med 2018;178:1645–58.
32. Grobbee EJ, van der Vlugt M, van Vuuren AJ, et al. Diagnostic yield of one-time colonoscopy vs one-time flexible sigmoidoscopy vs multiple rounds of mailed fecal immunohistochemical tests in colorectal cancer screening. Clin Gastroenterol Hepatol 2019;18(3):667–75.e1.
33. Nieuwenburg SAV, Vuik FER, Kruip M, et al. Effect of anticoagulants and NSAIDs on accuracy of faecal immunochemical tests (FITs) in colorectal cancer screening: a systematic review and meta-analysis. Gut 2019;68(5):866–72.
34. Brenner H, Calderazzo S, Seufferlein T, et al. Effect of a single aspirin dose prior to fecal immunochemical testing on test sensitivity for detecting advanced colorectal neoplasms: a randomized clinical trial. JAMA 2019;321:1686–92.

35. Robertson DJ, Lee JK, Boland CR, et al. Recommendations on fecal immuno-chemical testing to screen for colorectal neoplasia: a consensus statement by the US multi-society task force on colorectal cancer. Gastroenterology 2017; 152:1217–37.e3.

36. Randel KR, Botteri E, Romstad KMK, et al. Effects of oral anticoagulants and aspirin on performance of fecal immunochemical tests in colorectal cancer screening. Gastroenterology 2019;156:1642–9.e1.

37. Grazzini G, Ventura L, Rubeca T, et al. Impact of a new sampling buffer on faecal haemoglobin stability in a colorectal cancer screening programme by the faecal immunochemical test. Eur J Cancer Prev 2017;26:285–91.

38. Doubeni CA, Gabler NB, Wheeler CM, et al. Timely follow-up of positive cancer screening results: a systematic review and recommendations from the PROSPR Consortium. CA Cancer J Clin 2018;68:199–216.

39. Corley DA, Jensen CD, Quinn VP, et al. Association between time to colonoscopy after a positive fecal test result and risk of colorectal cancer and cancer stage at diagnosis. JAMA 2017;317:1631–41.

40. von Karsa L, Patnick J, Segnan N, et al. European guidelines for quality assur-ance in colorectal cancer screening and diagnosis: overview and introduction to the full supplement publication. Endoscopy 2013;45:51–9.

41. Jetelina KK, Yudkin JS, Miller S, et al. Patient-reported barriers to completing a diagnostic colonoscopy following abnormal fecal immunochemical test among uninsured patients. J Gen Intern Med 2019;34(9):1730–6.

42. Selby K, Baumgartner C, Levin TR, et al. Interventions to improve follow-up of positive results on fecal blood tests: a systematic review. Ann Intern Med 2017; 167:565–75.

43. Godber IM, Benton SC, Fraser CG. Setting up a service for a faecal immuno-chemical test for haemoglobin (FIT): a review of considerations, challenges and constraints. J Clin Pathol 2018;71:1041–5.

44. Toes-Zoutendijk E, Bonfrer JMG, Ramakers C, et al. Quality monitoring of a FIT-based colorectal cancer screening program. Clin Chem 2019;65:419–26.

45. Fraser CG, Allison JE, Halloran SP, et al. A proposal to standardize reporting units for fecal immunochemical tests for hemoglobin. J Natl Cancer Inst 2012;104: 810–4.

46. Cheng C, Ganz DA, Chang ET, et al. Reducing rejected fecal immunochemical tests received in the laboratory for colorectal cancer screening. J Healthc Qual 2019;41:75–82.

47. Senore C, Basu P, Anttila A, et al. Performance of colorectal cancer screening in the European Union Member States: data from the second European screening report. Gut 2019;68:1232–44.

48. Schreuders EH, Ruco A, Rabeneck L, et al. Colorectal cancer screening: a global overview of existing programmes. Gut 2015;64:1637–49.

49. Liang PS, Wheat CL, Abhat A, et al. Adherence to competing strategies for colo-rectal cancer screening over 3 years. Am J Gastroenterol 2016;111:105–14.

50. Jensen CD, Corley DA, Quinn VP, et al. Fecal immunochemical test program per-formance over 4 rounds of annual screening: a retrospective cohort study. Ann Intern Med 2016;164:456–63.

51. Zorzi M, Hassan C, Capodaglio G, et al. Long-term performance of colorectal cancerscreening programmes based on the faecal immunochemical test. Gut 2018;67:2124–30.

52. Knudsen AB, Zauber AG, Rutter CM, et al. Estimation of benefits, burden, and harms of colorectal cancer screening strategies: modeling study for the US preventive services task force. JAMA 2016;315:2595–609.
53. Buskermolen M, Cenin DR, Helsingen LM, et al. Colorectal cancer screening with faecal immunochemical testing, sigmoidoscopy or colonoscopy: a microsimulation modelling study. BMJ 2019;367:l5383.
54. Zorzi M, Fedeli U, Schievano E, et al. Impact on colorectal cancer mortality of screening programmes based on the faecal immunochemical test. Gut 2015;64:784–90.
55. Chiu HM, Chen SL, Yen AM, et al. Effectiveness of fecal immunochemical testing in reducing colorectal cancer mortality from the One Million Taiwanese Screening Program. Cancer 2015;121:3221–9.
56. van Roon AH, Wilschut JA, Hol L, et al. Diagnostic yield improves with collection of 2 samples in fecal immunochemical test screening without affecting attendance. Clin Gastroenterol Hepatol 2011;9:333–9.
57. Guittet L, Bouvier V, Guillaume E, et al. Colorectal cancer screening: why immunochemical faecal occult blood test performs as well with either one or two samples. Dig Liver Dis 2012;44:694–9.
58. Hernandez V, Cubiella J, Gonzalez-Mao MC, et al. Fecal immunochemical test accuracy in average-risk colorectal cancer screening. World J Gastroenterol 2014;20:1038–47.
59. Wong MC, Ching JY, Chan VC, et al. Diagnostic accuracy of a qualitative fecal immunochemical test varies with location of neoplasia but not number of specimens. Clin Gastroenterol Hepatol 2015;13:1472–9.
60. Schreuders EH, Grobbee EJ, Nieuwenburg SAV, et al. Multiple rounds of one sample versus two sample faecal immunochemical test-based colorectal cancer screening: a population-based study. Lancet Gastroenterol Hepatol 2019;4:622–31.
61. Passamonti B, Malaspina M, Fraser CG, et al. A comparative effectiveness trial of two faecal immunochemical tests for haemoglobin (FIT). Assessment of test performance and adherence in a single round of a population-based screening programme for colorectal cancer. Gut 2018;67:485–96.
62. de Klerk CM, Wieten E, van der Steen A, et al. Participation and ease of use in colorectal cancer screening: a comparison of 2 fecal immunochemical tests. Am J Gastroenterol 2019;114:511–8.
63. de Klerk CM, Vendrig LM, Bossuyt PM, et al. Participant-related risk factors for false-positive and false-negative fecal immunochemical tests in colorectal cancer screening: systematic review and meta-analysis. Am J Gastroenterol 2018;113:1778–87.
64. Auge JM, Pellise M, Escudero JM, et al. Risk stratification for advanced colorectal neoplasia according to fecal hemoglobin concentration in a colorectal cancer screening program. Gastroenterology 2014;147:628–36.e1.
65. Chiu HM, Ching JY, Wu KC, et al. A risk-scoring system combined with a fecal immunochemical test is effective in screening high-risk subjects for early colonoscopy to detect advanced colorectal neoplasms. Gastroenterology 2016;150:617–625 e3.

The Case for High-Quality Colonoscopy Remaining a Premier Colorectal Cancer Screening Strategy in the United States

Douglas K. Rex, MD

KEYWORDS

- Colonoscopy • Colorectal cancer screening • Colorectal cancer • Colorectal polyps
- Colorectal adenomas

KEY POINTS

- Fecal blood testing trials, flexible sigmoidoscopy trials, cohort and case-control studies, and studies on the impact of the adenoma detection rate on interval cancer all indicate that colonoscopy effectively reduces colorectal cancer incidence and mortality. This includes right-sided cancer, and protection in the screening setting.
- Colonoscopy has improved substantially over the past 2 decades as a result of technical advances and a quality movement.
- In the opportunistic setting, the long interval protection (10 years) provided by negative screening colonoscopy plays a critical role in maintaining screening adherence.
- New developments that could further enhance detection include aligning financial incentives with detection and introduction of artificial intelligence programs that enhance detection.
- Advances in colonoscopy performance will make screening intervals of 15 to 20 years safe in the near future.

INTRODUCTION

Colonoscopy is the most powerful cancer prevention tool in clinical medicine. Case control and cohort studies (see later in this article) show that average performance of colonoscopy in the United States and Germany results in a greater than 80% reduction in left-sided colon cancer incidence, and a 40% to 60% reduction in right-sided

This work was supported by a gift from Scott Schurz and his children to the Indiana University Foundation in the name of Douglas K. Rex, MD.
Division of Gastroenterology/Hepatology, Indiana University School of Medicine, 550 North University Boulevard, Suite 4100, Indianapolis, IN 46202, USA
E-mail address: drex@iu.edu

Gastrointest Endoscopy Clin N Am 30 (2020) 527–540
https://doi.org/10.1016/j.giec.2020.02.006
1052-5157/20/© 2020 Elsevier Inc. All rights reserved.

incidence.[1–8] Colonoscopy performance is highly operator dependent,[9–12] and high-quality colonoscopy produces greater protection against cancer than low-quality technical performance.[13–17] In the United States, colorectal cancer (CRC) incidence rates have been declining since 1975, and in 1985 there was a surge in lower bowel endoscopy in association with the diagnosis of President Reagan's colon cancer. Since 2001, when Medicare began coverage for screening colonoscopy, incidence rates of colon cancer have been declining by approximately 3% per year in persons older than 50, and there was a 30% decline in overall incidence in the first decade of the twenty-first century.[18] Much of the incidence decline can be attributed to the extensive and widespread use of screening, surveillance, and diagnostic colonoscopy across the United States.[18] Recently, declines have been documented in other Western countries in persons older than 50,[19] and these declines have occurred at the same time that CRC incidence rates have risen in persons younger than 50.[19] There is clear evidence of a birth cohort effect, indicating as yet undetermined environmental factors are driving the increasing incidence rate in persons younger than 50.[20,21] However, the divergence in incidence trends between younger and older persons, in the context of a general absence of screening in younger persons compared with older persons, hardly escapes notice.

Screening experts are widely aware that no randomized controlled trial of colonoscopy versus no screening or versus other screening methods have been completed. As a principle, it is accepted that CRC screening works, based on randomized controlled trials performed with guaiac-based fecal occult blood testing (gFOBT),[22–24] and flexible sigmoidoscopy.[25–28] Multiple lines of evidence from several types of clinical studies support the conclusion that colonoscopy also effectively prevents CRC incidence and mortality (see later in this article). Several trials are currently being conducted of colonoscopy versus other strategies,[29,30] primarily fecal immunochemical testing (FIT), but the results of these studies are not yet available.

Currently, much of the world is turning its attention to FIT as the primary means of CRC screening. Although no randomized controlled trials support FIT, its superior performance characteristics compared with gFOBT, including better cancer and advanced adenoma sensitivity,[31] and better adherence to screening,[32] indicate that FIT is an excellent approach to screening. FIT has low cost, and the FIT test included in the current commercially available FIT-fecal DNA test accounts for much of that test's cancer and adenoma sensitivity, although none of its sensitivity for sessile serrated polyps.[33] FIT and colonoscopy are each cost-effective strategies, and FIT virtually always performs well in cost-effectiveness analyses.[32,34] Both colonoscopy and FIT dominate the FIT-fecal DNA test, in that they are both more effective and cost-effective.[35]

Although FIT is effective and cost-effective for screening, it is not a clear first choice for screening in the United States. Early results of screening studies from Europe suggest that FIT on an annual or biannual basis is a better approach to screening than colonoscopy because of higher adherence rates. However, extrapolating these results to the United States must be considered in the context of the United States already having much greater penetration of screening colonoscopy than is the case for nearly every other country in the world.[19] Thus, in the United States, where screening adherence already exceeds 60%,[36,37] and where colonoscopy dominates screening, 2 different questions arise: first, what screening approach will produce gains in adherence above 60% in the general population; and second, will conversion to FIT as a primary form of screening shift a large segment of the population that has already undergone colonoscopy or would be willing to undergo colonoscopy away from colonoscopy and to FIT?

These questions must be considered in light of the one-time effectiveness of colonoscopy being substantially greater than FIT.[30] Thus, for patients who adhere to screening, colonoscopy detects more cancers than FIT, more advanced adenomas, and more total adenomas.[30] In the United States, most colonoscopy is performed in the opportunistic setting, rather than the organized setting.[38] The opportunistic setting refers to the office-based physician-patient interaction and discussion about screening.[34] Opportunistic screening often occurs in the absence of navigation and support systems that facilitate completion of annual or biannual FITs, and in the opportunistic setting, adherence to fecal-based testing falls off rapidly.[39] Countries and health care systems that endorse screening based on gFOBT or FIT use organized national screening-based programs in which screenees are repeatedly invited to complete testing, and may have the mailed invitation accompanied by a mailed FIT kit.[38] Navigators are often available to facilitate completion of colonoscopy in patients with positive FIT in the organized setting.

Given the US general reliance on opportunistic screening, the issue of how screening is offered in the physician-patient discussion becomes critical. Many experts advocate the multiple options approach, in which patients are given the choice of at least 2 tests.[34] Based on effectiveness and cost-effectiveness, these 2 tests should logically be colonoscopy and FIT in most settings.[34] Multiple options for testing leads to high rates of adherence but without detailed instruction and explanation of alternatives, patients often choose FIT because of the ease of performance relative to colonoscopy.[40,41] There is a widespread acceptance by many guidelines that multiple options offers of screening is the best way to proceed.[22,42] However, several randomized controlled trials, and to my knowledge all randomized controlled trials that have addressed the topic, indicate that sequential testing offers adherence rates that are equally as high as multiple options testing, but result in a higher percentage of patients undergoing the screening test with greater single time effectiveness.[41,43–45] Sequential testing refers to offering a single test to patients first, usually colonoscopy, and if they decline, offering a second test, usually FIT. Thus, in the opportunistic setting, where adherence to annual or biannual FIT may fall off rapidly, sequential offers of testing maximize single-time effectiveness, while simultaneously maximizing adherence.

Going forward, it should be recognized that none of the current randomized controlled trials comparing colonoscopy with FIT use an arm of sequential testing. Several of these studies are from outside the United States. The only study being performed in the United States is a Department of Veterans Affairs study.[29] Thus, given the already high penetration of screening colonoscopy in the United States, and the widespread reliance on opportunistic screening, it seems very reasonable to argue that continued reliance on a sequential approach of offering colonoscopy first, and noncolonoscopic screening, particularly FIT, as the alternative if colonoscopy is declined, remains a viable and potentially superior approach to CRC screening in the United States[34]

POTENTIAL TECHNICAL DISRUPTIONS TO SCREENING COLONOSCOPY

Colonoscopy has several suboptimal features as a screening test, including its invasiveness, need for bowel preparation, cost, and risk for complications.[34] Thus, it is certainly susceptible to an advance in screening technology that could disrupt the screening role of colonoscopy through superior effectiveness, noninvasive character, and acceptable cost-effectiveness. So far, such a disruption has not clearly occurred in US practice, and colonoscopy has preserved its screening, surveillance, diagnostic, and therapeutic roles.

At least 2 factors have prevented the disruption of screening colonoscopy in the United States. First, advances in the technology of alternative tests have simply not been sufficient to provide a clear-cut disruption. Certainly FIT is a more effective and easier test to undergo than gFOBT, but it remains a stool-based test that should be repeated annually or biannually.[32] The FIT-fecal DNA test is more sensitive than FIT,[33] but substantially less specific,[33] and consistently less cost-effective.[35,46] The first blood test available, Septin-9 from Epigenomics, has almost no features to support its use other than it is a blood test. It has modest sensitivity for cancer, no sensitivity for precancerous lesions, poor specificity, and poor cost-effectiveness.[34] Thus, each potentially disruptive technology must have its performance characteristics and cost-effectiveness evaluated in detail.

At the same time that new technologies have reached the marketplace and clinical availability, colonoscopy as a technology has improved dramatically. Probably the most important development has been the quality movement, with the development of the adenoma detection rate (ADR),[47] its validation,[13,14] and its increasingly widespread use.[48] Technical advances include high-definition optics[49] and alternative imaging platforms such as electronic chromoendoscopy,[50] the development of add-on mucosal exposure devices such as Endocuff Vision,[51–53] and the rapid emergence of artificial intelligence systems to assist detection,[54] and diagnosis.[55] Arguably, the advances in technology and quality of performance in colonoscopy can be seen in the relative courses of colonoscopy and computed tomography (CT) colonography or virtual colonoscopy. Two decades ago it seemed that CT colonography performance could essentially equal colonoscopy for detection of large polyps,[56] whereas recent trials consistently show colonoscopy resoundingly outperforming CT colonography, particularly for detection of flat and serrated lesions.[57,58]

Thus, although alternative screening approaches have appeared and continue to be developed, they have failed to rise to the level of disrupting screening colonoscopy particularly in the opportunistic setting. As colonoscopy technology continues to improve, colonoscopy, and particularly high-quality colonoscopy, is likely to set even higher performance bars. Eventually, this will result in protective intervals after negative colonoscopy that are longer than 10 years, longer post-polypectomy surveillance intervals for much of the adenoma cohort, and further reductions in CRC incidence and mortality.

ADVANTAGES AND DISADVANTAGES OF COLONOSCOPY AS A SCREENING STRATEGY
Advantages of Colonoscopy as a Screening Strategy

Colonoscopy has several significant advantages over other screening tests that have contributed substantially to its position as the dominant US CRC screening test (**Box 1**). First, it is widely recognized that it has unmatched performance for detection of precancerous lesions, and exceeds most other tests for detection of cancer. Although both physicians and patients in the United States tend to place undue importance on the significance of small and diminutive adenomas as potentially precancerous lesions, superiority of colonoscopy for detection of advanced nonmalignant lesions also exceeds all other screening tests.[34] Efficacy is widely viewed as an important attribute of colonoscopy. Second, the test is performed generally with sedation, and patients are more willing to repeat the test compared with unsedated flexible sigmoidoscopy.[59] The concept of evaluating only part of the colon in an unsedated setting is a concept that has led to the near disappearance of flexible sigmoidoscopy as a screening test in the United States.[60]

Box 1
Advantages and disadvantages of an average risk colorectal cancer screening test

Advantages:
- gold standard sensitivity for both adenomas and serrated class lesions
- single session diagnosis and treatment
- longest lasting protection against colorectal cancer

Disadvantages
- requires bowel preparation
- risk of complication associated with insertion (perforation, splenic injury)
- operator dependence
- high procedural charges, particularly by hospitals

Disadvantages of Colonoscopy as a Screening Strategy

A principal disadvantage of colonoscopy is the need for full bowel preparation. Many patients view bowel preparation for colonoscopy as the largest deterrent, including persons who have not previously undergone colonoscopy.[61] Low-volume preparations improve tolerability,[62] and the emergence in the near future of a safe pill-based preparation (based on sodium sulfate)[63] as well as for the future entry of bowel preparation incorporated into food products[64] hold promise for improving tolerability.

Colonoscopy also has the disadvantage of a higher complication rate for screening. Most bleeding complications are related to polypectomy, and therefore may not be avoidable by other screening strategies to the extent that they effectively identify advanced lesions, which account for a disproportionate percentage of post-polypectomy bleeding events because of their size. Cold snaring of lesions up to 1 cm in size,[65] abandonment of hot forceps for diminutive polyps,[66–69] the use of prophylactic clip closure for endoscopic mucosal resection defects ≥ 20 mm in size in or proximal to the hepatic flexure,[70,71] are important steps that can reduce complication rates. Diagnostic complications from colonoscope insertion, including rupture perforations of the rectosigmoid and splenic injuries are the most problematic.[72] Effective measures to reduce them include strict adherence to not pushing forcibly against fixed resistance, conversion from air to water filling whenever a difficult sigmoid colon is encountered to avoid barotrauma injury, and limited application of forceful torque in loop creation and reduction (to reduce splenic injury).

The operator dependence of colonoscopy technical performance is problematic. Systematic training in optimal detection and resection methods, widespread measurement and recording of ADR, and willingness of patients to investigate whether and what evidence of quality performance exists for a prospective colonoscopist can all contribute to reduced operator dependence.[34]

A fourth problem in US colonoscopy is high procedural charges, most often and most variable from hospital-based facility fees. Both private insurers and the federal government may charge copays or not based on whether a procedure is "preventive" or whether polypectomy is performed. In my experience, insurers consistently blame providers when patients complain about copays, and tell patients that their procedure was "coded wrong" or "not coded as preventive." There is no actual code for "preventive," and nearly all colonoscopic procedures (screening, surveillance, and diagnostic) are preventive procedures to the extent that they lead to removal of precancerous lesions. The policies place providers in the awkward situation of patients demanding procedures be labeled screening, even when they are clearly not screening procedures. Further, the concept of shifting costs to patients because a polyp was detected is particularly disingenuous. Although the American health care system may lead to some freedom of choice and wide availability of services, it lacks the price transparency characteristic of true markets. Further, hospitals are incentivized to establish ever larger health delivery systems that are essentially artificially fixed prices at levels far above costs. These are issues that clearly impact the real world cost-effectiveness of screening colonoscopy.

Box 1 summarizes the advantages and disadvantages of screening colonoscopy in the United States.

EVIDENCE THAT SCREENING COLONOSCOPY EFFECTIVELY REDUCES COLORECTAL CANCER AND RIGHT-SIDED COLON CANCER
Statement of the Problem

Currently, we already know that flexible sigmoidoscopy prevents left-sided colon cancer incident events and mortality based on randomized controlled trials comparing flexible sigmoidoscopy to no screening.[26,27,73,74] It seems reasonable to conclude that colonoscopy will also prevent left-sided cancer, but the issue of whether colonoscopy prevents right-sided cancer is critical because no randomized controlled trials of colonoscopy versus no screening or another screening test have yet been completed. What is the evidence that colonoscopy prevents incident CRC, and specifically prevents right-sided cancer (**Box 2**)?

Evidence from Flexible Sigmoidoscopy Randomized Trials

The US Prostate, Lung, Colorectal, and Ovary (PLCO) trial[27] used relatively liberal flexible sigmoidoscopy findings as an indication for colonoscopy. In the PLCO arm screened by flexible sigmoidoscopy, 22% of subjects were referred to colonoscopy, and the screened arm incurred a significant 14% reduction in the risk of right-sided cancer.[27] Other randomized trials with less liberal criteria for flexible sigmoidoscopy findings that would generate a colonoscopy, had a smaller percentage of patients in the screened arm undergo colonoscopy, and failed to demonstrate a reduction in right-sided cancer from flexible sigmoidoscopy screening.[26]

Adenoma Cohorts

Multiple adenoma cohorts have been shown to have a reduced incidence and mortality[75–82] from CRC after adenoma resection, and compared with reference populations, or to portions of the cohort with no adenomas. However, data are limited with regard to the risk of proximal versus distal cancer after adenoma resection.

Case-Control and Cohort Studies

A number of case-control and cohort studies[1,2,4–7,79,83–86] have evaluated the impact of colonoscopy on colorectal incidence and mortality, and often in a site-specific

---

Box 2
Types of evidence supporting effect of colonoscopy on colorectal cancer incidence and mortality (see text for references)

- US population trends in incidence and mortality
- reductions in right-sided cancer in flexible sigmoidoscopy trials
- incidence reductions in randomized trials of guaiac fecal occult blood testing
- incidence and mortality reductions in case-control studies
- studies of impact of variable detection on interval cancer incidence and mortality

ashion. Although original studies from Canada[6,83] did not identify a risk reduction in he right colon compared with the general population, studies from both the United States and Germany demonstrated ≥80% reduction in left-sided cancer and 40% o 60% reductions in right-sided cancer after colonoscopy.[1,4,5,7] Comparisons to he general population risk may not be the most informative, because colonoscoped populations often contain symptomatic patients with a higher baseline prevalence of CRC compared with the general population. Thus, case-control studies of screening populations have shown reductions of ≥80% in right-sided colon cancer risk[5] compared with the general population. Thus, case-control and cohort evidence indicates that high-quality screening colonoscopy is associated with a substantial reduction of both overall and right-sided CRCs.

Studies of Variable Performance

Studies on the impact of variable performance of colonoscopy and the risk of interval cancer also shed light on whether colonoscopy is generally effective. Thus, if colonoscopy in general does not impact the risk of CRC, then there should be no effect of variable performance on CRC risk. In fact, all studies of the impact of ADR on interval cancer risk have shown variation, with higher ADR associated with lower risk.[13–17] In particular, in the study with the greatest number of interval cancers, ADR had a similar impact on the risk of both proximal and distal CRC.[14] Collectively, these data strongly indicate that colonoscopy and polypectomy effectively reduce CRC incidence, including in the right colon. They render the concept of a screening trial of colonoscopy to no colonoscopy moot from the perspective of whether colonoscopy is effective, although the magnitude of the impact remains uncertain. Further, it remains uncertain whether super high detection of both adenomas and serrated lesions can eliminate or all but eliminate subsequent CRC risk. Certainly, there could be particularly biologically aggressive cancers, for example, signet ring cell cancers and certain poorly differentiated cancers that would defy prevention by even the most careful colonoscopy performed at long intervals.

All of the studies cited previously reflect average performance of colonoscopy. In some instances, average performance appears better in some countries than others. Thus, studies from the United States and Germany have consistently shown better protection against right colon cancer[1,4,5,7,84] than was achieved in initial studies from Canada. Within Canada, however, there is evidence that endoscopists with higher cecal intubation rates protect against right-sided colon cancer better than those with low cecal intubation rates,[87] and that gastroenterologists provide better protection than surgeons.[88] Indeed, within the United States, there is evidence that gastroenterologists have higher ADRs[89] and provide better cancer protection than nongastroenterologists.[1,90,91] This means there is still a substantial opportunity for better cancer protection through continuous quality improvement in colonoscopy. If the operator dependence of colonoscopy can be reduced by quality improvement, the protective effect of colonoscopy will be increased. This will create the potential and eventually the recommendation for longer intervals between normal screening examinations, such as 15 to 20 years, or potentially once-in-a-lifetime examinations. Longer intervals between screening and surveillance examinations will further enhance the cost-effectiveness of colonoscopy relative to other screening tests, which for the foreseeable future will almost certainly continue to require repeat testing at much shorter intervals. Several developments that could further enhance the effectiveness and cost-effectiveness of colonoscopy are described in the following section.

POTENTIAL ROUTES TO IMPROVED EFFECTIVENESS AND COST-EFFECTIVENESS OF SCREENING COLONOSCOPY

Change Financial Incentives for Colonoscopy

Currently, financial incentives for the performance of colonoscopy are obviously ineffective at enhancing quality. Colonoscopists in the United States are rewarded for removing the first polyp, and for performing colonoscopy without reference to their ADRs, and for performing colonoscopy frequently. Alternative approaches would be to pay endoscopists on a scaled rate according to their ADR. To enhance specificity payment would be made only for confirmed adenomas, sessile serrated polyps, or traditional serrated adenomas, or in a resect and discard paradigm for photographically documented precancerous lesions.[92] Polypectomy would not be paid for the removal of ≤5 mm hyperplastic polyps. Surveillance intervals would be stratified according to ADR. Thus, an endoscopist with an ADR ≥45% would be allowed to bring patients with 1 to 2 diminutive adenomas back in 10 to 15 years. The cost savings to payers for fewer colonoscopies would easily overcome increased payments based on ADR. Endoscopists would be incentivized to increase ADR, and expand surveillance intervals. Consistent use of appropriate screening and surveillance intervals would be rewarded by payers.

Public Education and Transparency

Although resources are available to facilitate patients acquiring an effective colonoscopy, and the US Multi-Society Task Force recommended that patients should ask their colonoscopist for their ADR,[35] anecdotal experience is that patients seldom do this. Almost certainly, patients are either unaware of the need to ask for an ADR, or they are unwilling to ask because of fear of negative reactions from the physician or other health care workers. Although asking about ADR is certainly encouraged, an alternative is to ask that the examination be video recorded, and a copy given to the patient to allow quality review. Another approach is for groups to publish the ADRs of individual endoscopists on a public Web site.[93] This type of exposure also improves endoscopist performance.[93]

Artificial Intelligence

Artificial intelligence (AI) programs that enhance detection[54] and allow endoscopic prediction of histology[55] have been developed and are likely to be clinically available in the near future. Initial detection programs highlight lesions exposed by the endoscopist. Ensuring effective exposure of mucosa on the proximal sides of folds could be facilitated by AI. This may require tracking of individual folds, recognition of shadowing by the fold, and real-time insistence on mucosal exposure of the proximal side of each tracked fold. The potential of combined polyp detection with mucosal exposure tracking has enormous implications for reducing the operator dependence of colonoscopic detection.

Expanded Intervals

There is already evidence that average colonoscopic performance of colonoscopy in Germany, and reasonable performance of colonoscopy in Poland, is associated with substantial reductions in CRC risk, extending to 15 to 20 years.[8] As noted previously, expansion of both intervals for screening colonoscopy in average-risk persons, and expansion of surveillance intervals in the low-risk adenoma cohort, when combined with high-quality detection, is associated with tremendous potential to improve the cost-effectiveness and appeal of colonoscopy.

SUMMARY

Screening colonoscopy remains the dominant screening strategy in the United States, partly because of its already high penetrance in the age-eligible screening population, but also because opportunistic screening is much more widespread in the United States than organized screening. Outside of organized screening, adherence to strategies that require repeated application at short intervals is quite difficult. Thus far, technical advances, such as the emergence of FIT, FIT-fecal DNA, and the first blood-based test for CRC screening, have been insufficiently effective or cost-effective to disrupt colonoscopy in any setting, particularly in the opportunistic setting. In the opportunistic setting, sequential offers of screening with colonoscopy first, and FIT reserved for patients who decline colonoscopy, remains an excellent approach to maximize application of the most effective single time test (colonoscopy) and simultaneously maximize adherence rates to screening. The position of screening colonoscopy relative to other screening strategies has been enhanced by widespread application of quality improvement measures and intense investigation and introduction of enhanced imaging platforms and mucosal exposure tools.

Additional gains in cancer prevention are expected based on further technical improvements in colonoscopy, the introduction of AI into lesion detection and mucosal exposure evaluation, and could be further enhanced by aligning financial incentives for colonoscopy with quality goals. Public education efforts beyond the budgets of gastrointestinal professional societies could substantially enhance patient demand for quality colonoscopy.

These factors, combined with the anticipated potential for expanded screening and surveillance intervals, underlie why colonoscopy remains a cornerstone of screening in the United States, and has the potential to remain so for the foreseeable future.

REFERENCES

1. Baxter NN, Warren JL, Barrett MJ, et al. Association between colonoscopy and colorectal cancer mortality in a US cohort according to site of cancer and colonoscopist specialty. J Clin Oncol 2012;30:2664–9.
2. Kahi CJ, Imperiale TF, Juliar BE, et al. Effect of screening colonoscopy on colorectal cancer incidence and mortality. Clin Gastroenterol Hepatol 2009;7:770–5 [quiz: 711].
3. Brenner H, Chang-Claude J, Seiler CM, et al. Protection from colorectal cancer after colonoscopy: a population-based, case-control study. Ann Intern Med 2011;154:22–30.
4. Doubeni CA, Weinmann S, Adams K, et al. Screening colonoscopy and risk for incident late-stage colorectal cancer diagnosis in average-risk adults: a nested case-control study. Ann Intern Med 2013;158:312–20.
5. Brenner H, Chang-Claude J, Jansen L, et al. Reduced risk of colorectal cancer up to 10 years after screening, surveillance, or diagnostic colonoscopy. Gastroenterology 2014;146:709–17.
6. Baxter NN, Goldwasser MA, Paszat LF, et al. Association of colonoscopy and death from colorectal cancer. Ann Intern Med 2009;150:1–8.
7. Nishihara R, Wu K, Lochhead P, et al. Long-term colorectal-cancer incidence and mortality after lower endoscopy. N Engl J Med 2013;369:1095–105.
8. Pilonis ND, Franczyk R, Wieszczy P, et al. 571-The predictive value of a high-quality single negative screening colonoscopy exceeds 15 years. Gastroenterology 2019;156. S-112–S-113.

9. Barclay RL, Vicari JJ, Doughty AS, et al. Colonoscopic withdrawal times and adenoma detection during screening colonoscopy. N Engl J Med 2006;355: 2533–41.
10. Chen SC, Rex DK. Endoscopist can be more powerful than age and male gender in predicting adenoma detection at colonoscopy. Am J Gastroenterol 2007;102: 856–61.
11. Imperiale TF, Glowinski EA, Juliar BE, et al. Variation in polyp detection rates at screening colonoscopy. Gastrointest Endosc 2009;69:1288–95.
12. Shaukat A, Oancea C, Bond JH, et al. Variation in detection of adenomas and polyps by colonoscopy and change over time with a performance improvement program. Clin Gastroenterol Hepatol 2009;7:1335–40.
13. Kaminski MF, Regula J, Kraszewska E, et al. Quality indicators for colonoscopy and the risk of interval cancer. N Engl J Med 2010;362:1795–803.
14. Corley DA, Jensen CD, Marks AR, et al. Adenoma detection rate and risk of colorectal cancer and death. N Engl J Med 2014;370:1298–306.
15. Shaukat A, Rector TS, Church TR, et al. Longer withdrawal time is associated with a reduced incidence of interval cancer after screening colonoscopy. Gastroenterology 2015;149:952–7.
16. Kaminski MF, Wieszczy P, Rupinski M, et al. Increased rate of adenoma detection associates with reduced risk of colorectal cancer and death. Gastroenterology 2017;153:98–105.
17. Lam A, Li Y, Gregory DL, et al. Sa1044 A comprehensive colonoscopy quality improvement program reduces interval colorectal cancer rates. Gastrointest Endosc 2019;89:AB151.
18. Siegel R, Desantis C, Jemal A. Colorectal cancer statistics, 2014. CA Cancer J Clin 2014;64:104–17.
19. Siegel RL, Torre LA, Soerjomataram I, et al. Global patterns and trends in colorectal cancer incidence in young adults. Gut 2019;68:2179–85.
20. Siegel RL, Fedewa SA, Anderson WF, et al. Colorectal cancer incidence patterns in the United States, 1974-2013. J Natl Cancer Inst 2017;109. https://doi.org/10.1093/jnci/djw322.
21. Wolf AMD, Fontham ETH, Church TR, et al. Colorectal cancer screening for average-risk adults: 2018 guideline update from the American Cancer Society. CA Cancer J Clin 2018;68:250–81.
22. Mandel JS, Bond JH, Church TR, et al. Reducing mortality from colorectal cancer by screening for fecal occult blood. Minnesota Colon Cancer Control Study. N Engl J Med 1993;328:1365–71.
23. Hardcastle JD, Chamberlain JO, Robinson MH, et al. Randomised controlled trial of faecal-occult-blood screening for colorectal cancer. Lancet 1996;348:1472–7.
24. Kronborg O, Fenger C, Olsen J, et al. Randomised study of screening for colorectal cancer with faecal-occult-blood test. Lancet 1996;348:1467–71.
25. Holme O, Bretthauer M, Fretheim A, et al. Flexible sigmoidoscopy versus faecal occult blood testing for colorectal cancer screening in asymptomatic individuals. Cochrane Database Syst Rev 2013:CD009259. https://doi.org/10.1002/14651858. CD009259.pub2.
26. Atkin WS, Edwards R, Kralj-Hans I, et al. Once-only flexible sigmoidoscopy screening in prevention of colorectal cancer: a multicentre randomised controlled trial. Lancet 2010;375:1624–33.
27. Schoen RE, Pinsky PF, Weissfeld JL, et al. Colorectal-cancer incidence and mortality with screening flexible sigmoidoscopy. N Engl J Med 2012;366:2345–57.

28. Brenner H, Stock C, Hoffmeister M. Effect of screening sigmoidoscopy and screening colonoscopy on colorectal cancer incidence and mortality: systematic review and meta-analysis of randomised controlled trials and observational studies. BMJ 2014;348:g2467.

29. Shaukat A, Robertson DJ, Dominitz J. CONFIRM-comparing colonoscopy and fecal occult testing. JAMA Intern Med 2017;177:889–90.

30. Quintero E, Castells A, Bujanda L, et al. Colonoscopy versus fecal immunochemical testing in colorectal-cancer screening. N Engl J Med 2012;366:697–706.

31. Rabeneck L, Chiu HM, Senore C. International perspective on the burden of colorectal cancer and public health effects. Gastroenterology 2019. https://doi.org/10.1053/j.gastro.2019.10.007.

32. Robertson DJ, Lee JK, Boland CR, et al. Recommendations on fecal immunochemical testing to screen for colorectal neoplasia: a consensus statement by the US Multi-Society Task Force on colorectal cancer. Gastrointest Endosc 2017;85:2–21.e3.

33. Imperiale TF, Ransohoff DF, Itzkowitz SH, et al. Multitarget stool DNA testing for colorectal-cancer screening. N Engl J Med 2014;370:1287–97.

34. Rex DK, Boland CR, Dominitz JA, et al. Colorectal cancer screening: recommendations for physicians and patients from the U.S. Multi-Society Task Force on Colorectal Cancer. Gastrointest Endosc 2017;86:18–33.

35. Naber SK, Knudsen AB, Zauber AG, et al. Cost-effectiveness of a multitarget stool DNA test for colorectal cancer screening of Medicare beneficiaries. PLoS One 2019;14:e0220234.

36. Joseph DA, King JB, Richards TB, et al. Use of colorectal cancer screening tests by state. Prev Chronic Dis 2018;15:E80.

37. Berkowitz Z, Zhang X, Richards TB, et al. Multilevel small-area estimation of colorectal cancer screening in the United States. Cancer Epidemiol Biomarkers Prev 2018;27:245–53.

38. Levin TR, Corley DA, Jensen CD, et al. Effects of organized colorectal cancer screening on cancer incidence and mortality in a large community-based population. Gastroenterology 2018;155:1383–91.e5.

39. Liang PS, Wheat CL, Abhat A, et al. Adherence to competing strategies for colorectal cancer screening over 3 years. Am J Gastroenterol 2016;111:105–14.

40. Inadomi JM, Vijan S, Janz NK, et al. Adherence to colorectal cancer screening: a randomized clinical trial of competing strategies. Arch Intern Med 2012;172:575–82.

41. Mehta SJ, Induru V, Santos D, et al. Effect of sequential or active choice for colorectal cancer screening outreach: a randomized clinical trial. JAMA Netw Open 2019;2:e1910305.

42. US Preventive Services Task Force, Bibbins-Domingo K, Grossman DC, Curry SJ, et al. Screening for colorectal cancer: US Preventive Services Task Force recommendation statement. JAMA 2016;315:2564–75.

43. Segnan N, Senore C, Andreoni B, et al. Randomized trial of different screening strategies for colorectal cancer: patient response and detection rates. J Natl Cancer Inst 2005;97:347–57.

44. Multicentre Australian Colorectalneoplasia Screening (MACS) Group. A comparison of colorectal neoplasia screening tests: a multicentre community-based study of the impact of consumer choice. Med J Aust 2006;184:546–50.

45. Scott RG, Edwards JT, Fritschi L, et al. Community-based screening by colonoscopy or computed tomographic colonography in asymptomatic average-risk subjects. Am J Gastroenterol 2004;99:1145–51.

46. Ladabaum U, Mannalithara A. Comparative effectiveness and cost effectiveness of a multitarget stool DNA test to screen for colorectal neoplasia. Gastroenterology 2016;151:427–39.e6.

47. Rex DK, Bond JH, Winawer S, et al. Quality in the technical performance of colonoscopy and the continuous quality improvement process for colonoscopy: recommendations of the U.S. Multi-Society Task Force on Colorectal Cancer. Am J Gastroenterol 2002;97:1296–308.

48. Peng M, Rex DK. Surveying ADR knowledge and practices among US gastroenterologists. J Clin Gastroenterol 2019. https://doi.org/10.1097/MCG.0000000000001188.

49. Subramanian V, Mannath J, Hawkey CJ, et al. High definition colonoscopy vs standard video endoscopy for the detection of colonic polyps: a meta-analysis. Endoscopy 2011;43:499–505.

50. Atkinson NSS, Ket S, Bassett P, et al. Narrow-band imaging for detection of neoplasia at colonoscopy: a meta-analysis of data from individual patients in randomized controlled trials. Gastroenterology 2019;157:462–71.

51. Chin M, Karnes W, Jamal MM, et al. Use of the Endocuff during routine colonoscopy examination improves adenoma detection: a meta-analysis. World J Gastroenterol 2016;22:9642–9.

52. Rex DK, Slaven JE, Garcia J, et al. Endocuff vision reduces inspection time without decreasing lesion detection in a randomized colonoscopy trial. Clin Gastroenterol Hepatol 2019. https://doi.org/10.1016/j.cgh.2019.01.015.

53. von Figura G, Hasenohrl M, Haller B, et al. Endocuff vision-assisted vs. standard polyp resection in the colorectum (the EVASTA study): a prospective randomized study. Endoscopy 2019. https://doi.org/10.1055/a-1018-1870.

54. Wang P, Berzin TM, Glissen Brown JR, et al. Real-time automatic detection system increases colonoscopic polyp and adenoma detection rates: a prospective randomised controlled study. Gut 2019;68:1813–9.

55. Byrne MF, Chapados N, Soudan F, et al. Real-time differentiation of adenomatous and hyperplastic diminutive colorectal polyps during analysis of unaltered videos of standard colonoscopy using a deep learning model. Gut 2019;68:94–100.

56. Pickhardt PJ, Choi JR, Hwang I, et al. Computed tomographic virtual colonoscopy to screen for colorectal neoplasia in asymptomatic adults. N Engl J Med 2003;349:2191–200.

57. IJspeert J, Tutein Nolthenius CJ, Kuipers EJ, et al. CT-colonography vs. colonoscopy for detection of high-risk sessile serrated polyps. Am J Gastroenterol 2016;111:516–22.

58. Cash BD, Fleisher MR, Fern S, et al. 479 a multicenter, prospective, randomized study comparing the diagnostic yield of colon capsule endoscopy versus computed tomographic colonography in a screening population. Results of the Topaz study. Gastrointest Endosc 2019;89:AB87–8.

59. Zubarik R, Ganguly E, Benway D, et al. Procedure-related abdominal discomfort in patients undergoing colorectal cancer screening: a comparison of colonoscopy and flexible sigmoidoscopy. Am J Gastroenterol 2002;97:3056–61.

60. Klabunde CN, Joseph DA, King JB, et al. Vital signs: colorectal cancer screening test use - United States, 2012. MMWR Morb Mortal Wkly Rep 2013;62:881–8.

61. Nicholson FB, Korman MG. Acceptance of flexible sigmoidoscopy and colonoscopy for screening and surveillance in colorectal cancer prevention. J Med Screen 2005;12:89–95.
62. Hassan C, East J, Radaelli F, et al. Bowel preparation for colonoscopy: European Society of Gastrointestinal Endoscopy (ESGE) Guideline - Update 2019. Endoscopy 2019;51:775–94.
63. Yang HJ, Park DI, Park SK, et al. Novel sulfate tablet PBK-1701TC versus oral sulfate solution for colon cleansing: a randomized phase 3 trial. J Gastroenterol Hepatol 2019. https://doi.org/10.1111/jgh.14826.
64. Rex DK, Levy CL, Bensen S, et al. Edible colon preparation shows excellent efficacy, safety and tolerability in a phase 2, randomized trial. Am J Gastroenterol 2016;111:S105.
65. Rex DK, Dekker E. How we resect colorectal polyps <20 mm in size. Gastrointest Endosc 2019;89:449–52.
66. Peluso F, Goldner F. Follow-up of hot biopsy forceps treatment of diminutive colonic polyps. Gastrointest Endosc 1991;37:604–6.
67. Komeda Y, Kashida H, Sakurai T, et al. Removal of diminutive colorectal polyps: a prospective randomized clinical trial between cold snare polypectomy and hot forceps biopsy. World J Gastroenterol 2017;23:328–35.
68. Weston AP, Campbell DR. Diminutive colonic polyps: histopathology, spatial distribution, concomitant significant lesions, and treatment complications. Am J Gastroenterol 1995;90:24–8.
69. Metz AJ, Moss A, McLeod D, et al. A blinded comparison of the safety and efficacy of hot biopsy forceps electrocauterization and conventional snare polypectomy for diminutive colonic polypectomy in a porcine model. Gastrointest Endosc 2013;77:484–90.
70. Pohl H, Grimm IS, Moyer MT, et al. Clip closure prevents bleeding after endoscopic resection of large colon polyps in a randomized trial. Gastroenterology 2019;157:977–84.e3.
71. Albeniz E, Alvarez MA, Espinos JC, et al. Clip closure after resection of large colorectal lesions with substantial risk of bleeding. Gastroenterology 2019;157:1213–21.e4.
72. Rex DK. Colonoscopic splenic injury warrants more attention. Gastrointest Endosc 2013;77:941–3.
73. Segnan N, Armaroli P, Bonelli L, et al. Once-only sigmoidoscopy in colorectal cancer screening: follow-up findings of the Italian Randomized Controlled Trial–SCORE. J Natl Cancer Inst 2011;103:1310–22.
74. Hoff G, Grotmol T, Skovlund E, et al. Risk of colorectal cancer seven years after flexible sigmoidoscopy screening: randomised controlled trial. BMJ 2009;338:b1846.
75. Winawer SJ, Zauber AG, Ho MN, et al. Prevention of colorectal cancer by colonoscopic polypectomy. The National Polyp Study Workgroup. N Engl J Med 1993;329:1977–81.
76. Loberg M, Kalager M, Holme O, et al. Long-term colorectal-cancer mortality after adenoma removal. N Engl J Med 2014;371:799–807.
77. Zauber AG, Winawer SJ, O'Brien MJ, et al. Colonoscopic polypectomy and long-term prevention of colorectal-cancer deaths. N Engl J Med 2012;366:687–96.
78. Click B, Pinsky PF, Hickey T, et al. Association of colonoscopy adenoma findings with long-term colorectal cancer incidence. JAMA 2018;319:2021–31.

79. Lee JK, Jensen CD, Levin TR, et al. Long-term risk of colorectal cancer and related death after adenoma removal in a large, community-based population. Gastroenterology 2019. https://doi.org/10.1053/j.gastro.2019.09.039.

80. Cottet V, Jooste V, Fournel I, et al. Long-term risk of colorectal cancer after adenoma removal: a population-based cohort study. Gut 2012;61:1180–6.

81. Coleman HG, Loughrey MB, Murray LJ, et al. Colorectal cancer risk following adenoma removal: a large prospective population-based cohort study. Cancer Epidemiol Biomarkers Prev 2015;24:1373–80.

82. Wieszczy P, Kaminski MF, Franczyk R, et al. Colorectal cancer incidence and mortality after removal of adenomas during screening colonoscopies. Gastroenterology 2019. https://doi.org/10.1053/j.gastro.2019.09.011.

83. Singh H, Nugent Z, Demers AA, et al. The reduction in colorectal cancer mortality after colonoscopy varies by site of the cancer. Gastroenterology 2010;139: 1128–37.

84. Samadder NJ, Pappas L, Boucherr KM, et al. Long-term colorectal cancer incidence after negative colonoscopy in the state of Utah: the effect of family history. Am J Gastroenterol 2017;112:1439–47.

85. Mulder SA, van Soest EM, Dieleman JP, et al. Exposure to colorectal examinations before a colorectal cancer diagnosis: a case-control study. Eur J Gastroenterol Hepatol 2010;22:437–43.

86. Singh H, Nugent Z, Mahmud SM, et al. Predictors of colorectal cancer after negative colonoscopy: a population-based study. Am J Gastroenterol 2010;105: 663–73 [quiz: 674].

87. Baxter NN, Sutradhar R, Forbes SS, et al. Analysis of administrative data finds endoscopist quality measures associated with postcolonoscopy colorectal cancer. Gastroenterology 2011;140:65–72.

88. Rabeneck L, Paszat LF, Saskin R. Endoscopist specialty is associated with incident colorectal cancer after a negative colonoscopy. Clin Gastroenterol Hepatol 2010;8:275–9.

89. Ko CW, Dominitz JA, Green P, et al. Specialty differences in polyp detection, removal, and biopsy during colonoscopy. Am J Med 2010;123:528–35.

90. Rex DK, Rahmani EY, Haseman JH, et al. Relative sensitivity of colonoscopy and barium enema for detection of colorectal cancer in clinical practice. Gastroenterology 1997;112:17–23.

91. Hassan C, Rex DK, Zullo A, et al. Loss of efficacy and cost-effectiveness when screening colonoscopy is performed by nongastroenterologists. Cancer 2012; 118:4404–11.

92. Rex DK, Hardacker K, MacPhail M, et al. Determining the adenoma detection rate and adenomas per colonoscopy by photography alone: proof-of-concept study. Endoscopy 2015;47:245–50.

93. Abdul-Baki H, Schoen RE, Dean K, et al. Public reporting of colonoscopy quality is associated with an increase in endoscopist adenoma detection rate. Gastrointest Endosc 2015;82:676–82.

Quality in Colorectal Cancer Screening with Colonoscopy

Philip Schoenfeld, MD, MSEd, MSc (Epi)*

KEYWORDS

- Quality indicators • Colonoscopy • Screening • Colon cancer

KEY POINTS

- In order to improve the effectiveness of colorectal cancer (CRC) screening with colonoscopy, appropriate quality indicators must be measured. These measures are associated with important outcomes, quantifiable, show variable performance among endoscopists, and can be improved with education.
- There is overuse of colonoscopy for CRC screening and colon polyp surveillance in low-risk patients. Therefore, the most important preprocedure quality indicator is frequency of scheduling colonoscopy at appropriate interval based on current guidelines.
- Adenoma detection rate (ADR) is the most important intraprocedure quality indicator because it is most closely associated with decreases in interval CRC. Mean withdrawal time greater than 6 minutes is associated with higher ADR.
- Postprocedure recommendations for timing of repeat colonoscopy are frequently shorter than recommended by guidelines. Providing guideline-consistent recommendation in greater than or equal to 90% of cases is the most important postprocedure quality indicator.

INTRODUCTION

Ultimately, the purpose of colorectal cancer (CRC) screening with colonoscopy is to prevent CRC while minimizing risks and costs for the patient. There are multiple strategies to meet these goals, which will be addressed in this article. These strategies emphasize the measurement of specific quality indicators. Why is this so important? To quote Peter Drucker, one of the great thinkers about business management, "If you can't measure it, then you can't improve it."

If we want to improve, then we must quantitatively measure our performance. Then, we can identify areas for improvement and implement appropriate strategies to meet numeric targets. It is not easy to create an environment focused on quality improvement. Many of the quality indicators described in this article are cumbersome to measure, and implementing protocols to improve may be hard to do. However, as a group,

Gastroenterology Section, John D. Dingell VA Medical Center, 4646 John R Street, Detroit, MI 48201, USA
* Corresponding author.
E-mail address: gidoc48105@gmail.com

Gastrointest Endoscopy Clin N Am 30 (2020) 541–551
https://doi.org/10.1016/j.giec.2020.02.014
1052-5157/20/Published by Elsevier Inc.

we need to do this because the evidence is quite clear that quality improvement facilitates our goal to minimize CRC with colonoscopy while minimizing costs and risks for the patient.

METHODOLOGY

The information in this article relies heavily on the multisociety position statement on "Quality Indicators for Colonoscopy,"[1] which I coauthored. Using this document, a list of quality indicators focused on colonoscopy for CRC screening in average-risk individuals, and colon polyp surveillance was created (**Box 1**). No new quality indicators are proposed in this article, although new data about measurement, quality improvement, and implementation strategies are discussed and referenced. Additional references are limited to position statements or guidelines from professional societies, which contain most of the existing data about quality indicators.[2–8] Quality indicators are stratified as preprocedure, intraprocedure, or postprocedure (see **Box 1**).

Most, but not all, of these quality indicators meet specific criteria. First, they are strongly associated with important outcomes (eg, prevention of CRC or decreasing

---

Box 1
Quality indicators for colorectal cancer screening/surveillance with colonoscopy

1. Informed consent is obtained, including discussions of risks associated with colonoscopy, and fully documented. Target greater than 98% of cases.

2. Colonoscopy is performed at the appropriate interval based on recommended postpolypectomy or post-CRC surveillance interval or 10-year interval between screening colonoscopy in average-risk patients with a normal complete colonoscopy and an adequate bowel cleansing. Target is greater than or equal to 90% of cases.

3. Adequate bowel preparation is achieved in order to follow recommended CRC screening or colon polyp surveillance intervals: Target is greater than or equal to 85% of cases. Quality of bowel preparation is documented. Target is greater than 98% of cases.

4. Cecum is intubated with appropriate photographic documentation of appendiceal orifice and ileocecal valve. Target is greater than or equal to 95% of CRC screening/colon polyp surveillance cases.

5. Mean withdrawal time is greater than or equal to 6 minutes for CRC screening colonoscopies without any endoscopic intervention. Withdrawal time is documented regardless of endoscopic intervention or indication.

6. Frequency of adenoma detection in asymptomatic, average-risk individuals undergoing their first CRC screening colonoscopy. Target is greater than 25% of cases. When assessed by gender, target is greater than or equal to 30% in men and greater than or equal to in women.

7. Frequency of colon perforation is less than 1:1000 during colonoscopy for CRC screening or colon polyp surveillance. Frequency of clinically important postpolypectomy bleeding is less than 1:100.

8. Repeat colonoscopy is recommended at the appropriate interval based on recommended guidelines for CRC screening/colon polyp surveillance guidelines. Target is greater than or equal to 90% of cases.

This is not a comprehensive list. It has been modified to focus on quality indicators associated with performance of colonoscopy for CRC screening and surveillance.

Adapted from Rex DK, Schoenfeld P, Cohen J, et al. Quality indicators in Colonoscopy. Gastrointestinal Endoscopy 2015; 81: 31-53; with permission.

the frequency of unnecessary colonoscopies). Also, you can measure these outcomes, and available data suggest wide variation in endoscopist performance. Finally, endoscopist performance can be improved with multiple interventions.

PREPROCEDURE INDICATORS

"Informed consent is the physician's legal requirement to disclose information to his or her patient and enables the patient to understand, evaluate, and authorize a specific... intervention."[2] Informed consent should be another opportunity to ensure that the patient has the necessary information to make an appropriate decision and to ask questions. It should not be approached as another routine "paperwork" task that needs to be completed before colonoscopy. Although there is no single "right" way to obtain informed consent, the following discussion provides additional guidance to do this before colonoscopy for CRC screening/surveillance.

Per the American Society for Gastrointestinal Endoscopy (ASGE) position statements,[2,3] appropriate informed consent before all endoscopic procedures include discussion of (1) the patient's pertinent medical diagnosis and test results; (2) the nature of the proposed procedure; (3) the reason that the procedure is being recommended; (4) the benefits of the procedure; (5) *the risks and complications of the procedure, including the relative incidence and severity, that would be material to the patient's decision-making process*; (6) reasonable alternatives to the proposed procedure; and (7) the potential consequences if the colonoscopy is declined (ie, informed refusal). Discussion of the sedation plan is also part of informed consent unless a separate anesthesia provider is providing sedation.

Ideally, the informed consent form should be designed specifically for colonoscopy instead of a generic ambulatory surgery/endoscopy unit form. This facilitates discussion with the patient. The quality of informed consent may also be an important issue if a colonoscopy complication occurs. The section on postprocedure quality indicators discusses the relative incidence and severity of colonoscopy complications. Although the ASGE position statement states that it is preferable that the endoscopist obtains informed consent, state and local regulations may not require this. Informed consent, documented sedation plan, and preprocedure history and physical examination all must be performed and documented before the procedure.

Endoscopists should document if the patient had a previous colonoscopy; date of prior colonoscopies; and the number, size, and histology of polyps found on prior colonoscopies. By completing this step, the endoscopist demonstrates that colonoscopy for CRC screening or colon polyp surveillance is being performed at the appropriate time.

New guidelines on colon polyp surveillance were published by the US Multi-Society Task Force on Colorectal Cancer in 2020.[6] The most important change is for individuals with 1 to 2 small (<10 mm) adenomas. Recommendation for repeat colonoscopy has been changed from 5 to 10 years to 7 to 10 years. Thus, repeat colonoscopy should be recommended for no sooner than 7 years in these patients as long as a complete colonoscopy with adequate bowel preparation was performed at baseline. For patients with 3 to 4 small adenomas, the recommendation has been changed from 3 years to a range of 3 to 5 years. These changes reflect additional data that the presence of small adenomas increases the risk of CRC minimally compared with individuals with a normal screening colonoscopy.

This is an important quality indicator because colonoscopy is frequently performed sooner than needed in patients with 1 to 2 small adenomas, patients with small hyperplastic polyps, or patients with a normal screening colonoscopy. For example, based on Medicare database studies, approximately 24% of average-risk individuals get repeat screening colonoscopy less than 7 years after a normal colonoscopy.[9] Survey studies demonstrate that this overuse is frequently because endoscopists choose to ignore guideline recommendations. They think that recommended intervals between colonoscopies are too long.[10] As discussed in other chapters of this edition of Gastrointestinal Endoscopy Clinics, there is overwhelming data that recommended intervals between procedures are appropriate and that interval CRC is rare as long as a complete colonoscopy with adequate bowel preparation was performed.[4,5] Also, the cost-effectiveness of colonoscopy for CRC screening is lost if colonoscopy is performed too frequently, and this practice exposes patients to unnecessary risks as well as inconveniencing them and their drivers/escorts.[4,5]

In order to minimize overuse of colonoscopy, endoscopists should get prior colonoscopy reports from other providers when feasible before scheduling colonoscopies. This is an additional administrative task that makes quality improvement difficult, but it is not insurmountable. Nurses or medical assistants should carefully discuss prior colonoscopies with the patient before scheduling colonoscopies in the open access setting. Protocols should outline the nature of these questions and processes to obtain records of previous colonoscopies. In addition, prospective studies should assess the frequency of overuse. Further research is needed about barriers to improving compliance with guideline recommendations, development of effective interventions to improve performance, and strategies for widespread implementation.

INTRAPROCEDURE QUALITY INDICATORS FOR COLORECTAL CANCER SCREENING/SURVEILLANCE WITH COLONOSCOPY

Bowel preparation is discussed in detail in a separate chapter. Nevertheless, several aspects of bowel preparation as a quality indicator should be emphasized (**Box 2**). Per the multisociety position statement on bowel preparation, if a patient has inadequate bowel cleansing, then repeat colonoscopy should be performed in less than or equal to 1 year. If a patient has adequate bowel cleansing, then a guideline-adherent recommendation for timing of repeat colonoscopy should be given.[7]

This is important for several reasons. First, multiple studies[1,7] demonstrate that endoscopists frequently recommend shortened intervals when the bowel preparation is "fair" based on the Aronchick scale. Specifically, repeat colonoscopy is recommended in 5 years (instead of 10 years) among patients with a normal screening colonoscopy, and repeat colonoscopy is recommended in 3 years (instead of 5–10 years) among individuals with 1 to 2 small adenomas.[11,12] Intuitively, this is an understandable change. If the bowel cleansing is "fair" and visualization of colonic mucosa is obscured, then adenomas could be missed. Therefore, by repeating colonoscopy earlier, missed adenomas can be found and resected before they grow into a colon cancer. The fallacy here is that interval CRC usually occurs before the repeat colonoscopy even if it is scheduled at a shorter interval! Based on the best available data from Veterans Affairs (VA) Cooperative Study 380, most interval CRCs occur within 48 months in patients with a normal screening colonoscopy. Interval CRC most commonly occurs within 24 months among individuals who had only 1 to 2 small adenomas on initial colonoscopy.[13] This is because most interval CRCs seem to arise from flat, large ($\geq$1 cm) adenomas or serrated polyps in the right side of the colon. Thus, if the bowel preparation is not adequate, then colonoscopy should be repeated in less than or equal to 1 year. Unfortunately, insurance may not reimburse for the second colonoscopy. This is quite problematic, and I do not have a good solution for this.

Box 2
Bowel cleansing before colonoscopy

1. Use split-dose bowel preparation with the second dose administered 4 to 6 hours before colonoscopy.[a]

2. In healthy, nonconstipated individuals, no specific regimen demonstrates clinically important improvements in quality of bowel cleansing.

3. Institute patient navigation to improve quality of bowel cleansing.[b]

4. Validated scales (eg, Boston Bowel Preparation Scale) should be used to assess quality of bowel cleansing. This standardizes assessment of bowel cleansing quality.

5. If a patient has an inadequate bowel preparation, then a split-dose, 4 L PEG-ELS should be prescribed for the next colonoscopy. Two-day clear liquid diets have not shown efficacy in these patients.

6. Past history of inadequate bowel preparation, current opioid use, current tricyclic antidepressant use, obesity (BMI $\geq$35), diabetes mellitus, and current laxative use for chronic constipation are risk factors for inadequate bowel preparation. Split-dose, 4 L PEG-ELS should be used in individuals with multiple risk factors.

7. If a patient has an inadequate bowel preparation, then repeat colonoscopy should be performed in less than or equal to 1 year. If a patient has an adequate bowel preparation, then a guideline-adherent recommendation for timing of repeat colonoscopy should be given.

Abbreviations: BMI, body mass index; PEG-ELS, polyethylene glycol electrolyte lavage solution.
 [a] Same-day dosing of bowel preparation is also acceptable. This approach may be especially attractive to patients scheduled for afternoon colonoscopy.
 [b] Trained patient navigators interact with the patient at multiple points before colonoscopy. This includes provision of written and oral instructions in the individual's native language when the colonoscopy is scheduled. Written instructions include photos, cartoons, or other visual tools. Patient navigators contact the patient 2 or more times by phone or mail to reinforce instructions and to address preprocedure questions.

Adapted from Kothari ST, Huang RJ, Shaukat A, et al. ASGE Review of Adverse Events in Colonoscopy. Gastrointest Endosc 2019; 90: 863-76; with permission.

What defines an "adequate" bowel preparation? Past guidelines[1,4,6,7] have defined adequate bowel preparation as cleansing adequate to see polyps greater than 5 mm. This is a subjective assessment. Personally, I recommend instituting the Boston Bowel Preparation Scale (BBPS).[14] With this validated scale, the cleanliness of the right-side, left-side, and transverse colon are graded separately on a 0 to 3 scale. Minimal training is required to achieve reliable and reproducible scores for grading cleanliness of a bowel segment. Most importantly, BBPS scores of 0 or 1 are associated with an increased risk of missed adenomas.[15] Therefore, the BBPS defines an adequate bowel cleansing as a score of 2 or 3 in each segment of the colon.

Several interventions should be emphasized to minimize inadequate bowel preparation. First, split-dose bowel preparation is the most important intervention to improve bowel cleansing. By splitting the dose, residual stool and chyme are cleansed from the right side of the colon. Do not forget that the second dose of the bowel preparation should be administered 4 to 6 hours before the colonoscopy. If it is delivered 8 hours or more before the colonoscopy, then the advantages of split prep are lost. Second, based on randomized controlled trials, there are no clinically important differences in quality of bowel cleansing with different bowel preparations.[7] However, these studies usually excluded patients with risk factors for poor bowel cleansing. Therefore, endoscopists should provide more intensive bowel preparation for patients with risk factors. History of inadequate bowel preparation on prior colonoscopy has the largest risk, whereas history of chronic constipation with current laxative use, current opioid use, obesity (body mass index [BMI] $\geq$35), diabetes mellitus, current tricyclic antidepressant use, and Parkinson disease are a partial list of other risk factors. There is inadequate data to recommend any specific regimen for these high-risk patients. Personally, I recommend using split-dose, 4 L polyethylene glycol electrolyte lavage solution (PEG-ELS) in patients with multiple risk factors and a split-dose, 6 L PEG-ELS (4:2 split) in patients with a history of inadequate cleansing with 4 L PEG-ELS. There is no published data about the effectiveness of the commonly used 2-day clear liquid diet for these patients.

The importance of cecal intubation is straightforward. Failure to complete colonoscopy by intubating the cecum is associated with higher rates of interval CRC in the ascending colon and cecum. Appropriate cecal intubation is defined as passing the distal tip of the scope past the ileocecal valve. Simply being able to visualize the cecum while the colonoscope is in the ascending colon is insufficient. The entire cecal mucosa should be visualized, and identification of the ileocecal valve and appendiceal orifice should be documented in the procedure report. Although the colonoscope is in the cecum, a photo of the appendiceal orifice should be obtained. Although the colonoscope is in the ascending colon, a photo of the ileocecal valve should be obtained. This should be done in every case. Notably, photographs are especially helpful if a malpractice suit is brought because an interval CRC occurs, and it is alleged that the colonoscopy was not completed. When calculating the cecal intubation rate, colonoscopies that are terminated because of an inadequate bowel preparation and colonoscopies that were undertaken only for a therapeutic intervention (eg, dilation of a malignant stricture) should not be included in the calculation.

In the seminal study by Barclay and colleagues,[16] endoscopists with a mean withdrawal time less than 6 minutes had lower adenoma detection rates (ADR) versus endoscopists with a mean withdrawal time greater than or equal to 6 minutes. This is unsurprising because it takes time to carefully inspect the colonic mucosa. For this quality measure, withdrawal time is measured using CRC screening colonoscopies without any endoscopic intervention colonoscopies.

Although withdrawal time is an important quality indicator, a couple of points deserve emphasis. First, withdrawal time less than 6 minutes may be adequate in patients with excellent bowel cleansing and colon anatomy that makes it easy to visualize the colon (eg, short colons with small haustra). Nevertheless, there are numerous anecdotal reports where a withdrawal time less than 6 minutes was equated with substandard care in malpractice claims for interval CRC. Second, ADR is the quality indicator most closely associated with minimizing interval CRC. Therefore, if an endoscopist has a very high ADR (eg, 40%), then their mean withdrawal time is not as important. However, for endoscopists with an ADR less than 25%, ensuring that the withdrawal time is greater than or equal to 6 minutes for every case may be a helpful intervention.

ADR is the number of average-risk individuals with at least one adenoma identified on their first screening colonoscopy divided by the total number of average-risk individuals who get their first screening colonoscopy during a specific interval, which is usually 6 or 12 month. In the seminal study by Corley and colleagues,[17] endoscopists with ADR less than 20% were twice as likely to experience an interval CRC complication compared with endoscopists with ADR greater than 32%. Also, for each 1% increase in ADR, the risk of interval CRC decreased by 3%. Therefore, measuring ADR and reporting it to endoscopists is crucial to identify poor performers, to initiate

---

Box 3
Improving adenoma detection rates

1. Use split-dose bowel preparation to improve bowel cleansing.

2. Upgrade to wide-angle, high-definition colonoscopes and monitors.

3. Perform "second look" in right side of colon.

4. Consider increasing withdrawal time to 8 to 10 minutes[a].

5. Attach cap device to distal tip of colonoscope to improve visualization of colonic mucosa.

6. Start measuring ADR for all endoscopists in hospital or ambulatory endoscopy site. Publicly report mean ADR for group and privately (or publicly) report ADR for each individual at 6- or 12-month intervals.

[a] When using wide-angle, high-definition colonoscopes and monitors, there is conflicting data about the utility of increasing withdrawal time to 8 to 10 minutes.

---

interventions to improve their ADR (**Box 3**), and to determine if these endoscopists can improve and achieve an adequate ADR.

When using ADR as part of a quality improvement project, several points deserve further emphasis. Ideally, ADR should be calculated from average-risk individuals getting their *first* screening colonoscopy. If an individual has a normal screening colonoscopy, then this person is actually less than average risk when he/she gets a repeat screening colonoscopy in 10 years. Second, if a colonoscopy is aborted because of poor bowel cleansing or because the cecum could not be reached, then this colonoscopy should not be included in the denominator. Third, serrated polyps, which have an incidence of approximately 10%,[18] are not included in this calculation. In the future, a separate serrated polyp detection rate may be added because large flat serrated polyps in the right side of the colon may be missed and grow into interval CRCs. Fourth, there is minimal data about an appropriate ADR among patients who get colonoscopy because of a positive fecal immunochemical test (FIT), although these patients are clearly higher than average risk. A recent study from the Chinese University of Hong Kong found an ADR of 53.6% for FIT + patients compared with an ADR of 37.5% for average-risk screening colonoscopy patients.[19] Finally, we need better research to determine the implementation of ADR as a quality indicator in hospital settings and ambulatory endoscopy centers.

There is virtually no data about the use of ADR as a quality indicator across the United States. Many gastroenterologists struggle with implementing ADR into their practices because it requires manual entry of polyp histology results into spreadsheets. This is particularly unfortunate because an effective tool to improve ADRs is to simply calculate and report ADRs.[20] This occurs simply because of the Hawthorne effect: individuals will modify their behavior if they know that they are being observed. It is simply imperative for endoscopists and their endoscopic facilities to institute measurement and reporting of ADR.

POSTPROCEDURE QUALITY INDICATORS FOR COLORECTAL CANCER SCREENING/ SURVEILLANCE WITH COLONOSCOPY

Colon perforation rates and postpolypectomy bleeding are so infrequent that these quality indicators cannot be adequately tracked over time. A single colon perforation will substantially change an endoscopist's colon perforation rate for a 6- or 12-month interval. Therefore, it is preferable for each colon perforation or postpolypectomy bleeding case to be reviewed by an adverse event committee. This approach may identify interventions to minimize the risk of complications.

The ASGE Standards of Practice Committee recently published their review of adverse events in colonoscopy along with meta-analyses about the frequency of perforations and postpolypectomy bleeding.[8] These data are quite helpful because informed consent forms should include the relative incidence and severity of these complications.

In the ASGE review and associated meta-analyses, the pooled rate of colon perforation was 5.8 per 10,000 colonoscopies (95% confidence interval [CI]: 5.7–6.0). This equates to 1 colon perforation per 1724 colonoscopies. The population-level perforation rates ranged from 1.6 per 10,000 to 11.9 per 10,000. This significant heterogeneity likely reflects differences in the patient populations (eg, number of patients with inflammatory bowel disease or complicated colonic strictures), indications for the procedure, and variable rates of endoscopic interventions, such as endoscopic mucosal resection (EMR). The average-risk CRC screening and colon polyp surveillance population should be a low-risk population for perforation, so the incidence of colon perforation could be lowered to 1 in 1500. Patients who undergo EMR should be excluded from this calculation because the risk of perforation as well as postpolypectomy bleeding is substantially higher.

The pooled rate of bleeding was 2.4 per 1000 colonoscopies (95% CI: 5.7–6.0). This equates to 1 episode of bleeding per 416 colonoscopies. The risk increases by 2.7% for every 1% increase in polyp resection rate. Additional data indicate that the risk of bleeding is approximately 1 in 100 when polypectomy is performed and is 0.6 per 1000 colonoscopies when no polypectomy is performed. Risk factors for postpolypectomy bleeding, including number of polyps removed, recent use of warfarin or other antithrombotic agents, polyps in the right side of the colon, and use of cold-snare versus hot-snare polypectomy, may also increase the rate of postpolypectomy bleeding.

Endoscopists may be tempted to recommend inappropriately short intervals between colonoscopies for multiple reasons, including fear of malpractice suits. The frequency of this practice varies among endoscopists. Medicare database studies[9] demonstrate the systematic overuse of colonoscopy for screening and polyp surveillance by some physicians. This overuse is not necessarily due to financial incentives. Data from VA databases[21] also show 16% of patients with normal screening colonoscopies, 26% with 1 to 2 small (<10 mm) adenomas, and even 29% with high-risk adenomas (≥3 adenomas or adenoma ≥10 mm or adenoma with high grade dysplasia). Endoscopists should remember that more colonoscopy does not necessarily equate to better care. Colonoscopy is our primary tool, but we should remember a famous quote by Abraham Maslow: "If the only tool you have is a hammer, then it's tempting to treat everything as if it were a nail." Although endoscopists may be quite stubborn and continue to perform colonoscopy earlier than recommended, this practice exposes patients to serious risks and eliminates the cost-effectiveness of colonoscopy for CRC screening.

Additional interventions to monitor this quality indicator must be identified and implemented. This will be especially important with the publication of new guidelines on colon polyp surveillance.[6] The interval between colonoscopies has been extended from 5 to 10 years to 7 to 10 years for individuals with 1 to 2 small adenomas. Also, patients with 3 to 4 small adenomas can wait up to 5 years before getting repeat colonoscopy. These changes reflect additional data that the presence of small denomas increases the risk of CRC minimally compared with individuals with a normal screening colonoscopy.

QUALITY INDICATORS FOR COLONOSCOPY AND MALPRACTICE CLAIMS

I am frequently asked if adherence to quality indicators will be useful in defense against malpractice claims. Therefore, he is providing a few thoughts about this when colonoscopy is performed for CRC screening or colon polyp surveillance. However, this general discussion is NOT legal advice. If your goal is to minimize malpractice risks, then appropriate advice from a lawyer should be sought.

Interval CRC, commonly defined as diagnosis of CRC before the next scheduled colonoscopy, and colon perforation are 2 of the most common malpractice claims brought against endoscopists. A successful malpractice claim should demonstrate that the standard of care was not met AND that the patient suffered harm because of this. The standard of care is commonly defined as "the type and level of care an ordinary, prudent, health care professional, with the same training and experience, would provide under similar circumstances in the same community." Documentation of adherence to quality indicators may help show that the standard of care was met.

With respect to preprocedure quality indicators, here are a couple of potential pitfalls. First, if a colonoscopy perforation (or any clinically significant complication) occurs, then it will be important to demonstrate that the colonoscopy was performed at the appropriate interval based on guidelines. This includes making a reasonable effort to get reports from previous colonoscopies performed by other providers. Second, if your informed consent form describes interval CRC and colon perforation as potential risks, including the relative incidence and severity of these complications, then it is more difficult for the patient to argue that he/she was not adequately informed.

Adherence to intraprocedure quality indicators is most helpful when an interval CRC occurs. The mere occurrence of interval CRC does not equate to substandard care. Colonoscopy is not 100% perfect at preventing CRC and your informed consent should state that this is a potential adverse event. However, inadequate bowel cleansing, failure to reach the cecum, withdrawal times that are too fast, and substandard ability to identify and remove adenomas are all associated with low ADR, missed adenomas, or interval CRC. Therefore, if you document that the bowel cleansing was adequate, prove that you reached the cecum (with photo documentation), document your withdrawal time for each individual case, and demonstrate that your mean withdrawal time is greater than or equal to 6 minutes and your adenoma detection rate is greater than or equal to 25%, then it is difficult to prove that your colonoscopy did not meet the standard of care.

Do not forget that the withdrawal time can be less than 6 minutes in an individual patient with excellent bowel cleansing and colon anatomy that makes it easy to visualize the colon. However, the withdrawal time should still be close to 6 minutes. You should be able to document a mean withdrawal time greater than or equal to 6 minutes, so you cannot be accused of systematically rushing to withdraw the colonoscope. Unfortunately, despite this definition for appropriate withdrawal time, there are numerous anecdotal reports where a withdrawal time less than 6 minutes was equated with substandard care in malpractice claims.

For postprocedure quality indicators, making a guideline-adherent recommendation for timing of repeat colonoscopy is important. If you recommend repeat colonoscopy in 3 years for a patient with inadequate bowel preparation, then you will be at risk if the patient develops CRC before the next colonoscopy. Alternatively, if an individual only has a single diminutive adenoma and you recommend repeat colonoscopy in 3 years, then you could be at risk. If the patient has any complication during the colonoscopy, then it could be argued that the procedure was unnecessary and only performed because of your recommendation. Because the complications of colonoscopy, including colon perforation and postpolypectomy bleeding, are uncommon, it will be difficult to accurately quantify an endoscopist's complication rate unless there is a clear pattern of frequent adverse events.

SUMMARY

Again, the purpose of CRC screening with colonoscopy is to prevent CRC while minimizing risks and costs for the patient. Tens of thousands of colonoscopies are performed each year to reduce CRC, and the rates of CRC among individuals older than or equal to 50 years have decreased substantially. Nevertheless, as a profession we should strive for continuous quality improvement. Most of the quality indicators in this article are ideal. They can be easily measured. Endoscopists vary in their ability to reach the numeric targets. They are associated with clinically important outcomes such as interval CRC, and endoscopists can improve with educational interventions.

Again, as Peter Drucker stated, "if you can't measure it, then you can't improve it." We now have appropriate quality indicators. Measurement can be a cumbersome process, such as ADR calculation and ensuring that patients get repeat colonoscopy at the appropriate interval. That is not an adequate reason to hold off on implementation. Future research should quantify implementation of these measurements, barriers, and incentives to start measuring quality indicators and identify more and better interventions to improve.

DISCLOSURE

Dr P. Schoenfeld has served as a consultant, advisory board member, and member of the speaker's bureau for Salix Pharmaceuticals, Inc. The views and opinions of the author expressed herein do not necessarily reflect those of the Deparment of Veterans Affairs.

REFERENCES

1. Rex DK, Schoenfeld P, Cohen J, et al. Quality indicators in colonoscopy. GastrointestEndosc 2015;81:31–53.
2. ASGE Standards of Practice Committee. Informed consent for GI endoscopy. GastrointestEndosc 2007;66:213–8.
3. Rizk M, Sawhney M, Cohen J, et al. Quality indicators common to all GI endoscopic procedures. Am J Gastroenterol 2015;110:48–59.
4. Rex DK, Johnson DA, Anderson JA, et al. The American College of Gastroenterology guideline for colorectal cancer screening. Am J Gastroenterol 2009;104(3) 739–50.
5. Lin J, Piper M, Perdue L, et al. Screeningfor colorectal cancer. updated evidence report and systematic review for the US Preventive Services task force. JAMA 2016;315:2576–94.
6. Gupta S, Lieberman D, Anderson JC, et al. Recommendations for follow-up after colonoscopy and polypectomy: a consensus update by the US Multi-Society Task Force on Colorectal Cancer. Gastroenterology 2020;91(3):463–85.e5.

7. Johnson DA, Barkun A, Cohen L, et al. Optimizing adequacy of bowel cleansing for colonoscopy: recommendations from the US multi-society task force on colorectal cancer. Am J Gastroenterol 2014;109:1528–45.

8. Kothari ST, Huang RJ, Shaukat A, et al. ASGEreview of adverse events in colonoscopy. GastrointestEndosc 2019;90:863–76.

9. Goodwin JS, Singh A, Reddy N, et al. Overuse of screening colonoscopy in the Medicare population. Arch Intern Med 2011;171:1335–43.

10. Saini SD, Nayak RS, Kuhn L, et al. Why don't gastroenterologists follow colon polyp surveillance guidelines? Results of a national survey. J ClinGastroenterol 2009;43:554–8.

11. Menees S, Elliott E, Govani S, et al. The impact of bowel cleansing on follow-up recommendations in average-risk patients with a normal colonoscopy. Am J Gastroenterol 2014;109:148–54.

12. Menees S, Elliott EE, Govani S, et al. Adherence to recommended intervals for surveillance colonoscopy in average-risk patients with 1 to 2 small (< 1 cm) polyps on screening colonoscopy. GastrointestEndosc 2014;79:551–7.

13. Lieberman D, Sullivan B, Hauser E, et al. Baseline colonoscopy findings associated with 10-year outcomes in a screening cohort undergoing colonoscopy surveillance. Gastroenterology 2020. https://doi.org/10.1053/j.gastro.2019.07.052.

14. Calderwood A, Schroy P, Lieberman D, et al. Boston bowel preparation scale scores provide a standardized definition of adequate for describing bowel cleanliness. GastrointestEndosc 2014;80:269–76.

15. Kluge M, Williams J, Wu C, et al. Inadequate Boston bowel preparation Scale scores predict the risk of missed neoplasia on the next colonoscopy. GastrointestEndosc 2018;87:744–51.

16. Barclay RL, Vicari JJ, Doughty A, et al. Colonscopic withdrawal times and adenoma detection during screening colonoscopy. N Engl J Med 2006;355:2533–41.

17. Corley DA, Jensen CD, Marks AR, et al. Adenoma detection rate and risk of colorectal cancer and death. N Engl J Med 2014;370:1298–306.

18. Anderson JC, Butterly L, Weiss J, et al. Providing data for serrated polyp detection rate benchmarks: an analysis of the New Hampshire Colonoscopy Registry. GastrointestEndosc 2017;85:1188–94.

19. Wong JCT, Chiu HM, Kim HS, et al. Adenoma detection rates in colonoscopies for positive fecal immunochemical tests versus direct screening colonoscopies. GastrointestEndosc 2019;89:607–13.

20. Kahi CJ, Ballard D, Shah A, et al. Impact of a quarterly report card on colonoscopy quality measures. GastrointestEndosc 2013;77:925–31.

21. Murphy C, Sandler R, Grubber J, et al. Underuse and overuse of colonoscopy for repeat screening and surveillance in the Veterans Health Administration. ClinGastroenterolHepatol 2016;14:436–44.

Multitarget Stool DNA for Average Risk Colorectal Cancer Screening

Major Achievements and Future Directions

John B. Kisiel, MD[a],*, Jason D. Eckmann, MD[b],
Paul J. Limburg, MD[a]

KEYWORDS

- Colorectal neoplasms/prevention and control • Colorectal neoplasms/diagnosis
- DNA • Neoplasm/analysis • Early detection of cancer/methods
- Colonoscopy/trends • Proximal colorectal neoplasia
- Precancerous conditions/diagnosis

KEY POINTS

- Multitarget stool DNA testing has been endorsed by the US Preventative Services Task Force as a first-line colorectal cancer screening test.
- The number of providers prescribing multitarget stool DNA testing and the number of patients completing the test have increased exponentially since its approval by the US Food and Drug Administration and Centers for Medicare & Medicaid Services.
- Adherence to multitarget stool DNA testing is approximately 70%; patients with positive multitarget stool DNA test results have high diagnostic colonoscopy completion rates.
- Positive predictive value for colorectal neoplasia in postapproval studies is high.
- The US Food and Drug Administration expanded multitarget stool DNA approval for use in patients 45 to 49 years of age. Next-generation multitarget stool DNA test prototypes portend even higher specificity.

INTRODUCTION: COLORECTAL CANCER SCREENING SAVES LIVES BUT IS UNDERUSED

Colorectal cancer (CRC) is the second leading cause of cancer-related death in the United States; an estimated 51,000 fatal cases occurred in 2019.[1] Both the incidence

[a] Division of Gastroenterology and Hepatology, Mayo Clinic, 200 First Street, Southwest, Rochester, MN 55905, USA; [b] Department of Internal Medicine, Mayo Clinic, 200 First Street, Southwest, Rochester, MN 55905, USA
* Corresponding author.
E-mail address: Kisiel.john@mayo.edu
Twitter: @DrJohnKisiel (J.B.K.); @JasonEckmannMD (J.D.E.); @limburg_paul (P.J.L.)

Gastrointest Endoscopy Clin N Am 30 (2020) 553–568
https://doi.org/10.1016/j.giec.2020.02.008
1052-5157/20/© 2020 The Author(s). Published by Elsevier Inc. This is an open access article under the CC BY-NC-ND license (http://creativecommons.org/licenses/by-nc-nd/4.0/).

and mortality of this disease can be reduced by screening.[1] However, despite these demonstrated benefits, CRC screening remains underused; approximately one-third of the screen-eligible population report nonadherence with current guidelines.[2] To assist patients and clinicians toward greater CRC screening participation, several national organizations such as the US Preventive Services Task Force (USPSTF) and Multi-Society Task Force recommend endoscopic, radiologic, and stool-based CRC screening test strategies beginning at age 50.[3,4] More recently, the American Cancer Society (ACS) has provided a recommendation to begin CRC screening at age 45.[5]

Of the endorsed screening tests, colonoscopy is the most often used in the United States[2]; reasons for preference include the simultaneous diagnosis and intervention for colorectal neoplasia (CRN). From an operator perspective, screening colonoscopy has several aspects actively targeted for improvement, including the need to increase sensitivity in the proximal colon[6–12] and decrease interoperator variability in colonoscopy quality.[13–16] From a patient perspective, test invasiveness, risk of complications, and the inconvenience of preparation, sedation, and time away from work are commonly cited as barriers to use.[17] Noninvasive screening modalities are endorsed as an alternative to colonoscopy for use in average risk patients. Of noninvasive tests, only guaiac-based fecal occult blood testing has been shown in randomized controlled trials to reduce CRC-related mortality, with modest benefit.[18–21] Dietary and medication interactions, poor performance in the proximal colon, and low adherence to the required annual screening program have reduced the use of this test.[22–2] Fecal immunochemical testing (FIT) overcomes some but not all of these limitations, leading to its inclusion in screening guidelines.[3,4] Relative to colonoscopy, FIT still has reduced sensitivity for right-sided and sessile serrated precursor lesions,[22,23,2] and similar to fecal occult blood testing, there is persistent poor adherence to required annual testing.[24,26–29] Other invasive (flexible sigmoidoscopy) and noninvasive (computed tomography colonography) are less widely used.

The multitarget stool DNA (mt-sDNA) assay (Cologuard, Exact Sciences, Madison WI) is the most recently endorsed noninvasive option for average-risk CRC screening.[3–5] The mt-sDNA screening is completed at home and requires no cathartic preparation, dietary modification, or medication restriction. Since receiving simultaneous US Food and Drug Administration (FDA) and Centers for Medicare and Medicaid Services (CMS) approval in August 2014, use of mt-sDNA testing has become widespread. Here, we describe the preclinical scientific development supporting mt-sDNA, highlight important achievements and real-world evidence since approval, and provide an outlook on future directions for mt-sDNA in clinical practice.

PRECLINICAL EVIDENCE AND BIOLOGICAL RATIONALE SUPPORT NONINVASIVE SCREENING BY STOOL DNA

The effectiveness of CRC screening as a whole is the product of test sensitivity, compliance, and access. Noninvasiveness and home testing enhances both compliance and access. Optimized sensitivity of noninvasive testing is centered on 2 important biologic observations. First, whereas tumor-associated bleeding can be used to detect CRC, such bleeding is intermittent. Ahlquist and colleagues[30] showed decades ago that asymptomatic persons with CRC had wide variability in stool hemoglobin concentrations (**Fig. 1**A). In contrast with hemoglobin, neoplastic colonocytes are exfoliated into the colon lumen at a more continuous and predictable rate. These cells show increased proliferation, decreased apoptosis, and altered intercellular adhesion. Consistent with these observations, cytokeratin staining was used to show that exfoliated colonocytes were much more abundant in the mucocellular layer overlying CRC

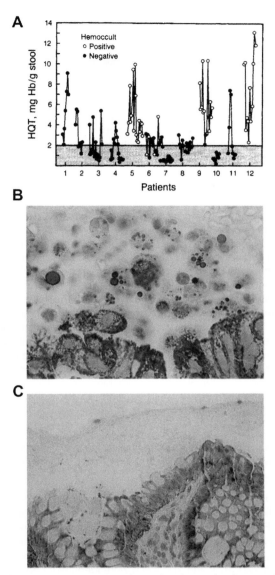

Fig. 1. Preclinical observations supporting the rationale to develop stool DNA testing. (*A*) Bleeding into stool from asymptomatic CRCs can be intermittent. (*B, C, cytokeratin immunostain*) Neoplastic cells and debris are continuously shed into the luminal mucocellular layer above (*B*) colon cancers and polyps, but not in (*C*) healthy control mucosae. HQT, HemoQuant. (*Adapted from* Ahlquist DA, McGill DB, Fleming JL, et al. Patterns of occult bleeding in asymptomatic colorectal cancer. Cancer 1989;63(9):1826-1830; and Ahlquist DA, Harrington JJ, Burgart LJ, et al. Morphometric analysis of the "mucocellular layer" overlying colorectal cancer and normal mucosa: relevance to exfoliation and stool screening. Human pathology 2000;31(1):51-57; with permission.)

tissue (**Fig. 1**B) compared with normal colorectal mucosa (**Fig. 1**C); tumor-exfoliated cells and cellular debris were also more consistently present in the mucocellular layer than erythrocytes.[31] Tumor-specific molecular features of CRN haven been widely studied and well-characterized over the last 4 decades. Of these, DNA abnormalities seemed to be the most stable in the harsh stool environment and were thus specifically targeted for noninvasive test development. Early attempts to develop a stool DNA panel assaying primarily mutations were limited by the heterogeneity of CRC.[32] However, DNA methylation-based panels were observed to be more broadly informative.[33]

For the mt-sDNA assay, marker selection studies ultimately led to a final panel that included DNA methylation (*NDRG4*, *BMP3*), DNA mutation (*KRAS*), and hemoglobin (by immunoassay) as well as a measure of total human DNA (*β-actin*) for clinical assay development.[34,35] To serve the needs of millions of screen-eligible persons, a high throughput automated assay system was designed. This system was tested in a multicenter case-control study of 93 CRC cases, 114 advanced precancerous lesions (APLs; adenomas with high-grade dysplasia, ≥25% villous features, or ≥1 cm in diameter; sessile serrated polyps ≥1 cm in diameter), and 796 healthy controls.[36] Quantitative output from the automated analytical platform was used to derive a multimarker logistic regression algorithm.

Locked-down and prespecified to the FDA before pivotal clinical testing, the mt-sDNA algorithm has 3 main components. The first is the logistic score, which is calculated from a logistic regression formula that uses group-level marker data to discriminate between patients with or without CRC or APLs. The second is the sum of scores, which combines the logistic score with individual marker scores to ensure that if the value from any DNA marker exceeds the 99.5th percentile among controls, the assay will yield a positive result. Third, there is a composite score, generated by subjecting the sum of scores to an exponential equation that generates an overall assay result ranging from 0 to 1000, with positive score threshold of 183 or greater. As designed and FDA approved, the mt-sDNA assay analysis platform does not provide independently interpretable marker data. This is because the algorithm yields higher sensitivity estimates than a single marker cutoff approach (positive assay result if ≥1 markers exceeds a set threshold) for both CRCs (98% vs 92%) and APLs (56% vs 49%).[36]

HIGH SENSITIVITY AND SPECIFICITY IN SCREENING STUDY SUPPORT US FOOD AND DRUG ADMINISTRATION AND CENTERS FOR MEDICARE AND MEDICAID SERVICES APPROVAL

The "DeeP-C" pivotal study (ClinicalTrials.gov identifier NCT01397747) was a cross-sectional investigation of mt-sDNA assay performance for the screening-setting detection of CRC and APLs in asymptomatic average risk persons, age 50 to 84, recruited from 90 sites in North America from June 2011 to November 2012.[37] Complete screening colonoscopy, mt-sDNA, and FIT data were available from 9989 participants. From these patients, 65 CRCs and 757 APLs were identified. Laboratory analyses and colonoscopy examinations were performed in blinded fashion, without prior knowledge of the comparator test results. Colonoscopy and associated histology were the reference standards for measurement of both mt-sDNA and FIT assay sensitivity and specificity. The primary outcome was to determine the sensitivity of mt-sDNA for CRC. The secondary outcomes included sensitivity for APL and noninferiority to FIT.

With respect to CRC detection, the sensitivity of the mt-sDNA assay both significantly exceeded the null hypothesis of 65% and was significantly higher than FIT (92.3% vs 73.8%; $P = .002$). Sensitivity for APLs was also higher in the mt-sDNA assay compared with FIT, both overall (42.4% vs 23.8%; $P<.001$) and in the APL subgroups of high-grade dysplasia (69.2% vs 46.2%; $P = .004$) and sessile serrated polyps greater than 1 cm in diameter (42.4% vs 5.1%; $P<.001$). Furthermore, mt-sDNA detection rates for highest risk polyp denominations by size increases proportionately

Fig. 2A). Specificities for the mt-sDNA assay and FIT were 87% and 95%, respectively, when non-advanced adenomas (AA) were considered among neoplasia negative results. Test specificity estimates made among patients with negative colonoscopy results were higher at 90% and 96%, respectively. It is important to emphasize that a point-in-time specificity of 90% for mt-sDNA translates into an annualized specificity of approximately 97% because the test is recommended at 3-year intervals, and this finding compares favorably with FIT specificity when test recommended each year. Additional supporting data for nonmarker assay components, technical specifications, and experiments detailing low cross-reactivity in stool samples from patients on various medications and other diseases, including cancers, can be found in the FDA Premarket Approval application (P130017).[38]

Based on these data and others, the FDA and CMS simultaneously approved the mt-sDNA in 2014; this medical device was the first to have completed the parallel approval process. As part of the FDA–CMS parallel review program, the CMS issued a National Coverage Determination, effective October 9, 2014, for mt-sDNA screening every 3 years in average-risk, asymptomatic, Medicare-eligible patients ages 50 to 85 years. The initial CMS reimbursement rate of $492.72 was set by CMS using a method that compared mt-sDNA with 3 existing tests on the Clinical Laboratory Fee Schedule. Subsequent CMS reimbursement is based on the volume-weighted median of private payer rates in accordance with the Protecting Access to Medicare Act of 2014.

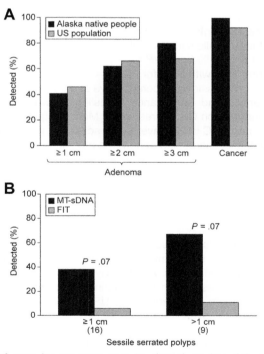

Fig. 2. Detection of CRN by mt-sDNA test in clinical studies. (*A*) mt-sDNA colorectal neoplasm detection rates by in the United States general and Alaska Native populations. (*B*) Comparison between mt-sDNA and FIT for sessile serrated polyp detection in Alaska Native people. (*Adapted from* Redwood DG, Asay ED, Blake ID, et al. Stool DNA Testing for Screening Detection of Colorectal Neoplasia in Alaska Native People. Mayo Clin Proc 2016;91(1):61-70; with permission.)

The test price of mt-sDNA also includes additional services beyond the collection processing, and reporting of the result. These include patient navigation support which has been shown to improve participation rates.[39,40] The patient navigation protocol begins with a telephone call from the support center describing mt-sDNA testing and sample collection. Next, a kit is mailed from Exact Sciences Laboratories (Madison, WI) to the patient. Until the kit is returned, telephone and mailed reminders are provided up to 3 times during the first 30 days after the test order. For incoming patient questions, telephone support from a human operator is available 24 hours per day, 365 days per year, with translation services available.

A SECOND SCREENING STUDY AND FAVORABLE BENEFITS TO HARMS SUPPORT US PREVENTATIVE SERVICES TASK FORCE ENDORSEMENT

The second major set of data on mt-sDNA performance in the screening setting was made available in early 2016. Redwood and colleagues[41] conducted a prospective cross-sectional study of asymptomatic Alaska Native adults aged 40 to 85 years undergoing screening or surveillance colonoscopy, the criterion standard; all received FIT and mt-sDNA. Among 435 patients in the screening group, CRC and APL detection rates were 50% for mt-sDNA and 31% for FIT ($P = .01$). Among all 661 patients under either screening or surveillance, the sensitivity of mt-sDNA increased with adenoma size and risk for progression, and it exceeded FIT sensitivity at all adenoma sizes. For example, mt-sDNA detected 62% of adenomas 2 cm or larger but only 29% were detected by FIT ($P = .05$). The overall adenoma and cancer detection rates by mt-sDNA were nearly identical between the 2 prospectively done screening studies (see **Fig. 2**A). For the 9 sessile serrated polyps larger 1 cm or larger, detection by mt-sDNA was 67% but only 11% by FIT ($P = .07$) (**Fig. 2**B). The point specificity for mt-sDNA was 93% compared with 96% for FIT ($P = .03$).[41]

The USPSTF also commissioned a comparative effectiveness modeling report from the Cancer Intervention and Surveillance Modeling Network to inform their 2016 updated recommendation on CRC screening.[42] Model outputs included the number of life-years gained and CRC deaths averted by screening participation for each modality. For the hypothetical screening cohort, the models also estimated total lifetime number of colonoscopies, the principal source of potential screening harm, and colonoscopy-specific complications related to gastrointestinal and cardiovascular events. **Table 1** displays the Cancer Intervention and Surveillance Modeling Network model outputs and the ratios of benefits to harms of 3 screening strategies: colonoscopy performed every 10 years, FIT performed annually, and mt-sDNA performed every 3 years. Although colonoscopy resulted in the most life-years gained and CRC deaths averted, this strategy also resulted in the greatest potential harms. Noninvasive CRC screening with FIT or mt-sDNA produced substantial gains with fewer estimated harms than colonoscopy. Additionally, because mt-sDNA testing is performed less frequently, it resulted in fewer lifetime colonoscopies than FIT.[3] Based on these data and others, the June 2016 USPSTF recommendation statement included mt-sDNA among several strategies for CRC screening.

CLINICAL MULTITARGET STOOL DNA TESTING USE IS RAPIDLY INCREASING AND ATTRACTING NEW COLORECTAL CANCER SCREENING PARTICIPATION

Since its commercial launch in late 2014, the number of tests completed has exceeded 3 million through September 2019, which closely parallels the rapid increase in providers enrolled to prescribe mt-sDNA (**Fig. 3**). Exact Sciences reported that 48% of mt-sDNA patients have not been screened for CRC before. This new-to-screening

Table 1
mt-sDNA screening results in fewer lifetime colonoscopies than FIT and has a superior benefit-to-harm ratio compared with colonoscopy

Modality	Life-Years Gained/ Complications (Ratio)	Life-Years Gained/ Colonoscopy (Ratio)	Deaths Averted[a]/ Complication (Ratio)	Deaths Averted[a]/ Colonoscopy (Ratio)
mt-sDNA	226/9 (25)	226/1714 (0.13)	20/9 (2.2)	20/1714 (0.01)
FIT	244/10 (24)	244/1757 (0.14)	22/10 (2.2)	22/1757 (0.01)
Colonoscopy	270/15 (18)	270/4049 (0.07)	24/15 (1.6)	24/4049 (0.006)

Values obtained by simulating a hypothetical cohort of 1000 persons participating in a screening program.
[a] Deaths attributable to CRC.

population includes those entering programmatic screening at age 50 as well as those who seem to have been previously nonadherent.[43]

Prince and colleagues[44] recently demonstrated increased use of mt-sDNA in previously nonadherent average-risk Medicare patients. Among a cohort of nearly 400 persons, 51% were found to have APLs at diagnostic colonoscopy after a positive mt-sDNA test. Notably, the rate of negative colonoscopy in the mt-sDNA–positive patients in this study was only 20%.[44] Moreover, in a detailed chart review at Mayo Clinic of nearly 2000 mt-sDNA–positive patients in the first 3 years of test availability, approximately 25% both had never received prior CRC screening and were over age 60, suggesting that mt-sDNA may be changing behaviors and attitudes toward participation in CRC screening.[45] Although it is difficult to imply causality, these

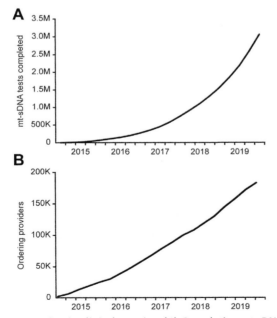

Fig. 3. Use of mt-sDNA testing in clinical practice. (*A*) Cumulative mt-sDNA tests completed over time and (*B*) providers who have enrolled to prescribe mt-sDNA. (*Courtesy of* Exact Sciences Corporation, Madison, WI.)

findings suggest that mt-sDNA is attracting previously nonadherent patients, a goal of great importance to public health efforts to reduce CRC-attributable mortality.

MULTITARGET STOOL DNA TESTING HAS A HIGH POSITIVE PREDICTIVE VALUE IN CLINICAL PRACTICE

In the largest cohorts of patients screened with mt-sDNA, 14% to 16% will have positive results.[37,45,46] For these patients, a diagnostic colonoscopy is required to exclude CRN. The adherence to diagnostic colonoscopy is thus critically important to the effectiveness of mt-sDNA testing. Estimates of adherence to diagnostic colonoscopy have to date ranged from 75% to 96%[44,46]; our analysis showed a diagnostic colonoscopy completion rate of approximately 90% in a large multipractice setting.[45] Nonadherence to recommended diagnostic colonoscopy is multifactorial and commonly related to patient aversion and medical comorbidities that might increase procedural risks, commonly from sedation or procedural intervention.[46] It is therefore critical that ordering providers provide education to patients before completing mt-sDNA testing to ensure the appropriate patients are selected. Regardless of the initial testing strategy, CRC screening should be discontinued in persons for whom colonoscopy poses an increased risk of harm.[47]

In a recent series, approximately two-thirds of patients were found to have at least 1 neoplastic lesion at diagnostic colonoscopy after positive mt-sDNA.[45] Among patients with CRN, 40% had at least 1 APL, and approximately 1% had CRC. Sessile serrated adenomas/polyps were detected in about one-half of patients with positive tests. Importantly, mt-sDNA testing in clinical practice seems to recapitulate clinical trial performance in detecting right-sided (proximal) neoplasia. In our multisetting practice, more than 50% of patients overall (and 80% of those with any neoplasm) were found to have proximal CRN at colonoscopy to evaluate positive mt-sDNA.[45] This high yield of proximal neoplasms is likely due to the infrequency of hemorrhage among these flat lesions[48] and the more continuous exfoliation of DNA markers during ongoing cellular turnover.[35] These data are consistent with a prior head-to-head observation that mt-sDNA is more sensitive than FIT for the detection of screen-relevant neoplasms proximal to the splenic flexure.[37]

These high point estimates for positive predictive value in clinical practice compared with clinical trials may reflect underlying differences in the populations being studied, or in differences in those opting to prescribe or complete the test. However, 2 additional mechanisms must be considered. Although mt-sDNA and FIT both increase post-test probability when the results are positive, data have emerged to show that endoscopist knowledge of a positive mt-sDNA test significantly increases withdrawal time and adenoma detection rate at diagnostic colonoscopy compared with blinded endoscopists from the same practice.[49] Moreover, recent data suggest that, although the yield of diagnostic colonoscopy is observed in all endoscopists in a large academic practice, the greatest improvement in polyp detection was seen in providers with the lowest baseline serrated polyp and adenoma detection rates.[50] This observation indicates that the improvement in the adenoma detection rate is not solely attributable to the increase in post–mt-sDNA probability, implying a change in colonoscopist behavior.

To date, real-world mt-sDNA performance and impact has largely been measured in single-center experiences. New data on mt-sDNA predictive value, screening adherence, and long-term health outcomes are anticipated to come from the prospective Voyage: Real-World Impact of the Multi-target Stool DNA Test on CRC Screening and Mortality study (ClinicalTrials.gov identifier NCT04124406). The Voyage study is currently recruiting toward a target of 150,000 adults prescribed mt-sDNA for routine CRC screening by their health care provider.

DISCORDANT MULTITARGET STOOL DNA TESTING AND COLONOSCOPY: AVOID FURTHER TESTING

Between 7% and 13% of patients tested with mt-sDNA will have a positive mt-sDNA test followed by a negative colonoscopy. There are recent data that provide clarity for patients and providers on the management of a false-positive mt-sDNA test result. In this situation, negative colonoscopy is defined according to the same standards used in the pivotal clinical trial of mt-sDNA. FDA labeling, therefore, defines true-positive mt-sDNA tests only when subsequent screening colonoscopy detected APL or CRC.[37] When positive mt-sDNA is followed by a diagnostic colonoscopy showing nonadvanced precursor lesions, mt-sDNA has most likely detected exfoliated DNA from a neoplasm falling below size-based criteria defined by epidemiology rather than biology. Next, providers must ensure that the diagnostic colonoscopy was high quality. Returning to the mt-sDNA clinical trials, only those with high-quality colonoscopy, defined as having good or excellent bowel preparation, photographic evidence of cecal intubation, and a withdrawal time of 6 or more minutes,[15] were included in primary analyses.[37,41]

The long-term follow-up of such patients found no increased risk of CRC in long-term follow-up of clinical study participants with negative colonoscopy after a positive mt-sDNA test result. A retrospective analysis of approximately 1000 patients with either false-positive or true-negative MT-sDNA tests found no increased rate of aerodigestive (lung and gastrointestinal tract) cancers after a median follow-up of 4 years.[41] Another prospective study evaluated 30 patients with initial false positive mt-sDNA testing after both colonoscopy and esophagogastroduodenoscopy (EGD), who underwent follow-up mt-sDNA, colonoscopy, and EGD 11 to 29 months later.[51] No neoplasms were found on EGD. APLs were found in 2 patients with persistently positive mt-sDNA, both in the proximal colon, and were found by endoscopists aware of the mt-sDNA test result. Although bowel preparation conditions from the index colonoscopy were not reported, the authors concluded that a more careful inspection at colonoscopy would likely have avoided missed colonic lesions.[51]

More recently, a multisite retrospective cohort study performed by Berger and colleagues[52] followed approximately 1200 DeeP-C study patients with negative colonoscopy for a median of 5 years, stratified by negative versus positive mt-sDNA test results. Although 16 aerodigestive cancer were diagnosed by individual chart review and cancer registry query, no increased incidence of aerodigestive cancers was observed in the positive mt-sDNA group (n = 5) versus the negative mt-sDNA group (n = 11) (P = .151). Aerodigestive cancer rates in those with positive mt-sDNA and negative colonoscopy were equivalent to the general population based on Surveillance, Epidemiology, and End Results Program data.[52] Therefore, based on the currently available evidence, guidelines advise that clinicians should not recommend repeat colonoscopy, EGD, or other further testing in patients with a positive mt-sDNA who have undergone a negative high-quality diagnostic colonoscopy and have no localizing signs or symptoms that would mandate evaluation.[4]

MULTITARGET STOOL DNA TESTING IS A COST-EFFECTIVE TEST FOR COLORECTAL CANCER PREVENTION

Triennial mtSDNA screening is a cost-effective strategy for reducing CRC incidence and mortality.[53,54] However, we challenge summative statements that mt-sDNA screening is an inefficient option compared with other strategies on the basis the existing model inputs for relative adherence to CRC screening for any modality an cost for FIT and colonoscopy are inconsistent with real-world observations. Neverthe less, there are existing data that suggest that the required thresholds for efficiency c mt-sDNA are already met. Naber and colleagues[53] proposed a threshold of greate than 30% adherence needed for mt-sDNA to be deemed cost effective relative t FIT adherence. A recent study of cross-sectional adherence in a large, national sampl (n = 368,494) of Medicare beneficiaries reported an mt-sDNA test completion rate c 71%.[55] This rate exceeds by 58% the modeled FIT screening adherence rate c 45%,[54] and is well above the proposed cost-effectiveness threshold from Nabe and colleagues.[53]

The cost inputs applied in the Naber study also do not allow for direct comparison across CRC screening strategies, nor do they account for the required programmati support and delivery of evidence-based interventions to achieve the desired hig levels of CRC screening participation.[56,57] As previously described, mt-sDNA is th only CRC screening option that includes nationwide patient navigation support t improve the overall experience and facilitate increased adherence. In our opinion, would be more financially informative and operationally applicable to better mode the combined clinical and nonclinical costs associated with each test. For example Ladabaum and Mannalithara[54] include the addition of $153 per cycle to each roun of FIT screening for patient support costs in their modeling analyses.

Existing modeling strategies are further limited by incomplete simulation of serrate neoplasia and adenoma progression,[53] nor do current input assumptions account fo variability in colonoscopy performance, such as operator dependency in the adenom detection rate, differential risk reduction for proximal versus distal neoplasia, and othe patient, polyp, and provider characteristics associated with missed and/or interval le sions[58,59] that can substantially affect the simulated outcomes of lifetime CR(screening and surveillance.

US FOOD AND DRUG ADMINISTRATION APPROVAL OF MULTITARGET STOOL DNA TESTING HAS BEEN EXPANDED TO YOUNGER PATIENTS

The 2018 ACS Colorectal Cancer Screening Guideline recommended that average risk CRC screening begin at age 45.[5] It included the use of mt-sDNA among othe stool-based noninvasive tests and structural examination approaches, dependin on patient preference and test availability.[5] The ACS based their recommendatio on increasing CRC incidence and mortality rates among patients under age 50,[6] and the results from microsimulation modeling, which suggested substantial gain in quality-adjusted life-years from CRC screening beginning at age 45.[5]

The ACS also expected that screening tests would perform similarly in adults age 45 to 49 compared with adults aged 50 or older. Data to support this assumptio have been lacking until recently. Through September 2018, there had been 224 completed mt-sDNA tests (through Exact Sciences Laboratories) in individual aged 45 to 49. Although it was unknown if these patients were at average risk only 7.4% (165/2241) had a positive result and 92.6% (2076/2241) had a negativ result. Although colonoscopy results are not available for either mt-sDNA–positiv or –negative patients, these proportions indicate that the specificity of mt-sDNA i this age group cannot be less than 92.6%, which is comparable with the specificit of patients aged 50 to 59 from the DeeP-C study.[37] This observation was included i the FDA decision in September 2019 to expand approval for mt-sDNA use in patient aged 45 to 84.[61]

After the label expansion, new data are beginning to address marker representation and specificity of mt-sDNA in patients aged 45 to 49. First, we conducted a retrospective study of DNA markers (*KRAS*, *BMP3*, *NDRG4*) included in the mt-sDNA assay to quantify and compare tissue marker levels in sporadic CRC cases and normal colon controls from patients in 45- to 49-year-old and 50- to 64-year-old age groups. DNA extracted from CRC tissue in the 45 to 49 (n = 90) and 50 to 64 (n = 96) age groups were compared with normal colon samples from adults aged 45 to 49 (n = 76) and 50 to 64 (n = 92). These samples were amplified by the Quantitative Allele-specific Real-time Target and Signal amplification assay, which is FDA approved for mt-sDNA. The Quantitative Allele-specific Real-time Target and Signal amplification products with *KRAS* mutations or *BMP3* and *NDRG4* methylation were not statistically different between cases of the younger versus older groups or between cases and controls.[62] A clinical study (ClinicalTrials.gov identifier NCT03728348) has also recently completed enrollment of more than 983 patients aged 45 to 49 at average risk for CRC. The primary end point—the specificity of the mt-sDNA test in the 45 to 49 age group in an average-risk population using colonoscopy with histopathology as the reference method—is anticipated to be reported in early 2020.

NEXT-GENERATION MULTITARGET STOOL DNA TESTING SHOWS HIGH SPECIFICITY

Next-generation mt-sDNA testing is also anticipated to have high specificity. Since the development of the mt-sDNA assay, next-generation sequencing has led to the discovery and development of hundreds of novel methylated DNA targets with strong association to CRC and precursor lesions.[63] To further improve CRC screening effectiveness, we conducted a blinded case-control study evaluating the accuracy of a mt-sDNA panel of novel, highly discriminant methylated DNA markers for CRC detection. Using a panel of 3 novel methylated DNA markers and FIT in archival stool samples from 117 CRC, 120 AA, 161 non-AA, and 327 controls, the cross-validated area under the curve was 0.97 for CRC and 0.84 for AA. At 92% (95% confidence interval, 88%–94%) specificity, the sensitivity of the panel was 92% (95% confidence interval, 86%–96%) for CRC.[64] These provocative results from next-generation mt-sDNA testing (mt-sDNA 2.0) will be prospectively validated in a large cross-sectional study, now open to enrollment. Clinical Validation of An Optimized Multi-Target Stool DNA (mt-sDNA 2.0) Test for Colorectal Cancer Screening "BLUE-C" (ClinicalTrials.gov identifier NCT04144738) will enroll up to 12,500 patients 40 years of age and older, who will complete the mt-sDNA 2.0 test and the commercially available FIT, followed by completion of a screening colonoscopy. Like the DeeP-C study, the results of the mt-sDNA screening test and FIT will not be provided to investigators,

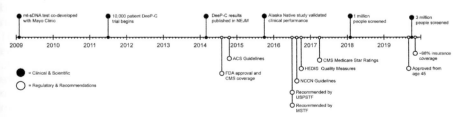

Fig. 4. Timeline of major milestones in mt-sDNA testing for CRC screening. FOBT, fecal occult blood test; HEDIS, Healthcare Effectiveness Data and Information Set; MSTF, US Multi-Society Task Force; NCCN, National Comprehensive Cancer Network; NEJM, *New England Journal of Medicine*.

and personnel performing the colonoscopy will also remain blinded to the results of the mt-sDNA 2.0 test results. Primary outcomes include the sensitivity and specificity of mt-sDNA 2.0 for CRC and secondary end points include sensitivity for AA, comparison with FIT, and specificity calculated from patients with non-neoplastic colonoscopy results.

SUMMARY

Although the scientific underpinnings of DNA-based CRC detection are now decades old, the last 10 years have seen rapid advancement of mt-sDNA from preclinical laboratory benchwork to wide dissemination in clinical practice (**Fig. 4**). Screen-setting studies have shown high sensitivity for CRC and APL by mt-sDNA, which is now included in major society guidelines and endorsed by USPSTF as a first-line CRC screening test. Uptake of mt-sDNA testing has increased exponentially since approval by the FDA and CMS. Emerging real-world data are encouraging. Adherence to mt-sDNA testing is approximately 70% and patients with positive mt-sDNA test results have high diagnostic colonoscopy completion rates in single-center studies. The positive predictive value for CRN in postapproval studies is high, possibly owing to increased endoscopist attention during diagnostic colonoscopy, as measured by withdrawal times and improvements in lesion detection rates. Patient with negative high-quality diagnostic colonoscopy after positive mt-sDNA do not seem to be at an increased risk for cancers of the gastrointestinal tract and do not require additional testing beyond what is directed by symptoms. The mt-sDNA test is cost effective in comparison with no screening and we anticipate that modeling studies that use more accurate inputs for CRC screening test costs and more accurately reflect the known variability in colonoscopy performance will show that mt-sDNA is efficient compared with other options. Based on high specificity of mt-sDNA in patients aged 45 to 49, the FDA recently expanded mt-sDNA approval to include this age range. A large cross-sectional study is now underway to validate the mt-sDNA 2.0 test, which is anticipated to maintain high sensitivity for CRC and APL and show even greater specificity than the first-generation mt-sDNA test.

DISCLOSURE

Mayo Clinic and Exact Sciences Corporation (Madison, WI) own intellectual property under which Dr J.B. Kisiel is listed as an inventor and may receive royalties in accordance with Mayo Clinic policy. Dr P.J. Limburg serves as Chief Medical Officer for Exact Sciences through a contracted services agreement with Mayo Clinic. Dr P.J. Limburg and Mayo Clinic have contractual rights to receive royalties through this agreement. Dr J.D. Eckmann has no conflicts to disclose.

REFERENCES

1. Siegel RL, Miller KD, Jemal A. Cancer statistics, 2019. CA Cancer J Clin 2019; 69(1):7–34.
2. Joseph DA, King JB, Richards TB, et al. Use of colorectal cancer screening tests by state. Prev Chronic Dis 2018;15:E80.
3. Bibbins-Domingo K. Colorectal cancer screening recommendations-reply. JAMA 2016;316(16):1717.
4. Rex DK, Boland CR, Dominitz JA, et al. Colorectal cancer screening: recommendations for physicians and patients from the U.S. Multi-Society task force on colorectal cancer. Gastroenterology 2017;153(1):307–23.

5. Wolf AMD, Fontham ETH, Church TR, et al. Colorectal cancer screening for average-risk adults: 2018 guideline update from the American Cancer Society. CA Cancer J Clin 2018;68(4):250–81.
6. Nishihara R, Wu K, Lochhead P, et al. Long-term colorectal-cancer incidence and mortality after lower endoscopy. N Engl J Med 2013;369(12):1095–105.
7. Xiang L, Zhan Q, Zhao XH, et al. Risk factors associated with missed colorectal flat adenoma: a multicenter retrospective tandem colonoscopy study. World J Gastroenterol 2014;20(31):10927–37.
8. Singh H, Nugent Z, Demers AA, et al. The reduction in colorectal cancer mortality after colonoscopy varies by site of the cancer. Gastroenterology 2010;139(4): 1128–37.
9. Kahi CJ, Hewett DG, Norton DL, et al. Prevalence and variable detection of proximal colon serrated polyps during screening colonoscopy. Clin Gastroenterol Hepatol 2011;9(1):42–6.
0. Baxter NN, Goldwasser MA, Paszat LF, et al. Association of colonoscopy and death from colorectal cancer. Ann Intern Med 2009;150(1):1–8.
1. Brenner H, Hoffmeister M, Arndt V, et al. Protection from right- and left-sided colorectal neoplasms after colonoscopy: population-based study. J Natl Cancer Inst 2010;102(2):89–95.
2. Lee JK, Jensen CD, Levin TR, et al. Long-term risk of colorectal cancer and related deaths after a colonoscopy with normal findings. JAMA Intern Med 2019;179(2):153–60.
3. Corley DA, Levin TR, Doubeni CA. Adenoma detection rate and risk of colorectal cancer and death. N Engl J Med 2014;370(26):2541.
4. Butterly L, Robinson CM, Anderson JC, et al. Serrated and adenomatous polyp detection increases with longer withdrawal time: results from the New Hampshire Colonoscopy Registry. Am J Gastroenterol 2014;109(3):417–26.
5. Barclay RL, Vicari JJ, Doughty AS, et al. Colonoscopic withdrawal times and adenoma detection during screening colonoscopy. N Engl J Med 2006;355(24): 2533–41.
6. Rex DK, Schoenfeld PS, Cohen J, et al. Quality indicators for colonoscopy. Gastrointest Endosc 2015;81(1):31–53.
7. Steinwachs D, Allen JD, Barlow WE, et al. National Institutes of Health state-of-the-science conference statement: enhancing use and quality of colorectal cancer screening. Ann Intern Med 2010;152(10):663–7.
8. Kronborg O, Fenger C, Olsen J, et al. Randomised study of screening for colorectal cancer with faecal-occult-blood test. Lancet 1996;348(9040):1467–71.
9. Faivre J, Dancourt V, Lejeune C, et al. Reduction in colorectal cancer mortality by fecal occult blood screening in a French controlled study. Gastroenterology 2004; 126(7):1674–80.
0. Scholefield JH, Moss SM, Mangham CM, et al. Nottingham trial of faecal occult blood testing for colorectal cancer: a 20-year follow-up. Gut 2012;61(7):1036–40.
1. Shaukat A, Mongin SJ, Geisser MS, et al. Long-term mortality after screening for colorectal cancer. N Engl J Med 2013;369(12):1106–14.
2. Haug U, Kuntz KM, Knudsen AB, et al. Sensitivity of immunochemical faecal occult blood testing for detecting left- vs right-sided colorectal neoplasia. Br J Cancer 2011;104(11):1779–85.
3. Hirai HW, Tsoi KK, Chan JY, et al. Systematic review with meta-analysis: faecal occult blood tests show lower colorectal cancer detection rates in the proximal colon in colonoscopy-verified diagnostic studies. Aliment Pharmacol Ther 2016; 43(7):755–64.

24. Fenton JJ, Elmore JG, Buist DS, et al. Longitudinal adherence with fecal occult blood test screening in community practice. Ann Fam Med 2010;8(5):397–401.

25. Zorzi M, Hassan C, Capodaglio G, et al. Divergent long-term detection rates of proximal and distal advanced neoplasia in fecal immunochemical test screening programs: a retrospective cohort study. Ann Intern Med 2018;169(9):602–9.

26. Jensen CD, Corley DA, Quinn VP, et al. Fecal immunochemical test program performance over 4 rounds of annual screening: a retrospective cohort study. Ann Intern Med 2016;164(7):456–63.

27. Liang PS, Wheat CL, Abhat A, et al. Adherence to competing strategies for colorectal cancer screening over 3 years. Am J Gastroenterol 2016;111(1):105–14.

28. Gellad ZF, Stechuchak KM, Fisher DA, et al. Longitudinal adherence to fecal occult blood testing impacts colorectal cancer screening quality. Am J Gastroenterol 2011;106(6):1125–34.

29. Cyhaniuk A, Coombes ME. Longitudinal adherence to colorectal cancer screening guidelines. Am J Manag Care 2016;22(2):105–11.

30. Ahlquist DA, McGill DB, Fleming JL, et al. Patterns of occult bleeding in asymptomatic colorectal cancer. Cancer 1989;63(9):1826–30.

31. Ahlquist DA, Harrington JJ, Burgart LJ, et al. Morphometric analysis of the "mucocellular layer" overlying colorectal cancer and normal mucosa: relevance to exfoliation and stool screening. Hum Pathol 2000;31(1):51–7.

32. Imperiale TF, Ransohoff DF, Itzkowitz SH, et al. Fecal DNA versus fecal occult blood for colorectal-cancer screening in an average-risk population. N Engl J Med 2004;351(26):2704–14.

33. Ahlquist DA, Sargent DJ, Loprinzi CL, et al. Stool DNA and occult blood testing for screen detection of colorectal neoplasia. Ann Intern Med 2008;149(7): 441–50. W481.

34. Zou H, Allawi H, Cao X, et al. Quantification of methylated markers with a multiplex methylation-specific technology. Clin Chem 2012;58(2):375–83.

35. Ahlquist DA, Zou H, Domanico M, et al. Next-generation stool DNA test accurately detects colorectal cancer and large adenomas. Gastroenterology 2012; 142(2):248–56 [quiz: e225–46].

36. Lidgard GP, Domanico MJ, Bruinsma JJ, et al. Clinical performance of an automated stool DNA assay for detection of colorectal neoplasia. Clin Gastroenterol Hepatol 2013;11(10):1313–8.

37. Imperiale TF, Ransohoff DF, Itzkowitz SH, et al. Multitarget stool DNA testing for colorectal-cancer screening. N Engl J Med 2014;370(14):1287–97.

38. Administration USFaD. FDA summary of safety and effectiveness data (SSED). 2014. Available at: http://www.accessdata.fda.gov/cdrh_docs/pdf13/P130017b. pdf. Accessed April 29, 2016.

39. Swartz R, Weiser E, Parks P, et al. Su1660 – colorectal cancer screening: compliance with multitarget stool DNA testing among Medicare beneficiaries. Gastroenterology 2019;156(6, Supplement 1):S601.

40. Dougherty MK, Brenner AT, Crockett SD, et al. Evaluation of interventions intended to increase colorectal cancer screening rates in the united states: a systematic review and meta-analysis. JAMA Intern Med 2018;178(12):1645–58.

41. Redwood DG, Asay ED, Blake ID, et al. Stool DNA testing for screening detection of colorectal neoplasia in Alaska native people. Mayo Clin Proc 2016;91(1): 61–70.

42. Knudsen AB, Zauber AG, Rutter CM, et al. Estimation of benefits, burden, and harms of colorectal cancer screening strategies: modeling study for the US Preventive Services Task Force. JAMA 2016;315(23):2595–609.

43. Finney Rutten LJ, Jacobson RM, Wilson PM, et al. Early adoption of a multitarget stool DNA test for colorectal cancer screening. Mayo Clin Proc 2017;92(5): 726–33.
44. Prince M, Lester L, Chiniwala R, et al. Multitarget stool DNA tests increases colorectal cancer screening among previously noncompliant Medicare patients. World J Gastroenterol 2017;23(3):464–71.
45. Eckmann J, Ebner D, Bering J, et al. Su1664 – high yield of total and right-sided colorectal neoplasia by multi-target stool DNA testing in average risk patients irrespective of prior screening. Gastroenterology 2019;156(6, Supplement 1): S602–3.
46. Daghestani A, Walker E, Mlinarevich N, et al. Mo1642 - diagnostic colonoscopy compliance following a positive multi-target stool DNA test in a colorectal cancer screening-resistant population. Gastroenterology 2018;154(6, Supplement 1): S-780.
47. Ko CW, Sonnenberg A. Comparing risks and benefits of colorectal cancer screening in elderly patients. Gastroenterology 2005;129(4):1163–70.
48. Sweetser S, Smyrk TC, Sinicrope FA. Serrated colon polyps as precursors to colorectal cancer. Clin Gastroenterol Hepatol 2013;11(7):760–7 [quiz: e754–65].
49. Johnson DH, Kisiel JB, Burger KN, et al. Multitarget stool DNA test: clinical performance and impact on yield and quality of colonoscopy for colorectal cancer screening. Gastrointest Endosc 2017;85(3):657–65.e1.
50. Ebner D, Eckmann J, Burger KN, et al. Sa1042 multi-target stool DNA testing enriches detection of colorectal neoplasia by colonoscopy but yield is influenced by baseline polyp detection rates. Gastrointest Endosc 2019;89(6, Supplement): AB149–50.
51. Cooper GS, Markowitz SD, Chen Z, et al. Evaluation of patients with an apparent false positive stool DNA test: the role of repeat stool DNA testing. Dig Dis Sci 2018;63(6):1449–53.
52. Berger BM, Kisiel JB, Imperiale TF, et al. Low incidence of aerodigestive cancers in patients with negative results from colonoscopies, regardless of findings from multitarget stool DNA tests. Clin Gastroenterol Hepatol 2019 [pii:S1542-3565(19) 30846-8].
53. Naber SK, Knudsen AB, Zauber AG, et al. Cost-effectiveness of a multitarget stool DNA test for colorectal cancer screening of Medicare beneficiaries. PLoS One 2019;14(9):e0220234.
54. Ladabaum U, Mannalithara A. Comparative effectiveness and cost effectiveness of a multitarget stool DNA test to screen for colorectal neoplasia. Gastroenterology 2016;151(3):427–39.e6.
55. Schwartz PH, Imperiale TF, Perkins SM, et al. Impact of including quantitative information in a decision aid for colorectal cancer screening: a randomized controlled trial. Patient Educ Couns 2019;102(4):726–34.
56. Paskett ED, Harrop JP, Wells KJ. Patient navigation: an update on the state of the science. CA Cancer J Clin 2011;61(4):237–49.
57. Wender RC, Doroshenk M, Brooks D, et al. Creating and Implementing a National Public Health Campaign: The American Cancer Society's and National Colorectal cancer roundtable's 80% by 2018 initiative. Am J Gastroenterol 2018;113(12): 1739–41.
58. Rex DK. Polyp detection at colonoscopy: endoscopist and technical factors. Best Pract Res 2017;31(4):425–33.

59. Singh S, Singh PP, Murad MH, et al. Prevalence, risk factors, and outcomes of interval colorectal cancers: a systematic review and meta-analysis. Am J Gastroenterol 2014;109(9):1375–89.

60. Siegel RL, Miller KD, Jemal A. Colorectal cancer mortality rates in adults aged 20 to 54 years in the United States, 1970-2014. JAMA 2017;318(6):572–4.

61. U.S. Food & Drug Administration. Cologuard Premarket Approval (PMA), supplement S029. Available at: https://www.accessdata.fda.gov/scripts/cdrh/cfdocs/cfpma/pma.cfm?id=P130017S029. Accessed March 7, 2020.

62. Limburg PMD, Mahoney DWMS, Ahlquist DMD, et al. Multi-target DNA aberrations in sporadic colorectal cancer tissues do not differ between younger and older patients: 273 [Abstract]. Am J Gastroenterol 2019;114(Supplement):S160.

63. Kisiel JB, Klepp P, Allawi HT, et al. Analysis of DNA methylation at specific loci in stool samples detects colorectal cancer and high-grade dysplasia in patients with inflammatory bowel disease. Clin Gastroenterol Hepatol 2019;17(5): 914–921 e915.

64. Domanico MP, Kisiel JMD, Gagrat Z, et al. Novel multi-target stool DNA marker panel yields highly accurate detection of colorectal cancer and premalignant neoplasia: 325 [Abstract]. Am J Gastroenterol 2019;114(Supplement):S191.

Update on Flexible Sigmoidoscopy, Computed Tomographic Colonography, and Capsule Colonoscopy

Seung Won Chung, MD[a], Seifeldin Hakim, MD[b],
Shaheer Siddiqui, MD[b], Brooks D. Cash, MD[b],*

KEYWORDS

- Sigmoidoscopy • Capsule colon • CT colonography • Virtual colonoscopy
- CRC screening

KEY POINTS

- Flexible sigmoidoscopy (FS) is a simple, safe endoscopic colorectal cancer (CRC) screening option that has proven to decrease CRC incidence and mortality.
- Computed tomographic colonography (CTC) is a noninvasive examination of the entire colon based on interpretation of images acquired with standard computed tomographic scanners of the insufflated colon. It requires specialized software for image processing and can depict the colon as a 2-dimensional or 3-dimensional structure. In expert hands, CTC accuracy approaches that of colonoscopy for the detection of polypoid lesions ≥6 mm.
- Colon capsule endoscopy (CCE) is an emerging CRC screening test candidate that has shown promising results for the detection of colorectal neoplasia compared with colonoscopy. It requires an aggressive bowel preparation and has recently shown superiority to CTC in a large randomized controlled trial.
- Neither CTC nor CCE is widely covered or approved for CRC screening by insurance companies or governmental programs, and their use for this indication remains minimal.
- Positive results with FS, CTC, or CCE should prompt timely performance of colonoscopy.

INTRODUCTION

In the context of colorectal cancer (CRC) screening and surveillance, colonoscopy is considered the gold-standard test, and the increasing availability and use of colonoscopy over the last 3 decades are widely recognized as one factor associated with the decreasing rates of CRC incidence and mortality that has been observed over this

[a] Department of Internal Medicine, 6431 Fannin Street, MSB 1.150, Houston, TX 77030, USA;
[b] Division of Gastroenterology, Hepatology, and Nutrition, 6431 Fannin Street, MSB 4.234, Houston, TX 77030, USA
* Corresponding author.
E-mail address: brooks.d.cash@uth.tmc.edu

Gastrointest Endoscopy Clin N Am 30 (2020) 569–583
https://doi.org/10.1016/j.giec.2020.02.009
1052-5157/20/© 2020 Elsevier Inc. All rights reserved.

time period. Colonoscopy is recommended as a CRC screening test in all major guide lines in the United States (US Preventative Services Task Force [USPSTF], Nation Comprehensive Cancer Network, American Cancer Society [ACS], and the US Multisc ciety Task Force on Colorectal Cancer Screening [USMSTF]) where it is explicit endorsed as a preferred (tier 1) test.[1–4] Colonoscopy is not without limitations, howeve that limit its universal application and uptake for CRC screening. Among commonly rec ommended CRC screening test options, colonoscopy is the most expensive and inva sive, requires sedation, and imparts a substantial time commitment by patients an others who must transport them for the procedure. One of the most important issue for patients considering colonoscopy is the requirement for a cathartic bowe preparation.

Despite its proven accuracy and value as a CRC screening test and its position a the preferred surveillance modality for patients with a personal history of colorect neoplasia, the issues mentioned above are frequently cited as reasons for nonadher ence with CRC screening in general. Therefore, it is important for patients and clini cians to recognize that there are multiple alternatives to colonoscopy for CRC screening. Several of these modalities, flexible sigmoidoscopy (FS), computed tomog raphy colonography (CTC), and colon capsule endoscopy (CCE), permit visualizatio the colonic lumen and identification of neoplasia, in contrast to other noninvasive CRC screening tests, such as high-sensitivity fecal occult blood testing (FOBT), fecal immu nochemical testing (FIT), and multitarget stool DNA. These tests are also included i existent CRC screening guidelines and, in the case of FS, FOBT, and FIT, are the pri mary CRC screening test in some systems and countries. This article provides a overview of the noncolonoscopic options for CRC screening that permit visualizatio of the colon lumen and detection of both CRC and colon polyps.

FLEXIBLE SIGMOIDOSCOPY

FS was the first endoscopic screening test that was shown to reduce CRC incidenc and mortality. Before the widespread use of colonoscopy for CRC screening, FS wa used alone and in combination with FOBT, with FS typically performed at 5-year inter vals and FOBT performed annually. FS examines the distal colon and, although the 60 cm FS can be advanced beyond the splenic flexure in some patients, the proxima extent of FS examination is typically the descending colon.[5] FS requires less bowe preparation compared with other structural examinations, typically 1 or 2 enemas and is usually performed without sedation. However, FS as a CRC screening tes has been less used over the past 2 decades in the United States, largely replaced by colonoscopy. In 2010, only 2.5% of adults 50 to 75 years old reported having FS for CRC screening, compared with 60% for colonoscopy.[6]

Four randomized control trials of FS have shown reduction in CRC incidence an mortality, and these studies have demonstrated remarkably consistent results despite diverse practice settings.[7–10] In the United States, the Prostate, Lung, Colo rectal, and Ovarian (PLCO) Cancer Screening Trial investigators showed significan decrease in the incidence of both distal (relative risk [RR] 0.71, 95% confidence inter val [CI] 0.64–0.80) and proximal (RR 0.86, 95% CI 0.76–0.97) CRC with FS.[9] A poole analysis of the PLCO, an Italian FS screening study (SCORE),[10] and the Norwegia Colorectal Cancer Prevention[8] trials showed reduction in CRC incidence by 21% and mortality by 27% with FS screening.[11] However, this analysis failed to demon strate a difference in CRC incidence or mortality in women 60 years of age or older possibly related to the increased incidence of proximal CRC in older women tha were not detected by FS. In an analysis conducted for recently updated CRC screening guidelines issued by the USPSTF, FS screening reduced overall CRC mortality by 27% over 12 years of follow-up (RR 0.73, 95% CI 0.66–0.82).[1] Importantly, distal CRC mortality was statistically significantly reduced with FS versus no screening (RR 0.63, 95% CI 0.49–0.84), but not for proximal CRC. In this analysis, the incidence of CRC was reduced by 21% (RR 0.70, 95% CI 0.75–0.85). Finally, a recent 17-year follow-up of the UK Flexible Sigmoidoscopy Screening Trial reported a 26% CRC incidence reduction (hazard ratio [HR] 0.74, 95% CI 0.70–0.80) and a 30% mortality reduction (HR 0.70, 95% CI 0.62–0.79).[12]

The recommended interval for CRC screening with FS is 5 years according to multiple different CRC screening guidelines.[1–4] The risks of FS are lower than the risks of colonoscopy.[13] The risk of bowel perforation is approximately 1 per 10,000 procedures, whereas the risk of major bleeding is 2 per 10,000.[7,13,14] Compared with colonoscopy, FS has negligible risk of cardiac or respiratory complications because no sedation is required, and the preparation is less intensive and not associated with fluid or electrolyte shifts. However, because FS is performed without sedation, patients can experience significant discomfort during the procedure, and the enemas required for FS preparation can be difficult for some patients to administer properly. Similar to other noncolonoscopy CRC screening tests, a positive FS result (defined as the identification of any colorectal neoplasia) should result in timely performance of a colonoscopy, which increases the cost and risk of CRC screening and may not be viewed favorably by patients. The PLCO trial found that the colonoscopy referral rate, based on the identification of any colorectal neoplasia on FS, was 23%.[9] Despite the low utilization of FS in the United States, its proven efficacy, relative ease, and low risk of adverse events make it an important CRC screening option for many patients throughout the world.

COMPUTED TOMOGRAPHY COLONOGRAPHY

CTC is a minimally invasive modality for examination of the colon and is also often referred to as virtual colonoscopy.[15] In 1994, during the 23rd annual meeting of the society of GI radiologists, Vining and colleagues[16] introduced CTC as an endoluminal fly-through video of the colon using images obtained from a multislice CT scanner (**Figs. 1–3**). Early studies of CTC were small and primarily proof of concept. Dachman and

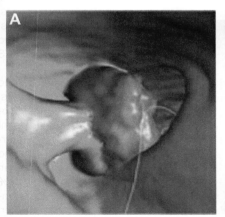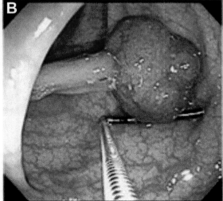

Fig. 1. Polyp detected with CTC and confirmed with colonoscopy. (A) 3D CTC image of a 12-mm pedunculated polyp and its (B) endoscopic correlate.

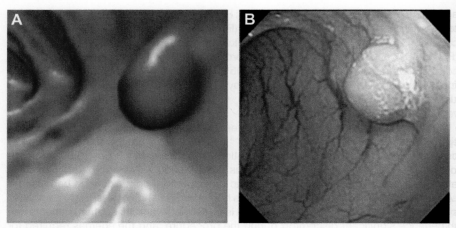

Fig. 2. Polyp detected with CTC and confirmed with colonoscopy. (A) 3D CTC image of a 4-mm polyp and its (B) endoscopic correlate.

colleagues[17] studied 44 patients with CTC after colonoscopy and calculated a polyp sensitivity of 83% and 100%, respectively, for 2 observers. Royster and colleagues[18] performed CTC in 20 patients after colonoscopy and found that CTC was able to identify all colon masses and 12 out 15 polyps greater than 6 mm in diameter. In 1997 Hara and colleagues[19] evaluated 70 average-risk patients undergoing CTC and, compared with regular CT or colonoscopy, found CTC to have 75% sensitivity for the detection of polyps greater than 10 mm. These initial small studies laid the groundwork for larger CTC feasibility studies.

Early feasibility studies of CTC were conducted in patients at increased risk of CRC based on personal/family history or positive results of previous screening tests, such as FS, FOBT, or FIT. In 1999, Fenlon and colleagues[20] reported the results of a prospective study of CTC compared with colonoscopy in 100 patients at increased risk of CRC. When polyps of all sizes were included, the per-patient sensitivity of CTC was 82% and the specificity was 84%. Performance characteristics of CTC were

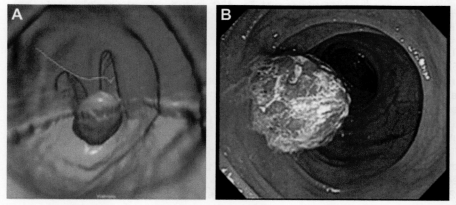

Fig. 3. Polyp detected with CTC and confirmed with colonoscopy. (A) 3D CTC image of a 10-mm polyp and its (B) endoscopic correlate.

ependent on polyp size, with sensitivity of 94% and specificity of 92% for the detec-
on of polyps between 6 and 9 mm in diameter, and for polyps ≥10 mm, the sensitivity
nd specificity were both 96%. Subsequent studies of CTC in high-risk patients
orroborated these results. Hara and colleagues[21] studied 237 patients with CTC
nd found the sensitivity of CTC for polyps ≥10 mm to be 78% to 100% with a spec-
icity of 90% to 93%. Fletcher and colleagues[22] studied 180 patients with similar con-
lusions (sensitivity 85.4%, specificity 93% for polyps >10 mm). Yee and colleagues[23]
valuated 300 patients (204 classified as having increased risk of CRC) and found CTC
ɔ have a sensitivity for polyps ≥10 mm of 100%. The UK SIGGAR trial consisted of 2
eparate arms involving symptomatic patients. One arm compared CTC against colo-
ιoscopy, and the other arm compared CTC with barium enema.[24,25] These compar-
ʒons showed CTC to be equivalent to colonoscopy and superior to barium enema for
ɪetection of large polyps and cancers.

After initial validation in high-risk patient groups, multiple pivotal clinical trials of CTC
s an average-risk CRC screening test were conducted. The first of these was pub-
shed in 2003 by Johnson and colleagues[26] and evaluated an increased-risk cohort
ɪf 703 adults, primarily because of a personal history of adenomatous polyps. In
ιis study, they found that CTC delivered a pooled sensitivity for large polyps of
ʌround 50%, although specificity was greater than 95%. Two additional large pro-
pective CTC trials involving low-risk patient cohorts, the first by Cotton and col-
ɜagues[27] and the second by Rockey and colleagues,[28] also produced
ɪisappointing results for CTC with per-patient sensitivity of CTC for large polyps of
·5% to 59% and specificity of 96%. It should be noted that all of the aforementioned
ɾials did not include true screening cohorts, used a primary 2-dimensional (2D) polyp
earch without oral contrast tagging and were subject to several additional technical
mitations related to insufficient colon cleansing and insufflation protocols, all of which
nay have impacted the findings.

A key event in CTC development was the 2003 publication by Pickhardt and col-
ɜagues[29] describing a large, multicenter Department of Defense (DoD) trial of
creening CTC compared with colonoscopy. Key differences of this trial compared
ʋith those of Johnson, Cotton, and Rockey included the size of the asymptomatic,
ιverage-risk adult cohort in the DoD study (n = 1233), the use of processing software
hat permitted primary 3-dimensional (3D) interpretation, the use of oral contrast
agging, segmental unblinding of CTC results during blinding colonoscopy, and stan-
ɪardized volume and pressure-regulated colonic insufflation. In this trial, CTC had a
ɜensitivity of 94% for large (≥1 cm) adenomas with a specificity of 96%. At a threshold
ɪf 6 mm, the sensitivity of CTC decreased to 89% with a specificity of 80%. In 2008,
he results of the American College of Radiology Imaging Network (ACRIN) National
ɔTC trial were published.[30] This trial was an even larger multicenter CTC trial involving
·531 average-risk screening subjects in which CTC demonstrated a sensitivity of 90%
or large adenomas and cancers, providing the additional validation to consider CTC a
ɾiable option for CRC screening. ACRIN also confirmed that there was no difference in
ɪerformance using either primary 2D or primary 3D imaging techniques, nor were
here significance differences between CTC vendor-specific software platforms. A
ʒubsequent study by Graser and colleagues[31] provided additional validation for
ɔTC compared with other CRC screening modalities. In this trial of 307 average-risk
ιdults, CTC showed high sensitivity (97%) for detecting advanced colorectal
ιeoplasia using a primary 3D interpretation, compared with low sensitivity for FIT
32%) and FOBT (20%). Mulhall and colleagues[32] incorporated 33 studies involving
ʒ393 patients and showed CTC to have a sensitivity of 85% to 93% for the detection
ɪf polyps ≥10 mm with a specificity of 97%. The sensitivity for detection of polyps

between 6 and 9 mm was 70% to 86% with a specificity of 86% to 93%. Sensitivity of CTC for the detection of CRC was found to be 96% in a metaanalysis by Halligan and colleagues,[33] whereas another metaanalysis from 2011 included 49 studies and found a sensitivity of CTC for CRC detection of 96.1% (compared with 94.7% for colonoscopy).[34]

Current recommendations for the performance of CTC recommend bowel preparation similar to that used with colonoscopy, with the addition of water-soluble contrast to tag residual colon contents for digital subtraction. There have been multiple trials evaluating "prepless" CTC, with most centered on the practice of ingesting some form of contrast agent that will permit digital subtraction during the postimage acquisition processing.[35–40] The results of these trials has been variable, with several of them demonstrating prepless or reduced prep CTC performance characteristics comparable to those obtained in larger prospective trials in which the colon was cleansed. There has been little published on the concept of prepless CTC in the last 5 to 8 years, however, and such an approach obviously precludes same-day colonoscopy, which may be preferable to patients.

Based on the accumulated evidence supporting CTC, in 2008, the ACS, in conjunction with a multidisciplinary consensus of the American College of Radiology (ACR) and the USMSTF, recommended CTC as a screening tool for CRC in the average-risk patient population.[41] At nearly the same time, CTC was given an indeterminate rating for CRC screening by the USPSTF.[42] Taking its lead from the USPSTF, the Centers for Medicare and Medicaid declined to cover CTC as a screening tool in 2009 and issued a national noncoverage decision.[43] However, in 2016, the USPSTF updated its guidelines and, based on accumulated evidence, included CTC in its recommendations for screening average-risk adults between 50 and 70 years of age for CRC.[1] Although local and national reimbursement issues have limited the widespread use of CTC as a screening tool, a handful of large centers of excellence adopted CTC for screening purposes.[15] The Colon Health Initiative was established in 2004 at the National Naval Medical Center in Bethesda, Maryland, and used CTC, along with other test options, to screen patients at average risk of CRC. President Obama actually underwent a screening CTC at this facility in 2010. The University of Wisconsin Medical Center in Madison, Wisconsin, offers CTC for average-risk CRC screening after achieving coverage decisions from local insurance payers. Both of these sites have published data based on their individually accumulated and pooled experience with screening CTC demonstrating that CTC is an accurate, acceptable, reproducible, and safe screening test that can improve compliance and patient satisfaction.[44–50]

Multiple issues surrounding CTC have generated considerable controversy. Current ACR recommendations suggest offering CTC surveillance in patients who are found to have polyps between 6 and 9 mm and not to report polyps that are less than 6 mm, because of the low specificity of CTC for small polyps.[51] Based on these recommendations, Hur and colleagues[52] conducted a modeling study of hypothetical patients with polyps between 6 and 9 mm divided into 2 groups. The WAIT group called for a repeat CTC in 3 years, and the COLO group consisted of immediate colonoscopy. Based on their assumptions and modeling, there were 79 deaths/100,000 and 773 cancers/100,000 in the WAIT group compared with 14 deaths/100,000 and 39 cancers/100,000 in the COLO group. Another controversial issue with CTC is the radiation exposure inherent in the examination. This concern, which was a prominent argument among CTC opponents, is largely theoretic and unproven. Based on best estimates of radiation-induced cancer risk, which is largely inferential, Brenner and Georgsson[53] concluded that the potential lifetime cancer risk from CTC performed at age 50 was 0.14% and 0.07% for CTC performed at age 70. In addition, increasing stringent dose reduction techniques for abdominal imaging and CTC have reduced the radiation delivery with this modality to an exceedingly small amount. Another area of controversy with CTC is the potential detection of extracolonic lesions that can result in significant additional diagnostic evaluations and costs. Although the complication rate of CTC is low, perforation has been described, although the reported rate of 0.009% represents a very low risk.[54]

Another area of controversy surrounding CTC is its ability to accurately detect flat and serrated polyps. Between 10% and 20% of CRC are estimated to develop from the serrated adenoma pathway, and optimal CRC screening tests should permit the detection of these lesions, because of their increased potential to develop into interval CRC.[55,56] Unfortunately, the detection rate of serrated lesions with CTC has not been well defined. Kim and colleagues[57] described the University of Wisconsin experience in their average-risk asymptomatic population of more than 8000 adults and found a prevalence of 3.1% for nondiminutive ($\geq$6 mm) serrated polyps. IJspeert and colleagues[58] compared CTC with colonoscopy for the detection of sessile serrated polyps (SSP). In this study, 1276 screening patients underwent colonoscopy and 982 underwent CTC. The prevalence of $\geq$1 high-risk SSP was 4.3% in patients undergoing colonoscopy compared with 0.8% for those in the CTC arm, suggesting that CTC missed most SSP, especially those that were flat or located in the proximal colon.

Guideline recommendations regarding CTC as a CRC screening test are variable. Current ACR indications for screening CTC include patients at average risk for colorectal neoplasia, patients with history of incomplete screening colonoscopy, or patients at increased risk of colonoscopy complications who need colorectal luminal imaging.[59] American College of Gastroenterology guidelines recommend CTC to be used in place of barium enema as a radiological alternative for screening of CRC if the patients decline colonoscopy or have incomplete colonoscopy.[60] The USPSTF and ACS guidelines include CTC as an acceptable CRC screening test for average-risk individuals.[1,3] Screening intervals for CTC in all of these guidelines are recommended to be 5 years. Current USMSTF guidelines include CTC as a tier 2 CRC screening test because of its low sensitivity for detection of polyps that are less than 6 mm as well as the aforementioned issues with CTC detection of flat polyps and SSP and the absence of evidence showing that CTC plays a major role in decreasing the incidence or mortality of CRC.[4]

COLON CAPSULE ENDOSCOPY

CCE is a relatively new diagnostic modality being explored for CRC screening. It is a minimally invasive procedure that does not require sedation, but does require complete bowel preparation, often more rigorous than that required for colonoscopy. CCE was introduced to the market in 2006 by Given Imaging (Yokneam, Israel) as a first-generation Pillcam Colon Capsule Endoscopy (PCCE I). PCCE I was initially designed as a capsule with a slippery surface and smooth edges designed to be swallowed by the patient. It measured 11 mm $\times$ 31 mm and had 2 cameras (one at either end of the capsule), and a light-emitting diode. Each camera had a 156° angle of view. This device captured 4 pictures per second and had a battery life of 10 to 11 hours. Similar to the well-established small bowel capsule endoscopy platform, images captured by the PCCE I were transmitted by a data recorder that the patient wore externally and were downloaded into a computer workstation for interpretation of images and data reporting (RAPID).

A second-generation PCCE was introduced in 2010 by Medtronic (Dublin, Ireland) with refinements designed to overcome the low sensitivity of PCCE I and was Food and Drug Administration (FDA) approved in 2014 (**Fig. 4**). PCCE II has a slightly different capsule design, data recorder, and a modified RAPID system. The capsule is slightly bigger in size than the PCCE I, measuring 11.6 mm × 31.5 mm. The 2 cameras have a wider angle of view than PCCE I, with each permitting a 172° angle, so that each capsule can provide a nearly 360° view. The PCCE II has a similar battery time of 10 hours, but the addition of an adaptive frame rate (AFR) conserves battery life and improves efficiency.[61] The AFR allows PCCE II to capture images at 14 frames per second when it is in the stomach, increasing to a rate of 35 frames per second when it is in motion, and decreasing to 4 frames per second when it is slow or stationary. The data recorder has a real-time viewer and bidirectional communication that send signals that alert patients to take additional cathartic to promote caudal movement of the capsule. The updated RAPID software also has a polyp size estimation function and flexible spectral imaging color enhancement to enhance the visualization of the surface mucosal pattern and vasculature.[62]

Exquisite colon preparation is crucial in CCE because it is not possible to use external adjuncts, such as endoscopic irrigation or digital subtraction of tagged residua, to cleanse the colon of retained debris during the procedure. Even a small amount of debris can interfere with CCE ability to identify colonic polyps. Of note, colonic preparation during CCE not only aims to achieve an adequate cleansing level but also is meant to distend the colonic wall with clean liquid to provide clear images as well as to promote capsule propulsion and excretion (**Fig. 5**).[63] The current European Society of Gastrointestinal Endoscopy guidelines recommend 4 L of polyethylene glycol solution administered in split doses (2 L the evening before the CCE procedure and 2 L on the day of the examination before capsule ingestion).[64] The purgative can also be combined with booster solution consisting of an osmotic or stimulant purgative. Booster solution should be given once the small bowel mucosa is identified on CCE, and a second dose of booster is recommended if the capsule is not excreted 3 hours after the first booster administration. The most commonly used booster solution in Europe is sodium phosphate solution; however, because of concerns surrounding sodium phosphate renal toxicity, trials in the United States have used osmotic purgatives as the booster.[65] It is important to note that in contrast to incomplete colonoscopy, incomplete CCE examination leaves the left colon uninvestigated.

CCE is minimally invasive and does not require sedation or anesthesia. It was reported in a recent metaanalysis that CCE was associated with an incidence of 4% (14/357) adverse events, most of which were rated as mild to moderate and judged to be related to bowel preparation (headache, nausea, vomiting, abdominal pain).[66] Difficulty swallowing the capsule occurred in less than 1%. Capsule retention occurred in less than 1% and required endoscopic or surgical removal. Other

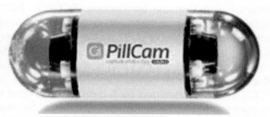

Fig. 4. PCCE II Colon Capsule. PCCE II capsule measuring 11.6 mm × 31.5 mm. The 2 cameras each permit a 172° angle. (© 2012 Medtronic. All rights reserved. Used with the permission of Medtronic.)

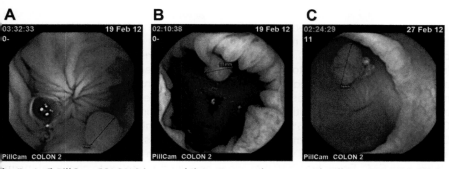

Fig. 5. *A–C)* PillCam COLON 2 images. *(A)* An 7-mm polyp seen with PillCam COLON 2. *(B)* An 1-mm polyp seen with PillCam COLON 2. *(C)* A 14-mm polyp seen with PillCam COLON 2. (© 2012 Medtronic. All rights reserved. Used with the permission of Medtronic.)

dverse events included technical failures owing to capsule or data recorder issues. Given the use of microwave used to transmit the data from the capsule to the recorder, pregnancy is considered a contraindication until further studies are available regarding safety in pregnancy. Like small bowel capsule endoscopy, known or suspected stricture or bowel obstruction is a contraindication given the high risk of capsule retention. MRI scanning should not be performed until the capsule is excreted from the gastrointestinal tract because of the metallic contents of the capsule. It is recommended to avoid CCE in patients with cardiac pacemakers and implantable defibrillators to avoid any potential interface between the devices.[63,65]

Multiple studies have demonstrated that CCE can be a useful adjunct for detecting colorectal neoplasia after incomplete colonoscopy, in patients with symptoms of colorectal neoplasia, or increased risk based on positive indirect CRC screening tests, such as FIT or FOBT.[67–76] More recently, several important studies have evaluated CCE as a screening test in patients at average risk for CRC. Rex and colleagues[77] examined the accuracy of CCE compared with colonoscopy for the detection of colorectal polyps in an average-risk screening population of 884 patients and found the sensitivity of CCE for conventional adenomas ≥ 6 mm and ≥ 10 mm to be 88% and 92%, respectively, with specificity of 82% and 95%, respectively. CCE sensitivity for detecting subjects with any polyp ≥ 6 mm and ≥ 10 mm when matched by colon segment was 81% and 80%, respectively, and the specificity was greater than 93% for both polyp size criteria. When matched by the entire colon, the sensitivity for detecting subjects with any polyp ≥ 6 mm and ≥ 10 mm was 87% and 85%, respectively, and the specificity was greater than 94%. Zavoral and colleagues[78] found the sensitivity of CCE for polyps ≥ 6 mm and ≥ 10 mm and adenomas ≥ 10 mm was 79% (95% CI 62%–91%), 88% (95% CI 62%–98%), and 100% (95% CI 72%–100%), respectively, in another study of CCE versus colonoscopy in an average-risk screening population (n = 225). The specificity for polyps ≥ 6 mm and ≥ 10 mm in this study was 97% (95% CI 94%–99%) and 99% (95% CI 97%–100%), respectively. Spada and colleagues[79] examined the accuracy of first- and second-generation CCE for the detection of colorectal polyps in a systematic review and metaanalysis and found that CCE-2 detected polyps ≥ 6 mm with 86% sensitivity (95% CI 82%–89%) and 58% sensitivity (95% CI 44%–70%). CCE-2 and detected polyps ≥ 10 mm with 87% sensitivity (95% CI 81%–91%) and 54% sensitivity (95% CI 29%–77%). In the average-risk screening population, CCE-2 had a specificity of 94.7% for polyps ≥6 mm and 98% for polyps ≥10 mm and identified all 11 invasive cancers detected by colonoscopy.

Cash and colleagues[80] reported the results of a large noninferiority study comparing CCE and CTC in patients at average risk for CRC. All patients (n = 261) were randomized to CCE or CTC and also underwent confirmatory blinded and, if necessary, unblinded colonoscopy. For the primary effectiveness assessment, the detection of polyps ≥6 mm, CCE demonstrated superior diagnostic yield and 2 to 3 times higher sensitivity across all polyp-matching methods compared with CTC (25.6% with CCE vs 8.6% with CTC; P = .99 for noninferiority). The accuracy of CCE versus CTC in the detection of polyps ≥6 mm was assessed in relation to confirmatory colonoscopy results with CCE demonstrating an accuracy of 64.2% versus 26.8% with CTC. For polyps ≥10 mm, when assessed in relation to confirmatory colonoscopy results, CCE had a higher sensitivity compared with CTC (66.7% vs 50.0%, respectively; P = .99 for noninferiority). Moreover, the observed 10.5% diagnostic yield of CCE for polyps ≥10 mm was similar to the 10.3% diagnostic yield of colonoscopy.

Disadvantages of CCE include (1) more aggressive bowel preparation compared with colonoscopy, (2) procedure completion rate (91%) less than colonoscopy (>95%), (3) divergent results regarding sessile serrated lesion detection, (4) limited to diagnosis only, and (5) lower sensitivity and specificity compared with colonoscopy.[61,63,77] The EGSE concluded that "CCE is a feasible, safe and appears to be accurate when used in average-risk individuals." However, US guidelines do not recommend CCE for routine CRC screening, and CCE is not FDA approved for this indication.

SUMMARY

Although colonoscopy is considered the gold-standard CRC screening test and is listed as a preferred modality in some guidelines, it is important to recognize that colonoscopy has limitations related to adherence, acceptability, cost, invasiveness, and availability that limit its universal application to the CRC screening population. For these reasons, it is important to have alternative CRC screening tests available. Offering patients a choice of screening options has been shown to increase CRC screening compliance.[81] Among the screening alternatives discussed in this article, FS has the most robust clinical data supporting its ability to decrease the incidence and mortality of CRC and is used as a preferred CRC screening test in multiple countries. Similar data are lacking for CTC and CCE; however, both of these tests permit visualization of the entire colon, which was one of the arguments that resulted in the emergence of colonoscopy over FS for CRC screening over the last 2 decades in the United States. It is important to recognize that, similar to other noncolonoscopy CRC screening tests, positive findings on FS, CTC, or CCE should result in timely performance of colonoscopy to confirm the findings and ideally permit resection of colorectal neoplasia. While there are convincing data regarding results, the accuracy of CTC as a CRC screening test in expert hands, questions regarding outside expert centers as well as its ability to detect subtle right-sided and flat lesions have limited its uptake. Positive data also support the continued development and investigation of CCE as CRC screening option, but the practical aspects of its cost, the intensive bowel preparation, and the time required for the procedure in terms of image acquisition, processing, and interpretation may affect its place among the various screening options if it is ultimately provided with a screening indication.

REFERENCES

1. Lin JS, Piper MA, Perdue LA, et al. Screening for colorectal cancer: updated evidence report and systematic review for the US Preventive Services Task Force. JAMA 2016;315:2576–94.
2. Provenzale D, Gupta S, Ahnen DJ, et al. NCCN guidelines insights: colorectal cancer screening, version 1.2018. J Natl Compr Canc Netw 2018;16:939–49.
3. Wolf AMD, Fontham ETH, Church TR, et al. Colorectal cancer screening for average risk adults: 2018 guideline update from the American Cancer Society. CA Cancer J Clin 2018;68:250–81.
4. Rex DK, Boland CR, Dominitz JA, et al. Colorectal cancer screening: recommendations for physicians and patients from the U.S. Multi-Society Task Force on colorectal cancer screening. Am J Gastroenterol 2017;112:1016–30.
5. Painter J, Saunders DB, Bell GD, et al. Depth of insertion at flexible sigmoidoscopy: implications for colorectal cancer screening and instrument design. Endoscopy 1999;31:227–31.
6. Health, United States, 2016. Hyattsville (MD): National Center for Health Statistics; 2017. Report No.: 2017-1232.
7. Atkin WS, Edwards R, Kralj-Hans I, et al. Once-only flexible sigmoidoscopy screening in prevention of colorectal cancer: a multicentre randomised controlled trial. Lancet 2010;375:1624–33.
8. Holme O, Loberg M, Kalager M, et al. Effect of flexible sigmoidoscopy screening on colorectal cancer incidence and mortality: a randomized clinical trial. JAMA 2014;312:606–15.
9. Schoen RE, Pinsky PF, Weissfeld JL, et al. Colorectal-cancer incidence and mortality with screening flexible sigmoidoscopy. N Engl J Med 2012;366:2345–57.
10. Segnan N, Armaroli P, Bonelli L, et al. Once-only sigmoidoscopy in colorectal cancer screening: follow-up findings of the Italian randomized controlled trial–SCORE. J Natl Cancer Inst 2011;103:1310–22.
11. Holme O, Schoen RE, Senore C, et al. Effectiveness of flexible sigmoidoscopy screening in men and women and different age groups: pooled analysis of randomised trials. BMJ 2017;356:i6673.
12. Atkin W, Wooldrage K, Parkin DM, et al. Long-term effects of once-only flexible sigmoidoscopy screening after 17 years of follow-up: the UK Flexible Sigmoidoscopy Screening Randomised Controlled Trial. Lancet 2017;389:1299–311.
13. Fisher DA, Maple JT, Ben-Menachem T, et al. Complications of colonoscopy. Gastrointest Endosc 2011;74:745–52.
14. Knudsen AB, Zauber AG, Rutter CM, et al. Estimation of benefits, burden, and harms of colorectal cancer screening strategies: modeling study for the US Preventive Services Task Force. JAMA 2016;315:2595–609.
15. Pickhardt PJ, Yee J, Johnson CD. CT colonography: over two decades from discovery to practice. Abdom Radiol (NY) 2018;43:517–22.
16. Vining DJ, Gelfand DW, Bechtold RE, et al. Technical feasibility of colon imaging with helical CT and virtual reality (abstr). AJR Am J Roentgenol 1994;162:104.
17. Dachman A, Kuniyoshi J, Boyle C, et al. CT colonography with three-dimensional problem solving for detection of colonic polyps. AJR Am J Roentgenol 1998;171:989–95.
18. Royster AP, Fenlon HM, Clarke PD, et al. CT colonoscopy of colorectal neoplasms: two-dimensional and three-dimensional virtual-reality techniques with colonoscopic correlation. AJR Am J Roentgenol 1997;169:1237–42.

19. Hara AK, Johnson CD, Reed JE, et al. Detection of colorectal polyps with CT colography: initial assessment of sensitivity and specificity. Radiology 1997;205: 59–65.

20. Fenlon HM, Nunes DP, Schroy PC, et al. A comparison of virtual and conventional colonoscopy for the detection of colorectal polyps. N Engl J Med 1999;341: 1496–503.

21. Hara AK, Johnson CD, MacCarty RL, et al. CT colonography: single- versus multidetector row imaging. Radiology 2001;219:461–5.

22. Fletcher JG, Johnson CD, Welch TJ, et al. Optimization of CT colonography technique: prospective trial in 180 patients. Radiology 2000;216:704–11.

23. Yee J, Akerkar GA, Hung RK, et al. Colorectal neoplasia: performance characteristics of CT colonography for detection in 300 patients. Radiology 2001;219: 685–92.

24. Atkin W, Dadswell E, Wooldrage K, et al. Computed tomographic colonography versus colonoscopy for investigation of patients with symptoms suggestive of colorectal cancer (SIGGAR): a multicentre randomised trial. Lancet 2013;381: 1194–202.

25. Halligan S, Wooldrage K, Dadswell E, et al. Computed tomographic colonography versus barium enema for diagnosis of colorectal cancer or large polyps in symptomatic patients (SIGGAR): a multicentre randomised trial. Lancet 2013; 381:1185–93.

26. Johnson CD, Harmsen WS, Wilson LA, et al. Prospective blinded evaluation of computed tomographic colonography for screen detection of colorectal polyps. Gastroenterology 2003;125:311–9.

27. Cotton PB, Durkalski VL, Benoit PC, et al. Computed tomographic colonography (virtual colonoscopy)–a multicenter comparison with standard colonoscopy for detection of colorectal neoplasia. JAMA 2004;291:1713–9.

28. Rockey DC, Poulson E, Niedzwiecki D, et al. Analysis of air contrast barium enema, computed tomographic colonography, and colonoscopy: prospective comparison. Lancet 2005;365:305–11.

29. Pickhardt PJ, Choi JR, Hwang I, et al. Computed tomographic virtual colonoscopy to screen for colorectal neoplasia in asymptomatic adults. N Engl J Med 2003;349:2191–200.

30. Johnson CD, Chen MH, Toledano AY, et al. Accuracy of CT colonography for detection of large adenomas and cancers. N Engl J Med 2008;359:1207–17.

31. Graser A, Stieber P, Nagel D, et al. Comparison of CT colonography, colonoscopy, sigmoidoscopy, and fecal occult blood tests for the detection of advanced adenoma in an average risk population. Gut 2009;58:241–8.

32. Mulhall BP, Veerappan GR, Jackson JL. Test performance of CT colonography: a systematic review of the literature and meta-analysis. Ann Intern Med 2005;142: 635–50.

33. Halligan S, Altman DG, Taylor SA, et al. CT colonography in the detection of colorectal polyps and cancer: systematic review, meta-analysis, and proposed minimum data set for study level reporting. Radiology 2005;237:893–904.

34. Pickhardt PJ, Hassan C, Halligan S, et al. Colorectal cancer: CT colonography and colonoscopy for detection—systematic review and meta-analysis. Radiology 2011;259:393–405.

35. Kitasaka OM, Suenaga MK, Takayama T, et al. Digital bowel cleansing free colonic polyp detection method for fecal tagging CT colonography. Acad Radiol 2009;16:486–94.

6. Linguraru MG, Zhao S, Van Uitert RL, et al. CAD of colon cancer on CT colonography cases without cathartic bowel preparation. Conf Proc IEEE Eng Med Biol Soc 2008;2008:2996–9.

7. Fletcher JG, Silva AC, Fidler JL, et al. Noncathartic CT colonography: image quality assessment and performance in a screening cohort. AJR Am J Roentgenol 2013;201:787–94.

8. Iannaccone R, Laghi A, Catalano C, et al. Computed tomographic colonography without cathartic preparation for the detection of colorectal polyps. Gastroenterology 2004;127:1300–11.

9. Jensch S, DeVries AH, Peringa J, et al. CT colonography with limited bowel preparation: performance characteristics in an increased risk population. Radiology 2008;247:122.

0. Nagata K, Okawa T, Honma A, et al. Full-laxative versus minimum-laxative fecaltagging CT colonography using 64-detector row CT: prospective blinded comparison of diagnostic performance, tagging quality, and patient acceptance. Acad Radiol 2009;16:780–9.

1. Levin B, Lieberman DA, McFarland B, et al. Screening and surveillance for the early detection of colorectal cancer and adenomatous polyps, 2008: a joint guideline from the American Cancer Society, the US Multi-Society Task Force on Colorectal Cancer, and the American College of Radiology. Gastroenterology 2008;134:1570–95.

2. Whitlock EP, Lin JS, Liles E, et al. Screening for colorectal cancer: a targeted, updated systematic review for the US Preventive Services Task Force. Ann Intern Med 2008;149:638–58.

3. Dhruva SS, Phurrough SE, Salive ME, et al. CMS's landmark decision on CT colonography—examining the relevant data. N Engl J Med 2009;360:2699–701.

4. Pickhardt PJ, Taylor AJ, Kim DH, et al. Screening for colorectal neoplasia with CT colonography: initial experience from the 1st year of coverage by third-party payers. Radiology 2006;241:417–25.

5. Cash BD, Riddle MS, Bhattacharya I, et al. CT colonography of a Medicare-aged population: outcomes observed in an analysis of more than 1400 patients. AJR Am J Roentgenol 2012;199:W27–34.

6. Cash BD, Stamps K, McFarland EG, et al. Clinical use of CT colonography for colorectal cancer screening in military training facilities and potential impact on HEDIS measures. J Am Coll Radiol 2013;10:30–6.

7. Pooler BD, Baumel MJ, Cash BD, et al. Screening CT colonography: multicenter survey of patient experience, preference, and potential impact on adherence. AJR Am J Roentgenol 2012;198:1361–6.

8. Kim DH, Pooler BD, Weiss JM, et al. Five-year colorectal cancer outcomes in a large negative CT colonography screening cohort. Eur Radiol 2012;22:1488–94.

9. Pickhardt PJ, Hain KS, Kim DH, et al. Low rates of cancer or high-grade dysplasia in colorectal polyps collected from computed tomography colonography screening. Clin Gastroenterol Hepatol 2010;8:610–5.

0. Smith MA, Weiss JM, Potvien A, et al. Insurance coverage for CT colonography screening: impact on overall colorectal cancer screening rates. Radiology 2017;284(3):717–24.

1. Zalis ME, Barish MA, Choi JR, et al. CT colonography reporting and data system: a consensus proposal. Radiology 2005;236:3–9.

2. Hur C, Chung DC, Schoen RE, et al. The management of small polyps found by virtual colonoscopy: results of a decision analysis. Clin Gastroenterol Hepatol 2007;5:237–44.

53. Brenner DJ, Georgsson MA. Mass screening with CT colonography: should the radiation exposure be of concern? Gastroenterology 2005;129:328–37.
54. Pickhardt PJ. Incidence of colonic perforation at CT colonography: review of existing data and implications for screening of asymptomatic adults. Radiology 2006;239:313–6.
55. Li D, Jin C, McCulloch C, et al. Association of large serrated polyps with synchronous advanced colorectal neoplasia. Am J Gastroenterol 2009;104:695–702.
56. Hassan C, Quintero E, Dumonceau JM, et al. Post-polypectomy colonoscopy surveillance: European Society of Gastrointestinal Endoscopy (ESGE) guideline. Endoscopy 2013;45:842–64.
57. Kim DH, Matkowskyj KA, Lubner MG, et al. Serrated polyps at CT colonography: prevalence and characteristics of the serrated polyp spectrum. Radiology 2016; 280:455–63.
58. IJspeert JE, Tutein Nolthenius CJ, Kuipers EJ, et al. CT colonography vs. colonoscopy for detection of high-risk sessile serrated polyps. Am J Gastroenterol 2016; 111:516–22.
59. Yee J, Kim DH, Rosen MP, et al. ACR appropriateness criteria colorectal cancer screening. J Am Coll Radiol 2014;11:543–51.
60. Rex DK, Johnson DA, Anderson JC, et al. American College of Gastroenterology guidelines for colorectal cancer screening 2009. Am J Gastroenterol 2009;104: 739–50.
61. Pasha SF. Applications of colon capsule endoscopy. Curr Gastroenterol Rep 2018;20(5):22.
62. Carter D, Eliakim R. PillCam colon capsule endoscopy (PCCE) in colonic diseases. Ann Transl Med 2016;4(16):307.
63. Han YM, Im JP. Colon capsule endoscopy: where are we and where are we going. Clin Endosc 2016;49(5):449–53.
64. Spada C, Hassan C, Galmiche JP, et al. Colon capsule endoscopy: European Society of Gastrointestinal Endoscopy (ESGE) Guideline. Endoscopy 2012;44(5): 527–36.
65. Tal AO, Vermehren J, Albert JG. Colon capsule endoscopy: current status and future directions. World J Gastroenterol 2014;20(44):16596–602.
66. Health Quality Ontario. Colon capsule endoscopy for the detection of colorectal polyps: an evidence-based analysis. Ont Health Technol Assess Ser 2015; 15(14):1–39.
67. Spada C, Hassan C, Barbaro B, et al. Colon capsule versus CT colonography in patients with incomplete colonoscopy: a prospective, comparative trial. Gut 2015;64(2):272–81.
68. Negreanu L, Babiuc R, Bengus A, et al. PillCam Colon 2 capsule in patients unable or unwilling to undergo colonoscopy. World J Gastroenterol 2013;5(11): 559–67.
69. Baltes P, Bota M, Albert J, et al. PillCam COLON 2 after incomplete colonoscopy– a prospective multi-center study. World J Gastroenterol 2018;24:3556–66.
70. Nogales O, Garcia-Lledo J, Lujan M, et al. Therapeutic impact of colon capsule endoscopy with PillCam COLON 2 after incomplete standard colonoscopy: a Spanish multicenter study. Rev Esp Enferm Dig 2017;109:322–7.
71. Morgan DR, Malik PR, Romeo DP, et al. Initial US evaluation of second-generation capsule colonoscopy for detecting colon polyps. BMJ Open Gastroenterol 2016; 3(1):e000089.
72. Spada C, Hassan CM, Munoz-Navas M, et al. Second-generation colon capsule endoscopy compared with colonoscopy. Gastrointest Endosc 2011;74:581–9.

73. Eliakim R, Yassin K, Niv Y, et al. Prospective multicenter performance evaluation of the second-generation colon capsule compared with colonoscopy. Endoscopy 2009;41:1026–31.
74. Romero C, Rodriguez de Miguel C, Serradesanferm A, et al. PillCam colon capsule for colorectal cancer screening: a prospective and comparative study with colonoscopy. Gastroenterology 2015;148(4S1):S759.
75. Holleran G, Leen R, O'Morain C, et al. Colon capsule endoscopy as possible filter test for colonoscopy selection in a screening population with positive fecal immunology. Endoscopy 2014;46:473–8.
76. Hagel AF, Gabele E, Raithel M, et al. Colon capsule endoscopy: detection of colonic polyps compared with conventional colonoscopy and visualization of extracolonic pathologies. Can J Gastroenterol Hepatol 2014;28(2):77–82.
77. Rex DK, Adler SN, Aisenberg J, et al. Accuracy of capsule colonoscopy in detecting colorectal polyps in a screening population. Gastroenterology 2015; 148:948–57.
78. Voska M, Zavoral M, Grega T, et al. Accuracy of colon capsule endoscopy for colorectal neoplasia detection in individuals referred for a screening colonoscopy. Gastroenterol Res Pract. 2019;2019:5975438.
79. Spada C, Pasha SF, Gross SA, et al. Accuracy of first- and second-generation colon capsules in endoscopic detection of colorectal polyps: a systematic review and meta-analysis. Clin Gastroenterol Hepatol 2016;14(11):1533–43.
80. Cash BD, Fleisher MR, Fern S, et al. A multicenter, prospective, randomized study comparing the diagnostic yield of colon capsule endoscopy versus computed tomographic colonography in a screening population. Results of the TOPAZ study. Gastrointest Endosc 2019;89:AB87–8.
81. Inadomi J, Vijan S, Janz NK, et al. Adherence to colorectal cancer screening: a randomized clinical trial or competing strategies. Arch Intern Med 2012;172: 575–82.

How Artificial Intelligence Will Impact Colonoscopy and Colorectal Screening

Dennis L. Shung, MD[a],
Michael F. Byrne, MA, MD (Cantab), FRCPC, MRCP[b],*

KEYWORDS

- Artificial intelligence • Colonoscopy • Value-based care

KEY POINTS

- Artificial intelligence can improve colonoscopy quality by detecting adenomatous polyps and decrease associated costs by classifying low-risk polyps that do not need removal.
- An integrated system with artificial intelligence can improve the provider experience by decreasing documentation burden through automating data entry for quality measures.
- Important limitations of the technology must be recognized, including the dataset features for algorithm development and integration into endoscopist workflow.
- Future directions include automatic assessment of polyp size and borders, histologic staging and personalized risk stratification.

INTRODUCTION

Colorectal cancer is a major cause of cancer-related death, and colonoscopy with complete resection of neoplastic lesions has been suggested to reduce both incidence and mortality of colorectal cancer.[1,2] Quality of colonoscopies in detecting malignancies varies, and outpatient colonoscopies in surgery centers cost the most for all procedures performed in ambulatory surgery centers, an estimated $3.2 billion in the United States in 2018.[3] In the American Board of Internal Medicine's "Choosing Wisely" campaign, one of the areas of endoscopic overuse is surveillance colonoscopy in individuals with low-risk polyps.[4] Payers are motivated to decrease unnecessary costs associated with colonoscopy.

Artificial intelligence (AI) is poised to transform clinical practice through machine learning, a method that overlaps computer science and statistics to create software programs that directly learn from patterns found in data input.[5]

[a] Section of Digestive Diseases, Department of Medicine, Yale School of Medicine, P.O. Box 208019, New Haven, CT 06520-8019, USA; [b] Division of Gastroenterology, Vancouver General Hospital, University of British Columbia, 5153 - 2775 Laurel Street, Vancouver, British Columbia, Canada
* Corresponding author.
E-mail address: michael.byrne@vch.ca

Gastrointest Endoscopy Clin N Am 30 (2020) 585–595
https://doi.org/10.1016/j.giec.2020.02.010
1052-5157/20/© 2020 Elsevier Inc. All rights reserved.

giendo.theclinics.com

AI adds value to colorectal cancer screening and surveillance by enhancing the visual abilities of the endoscopist to find precancerous polyps and classify polyps that do not need to be removed. Currently, the state of AI in colonoscopy consists of software running supervised machine learning algorithms to specifically find polyps or to classify them. In the future, we anticipate a fully integrated system that will provide decision support for assessing depth of invasion, and possibly even integrating genotypic and other data to provide personalized risk assessments for colon cancer.

ARTIFICIAL INTELLIGENCE PROMOTES VALUE IN COLORECTAL CANCER SCREENING AND SURVEILLANCE

Value in health care has been defined as improvement in quality or decrease in cost.[6] Colonoscopy as a preventive measure to completely remove neoplastic lesions holds value for public health in preventing colorectal cancer.[1] However, this is dependent on the quality of the procedure in finding all precancerous lesions, which can be reflected with adenoma detection rates (ADRs).[7] One study has suggested that increase of 1% in ADR leads to a 3% decreased risk of interval colorectal cancer.[7] AI in colonoscopy can potentially improve the quality of the procedure through computer-aided detection (CADe) to increase the adenoma detection rate.

Costs can be managed by expert judgment to avoid removing low-risk polyps unnecessarily, proposed in the Preservation and Incorporation of Valuable endoscopic Innovations (PIVI) by guidelines from the American Society for Gastrointestinal Endoscopy for optic biopsy of diminutive polyps.[8] AI can decrease the costs related to unnecessary polyp removal through computer-aided diagnosis (CADx), as implemented by either a resect-and-discard or diagnose-and-leave strategy.

The technology that has advanced CADe into real-world implementation is deep learning through neural networks, a branch of machine learning that discovers features that are meaningful through large amounts of data. This contrasts with earlier methods, when algorithms were built by a human selecting features thought to be meaningful (recently summarized in a review by Ahmad and colleagues[9]).

For deep learning-driven CADe alone, there are 3 recent prospective validation studies.[10–12] (**Table 1**).

For CADx alone, machine learning models have been used in 6 prospective validation studies, which test different modalities: magnifying narrow band imaging (NBI),[13,14] endocytoscopy,[15] laser-induced fluorescence spectroscopy,[16,17] and autofluorescence endoscopy.[18] (**Table 2**).

Both CADe and CADx have been integrated for fully automated polyp detection and immediate characterization in real time in a recent study trained a convolutional neural network using a training set of 223 polyp videos (60,089 frames) and validated the algorithm on 40 videos (106 polyps) with sensitivity 98% and specificity of 83% for identifying adenomas.[19]

An obvious limitation of the technology is that the algorithm cannot detect polyps that are not in the visual field of the colonoscope and performance may vary based on quality of inspection. Furthermore, other factors such as the speed of withdrawal and bowel preparation can also affect algorithm performance. This of course is not unique to AI, but applies to other devices such as forms of virtual chromoendoscopy.

Finally, a group recently presented (in abstract form) a system that decreases documentation burden by automating the input of quality measures based on image recognition (time of insertion, cecal intubation time, withdrawal time, tool use and intervention via Current Procedural Terminology codes and preparation quality via

Table 1
Deep learning computer-aided detection with validation on colonoscopy videos with histologically confirmed polyps

Study	Methods	Training Dataset	Validation Dataset	Sensitivity (per Image Frame), %	Specificity, %	Area Under the Receiver Operator Curve
Wang et al,[10] 2018	Convoluted Neural Networks	5545 images	138 videos	91.6		
Misawa et al,[11] 2018	Convoluted Neural Networks	73 colonoscopy videos divided into short videos: training (411 videos)	Testing (135 videos)	90.0	63.3	0.87
Urban et al,[12] 2018	Convoluted Neural Networks	8641 images	9 videos	93.0	93.0	

Boston Bowel Preparation Scale).[20] They deployed an approach with 7 separate convoluted neural networks with live feedback during the procedure.

INTEGRATION INTO CLINICAL PROCESSES DIRECTLY AFFECTS ADOPTION OF MACHINE LEARNING PRODUCTS

Clinical integration is key, particularly in the fast-paced world of colonoscopy, and special considerations must be taken to ensure that the product enhances clinical care. As a baseline, machine learning products should provide a fully automate diagnostic workflow during colonoscopy that detects and characterizes polyps in real time. A recent model that does both was tested on 215 colonoscopy videos in which the model detected and tracked individual polyps while also providing an estimate for the histology via optical biopsy.[21] In addition, the product should not unnecessarily prolong procedures, overwhelm practitioners with false positives, or become a distraction that adversely affects the ability of practitioners to perform the procedures well. These models function as clinical decision support, and must consider how explainable the model is to providers, the usability of the product during clinical care, how the information is delivered to the providers and how the product increases or decreases the time necessary to provide clinical care.[22] The ultimate goal is to enhance the providers' performance; for colonoscopy, improving efficiency for endoscopists is a priority for quality care.[23]

Most proposed measures for efficiency include an element of time. This is particularly relevant in high-volume endoscopy centers, where the number of cases that can be performed directly affects the revenue of the center. Algorithms used must therefore seek to decrease the amount of time it takes for colonoscopies to be performed with the same level of quality (eg, with no decrease in the adenoma detection rate).

Successful integration also requires adequate study of the human factors and perception of the product, including robust educational programming and training, ongoing user feedback regarding confidence in the tool, and logistical issues

Table 2
Machine learning computer-aided diagnosis with validation on captured images of polyps

Study	Setting	Methods (with # Features)	Training Dataset	Validation Dataset, no. Polyps	Sensitivity, %	Specificity, %
Chen et al,[14] 2018	Magnifying NBI	Deep Neural Network	2157 polyps	284	96.3	78.1
Kominami et al,[13] 2016	Magnifying NBI	Support Vector Machines (SVM) (128 features)	2247 polyps at maximal magnifying NBI	118	95.9	93.3
Mori et al,[15] 2017	Endocytoscopy	SVM (312 features)	61,925 endocytoscopic images	466	91.3 – 93.8	88.7 – 91.0
Rath et al,[16] 2016	Laser-induced fluorescence spectroscopy	WavStat4 – Linear Discriminant Analysis	Not reported	137	81.8	85.2
Kuiper et al,[17] 2015	Laser-induced fluorescence spectroscopy	WavStat4 – Linear Discriminant Analysis	Not reported	207	85.3	58.8
Aihara et al,[18] 2013	Autofluorescence endoscopy	Unknown	103 polyps	102	94.2	88.9

egarding its use. For example, training should not only teach providers how to use the product but also educate providers on how to adjudicate recommendations that may not agree with their clinical experience or impression. An ongoing challenge specific to deep learning is the "black box" nature of the deep learning algorithms, which limit the ability to explain how the algorithm came up with specific recommendations.

MACHINE LEARNING PRODUCTS REQUIRE RIGOROUS VALIDATION

When working with deep learning or other machine learning products, it is essential to ensure that the models are appropriately tested, or validated.[24] Because the model learns from the available data, the data used to train the models should never be used to evaluate the model performance. Validation of the model using new data allows for the best measure of the model's true performance, or generalizability. Ideally this would proceed in a well-designed, adequately powered prospective randomized controlled trial with real-time use of the machine learning models during colonoscopy versus colonoscopy without AI.[25–27] An alternative strategy proposed is a random tandem randomized controlled trial, which would theoretically be better because each patient would serve as his or her own control group.

The only randomized controlled trial to date for CADe was performed in China, an open, nonblinded trial of diagnostic colonoscopy with or without assistance of a real-time polyp detection system running a convoluted neural network in real time. In the trial, 1058 patients were included with 536 controls and 522 with the AI intervention. The intervention arm demonstrated significantly improved adenoma detection rate (29.1% vs 20.3%, $P<.001$) and significantly higher withdrawal time (6.9 vs 6.4 minutes, $P<.001$) that became equivalent after excluding biopsy time (6.18 vs 6.07 minutes, $P = .15$). They reported a total of 39 false alarms in the intervention arm, which averaged to 0.075 false alarms per colonoscopy.

Despite carefully designed experiments to test model performance, in real-world application deep learning models may be limited by model bias and model interoperability stemming from the limitations of the training data.[28] For example, if the training data for a polyp detection model were predominantly in East Asian patients with a specific brand of endoscope, the model may not be perform well in a white-predominant population with a different brand.

In addition, the issues of safety, reliability, and demonstrated improvement from the standard of care are key issues that go beyond validation on new datasets. To reassure providers that the tool is both safe and reliable, parallel processes should be in place to identify and deal with errors.[22] This emphasizes the importance of continuous maintenance and monitoring, which has been addressed by the Food and Drug Administration (FDA) in a recent whitepaper detailing the regulatory framework for updating software as medical devices.

MACHINE LEARNING PRODUCTS FACE REGULATORY, LEGAL, AND ETHICAL CHALLENGES

Regulatory rules vary from country to country, but are required before implementation of these algorithms for clinical care. In the United States, the FDA has drafted a framework for streamlined review under the term software as medical devices (SaMD).[29–31] This is defined by the International Medical Device Regulators Forum as "software intended to be used for one or more medical purposes that perform these purposes without being part of a hardware medical device." The proposed risk-based regulatory framework for SaMD outlines categories of regulation based on severity of health care condition or situation (critical, serious, and nonserious) and significance of information provided by the software to the health care decision (for treatment or diagnosis, to drive clinical management, or to inform clinical management). This framework is adopted from the International Medical Device Regulators Forum and shared by the European Union Medical Device Regulation and Canadian Draft Guidance Document for Software as a Medical Device.[32] The 3 risk classes are as follows: Class I (low risk), Class II (divided into IIA and IIB), and Class III (highest risk) with exemptions for classes I and II from 510(k) requirements either by specific FDA exemption or if they were legally marketed before the enactment of Medical Device Amendments on May 28, 1976. Classes I and II require a 510(k), which is a premarket submission that demonstrates that the device is at least as safe and effective as an existing legally marketed device. For Class III, a premarket approval application to demonstrate safety and effectiveness, which includes clinical trial data with study protocols, safety and effectiveness data, adverse reactions and complications, device failures and replacements, patient information, complaints, all subject data, and all statistical analyses (**Table 3**).

Furthermore, manufacturers must manage patient risks throughout the entire product lifecycle, mainly to ensure safety and effectiveness. The updated strategy includes SaMD Prespecifications, or "what" the algorithm is intended to learn, and an algorithm change protocol, or "how" the algorithm will learn while maintaining safety and efficacy.[30]

An example for colonoscopy is as follows:

1. Polyp Detection and Classification SaMD for Adenomatous Polyps

Description of SaMD: An AI/ML application intended for average risk patients presenting for screening and surveillance colonoscopy. The images from the colonoscopy video are processed and analyzed to detect polyps in the visual field throughout the colon. When an image is captured, it will be classified to be adenomatous or nonadenomatous with a percentage risk generated to indicate the probability of being adenomatous. This SaMD application will improve polyp detection and help guide decisions for low-risk polyps to be resected and discarded or left in.

SaMD Prespecifications:
- Modify the algorithm to ensure consistent performance across different levels of bowel preparation
- Reduce false alarm rates while maintaining sensitivity to polyps

Algorithm Change Protocol: For these modifications, the algorithm change protocol includes detailed methods for database generation, reference standard labeling, and

Table 3
Software as medical device (SaMD) category risk-based classification

State of Health Care Situation or Condition	Significance of Information Provided by SaMD to Health Care Decision		
	Treat or Diagnose	**Drive Clinical/ Patient Management**	**Inform Clinical/Patient Management**
Critical	III	III	I or II[b]
Serious	II or III[a]	II or III[a]	I or II[b]
Nonserious	I or II[b]	I or II[b]	I or II[b]

[a] Class III if an erroneous result could lead to immediate danger.
[b] Class II if the software is intended to image or monitor a physiologic process or condition. Class I under Rule 12.

comparative analysis along the performance requirements, including sensitivity and specificity, and statistical analysis plan. The manufacturer follows good machine learning practices.

In Japan, this has been studied by the Pharmaceuticals and Medical Devices Agency.[33] Of note, Japan's regulatory agency has recently approved the first AI-assisted endocytoscopy product was approved without a prospective randomized controlled trial.

Legal

The framework for legal responsibilities has not been established, and in a sensitive field such as medicine, the possibility of error in health care decisions made in part with the help of algorithms may expose providers to unanticipated liability (eg, for misdiagnosis of a low-risk polyp that becomes interval cancer).[24] Modifications to malpractice insurance, informed consent for the use of AI, and contingency plans should be in place to mitigate risk. Unfortunately, due to the absence of real-world use of AI in health care, there is limited precedent to draw on to provide guidance for patients, providers, or health care systems.

Ethics and Data Security

Respect for autonomy

AI applications in colonoscopy require a large volume of images and videos to develop, validate, and maintain performance. Because of the insatiable appetite for data, patient privacy and data security are key issues that should be thoughtfully addressed.

Patient privacy has traditionally been maintained through the system of individual patient consents, which has been argued to be prohibitively restrictive for purposes of AI research. A proposed solution is a "broad consent" policy, in which patients allow multiple secondary uses of their fully anonymized health data.[34]

Data security covers both maintenance of secure databases and also ensuring secure sharing and transfer across institutions and organizations. Data breaches could undermine patient privacy and the patient-physician relationship. Secure cloud computing solutions have been proposed and developed by commercial entities and electronic health record companies, but data harmonization and interoperability across systems remains a particular challenge.

Nonmaleficence

Deployment of AI applications in colonoscopy could result in mistakes that lead to interval cancers or overutilization by performing unnecessary biopsies. High-risk polyps could be wrongly classified as benign, and polyp detection could either miss a cancerous lesion or result in additional unnecessary biopsies of benign lesions. Furthermore, the phenomenon of "automation bias," in which providers trust AI decisions even if they are incorrect, may lead to overreliance on the technology and deskilling of the endoscopists.[35] Proper education and training of providers on the limitations of the AI technology is critical before widespread deployment. Accountability also should be considered in the event that a mistake is made when using the AI application, possibly titrated to the degree of autonomy accorded to the application.

Beneficence

To ensure that AI applications in colonoscopy act for the best interest of the patient, its recommendations should be taken into clinical context. One suggestion has been a new workflow that may incorporate the use of multidisciplinary meetings to review lesions characterized by the AI system and discuss the best approach for treatment.[34]

Justice

AI applications in colonoscopy may concentrate the benefits in wealthier systems and have data bias that do not include patients from low-resource settings. The expense of computational infrastructure to store data and deploy AI applications for colonoscopy may lead to a disparity in treatment between wealthy and poorer health systems. In addition, patients in low-resource settings may not have their data incorporated into the AI applications, leading to underrepresentation that may lead to poorer performance even if deployed for their care. To promote widespread uptake, funding of prospective trials should include earmarked funds to provide a basic level of infrastructure for every center. Furthermore, careful validation of the AI applications in multiple settings is important to ensure that the performance is consistent for all patients.

DATA LABELING IS A KEY LIMITATION TO DEVELOPING AND MAINTAINING MACHINE LEARNING PRODUCTS

The greatest limitation for the current models being developed is the need for large volumes of labeled datasets, commonly known as "ground truth." In the case of colonoscopy, the ground truth is either human annotation that the polyp is present, or pathologic diagnosis of a polyp adjudicated by multiple graders. In particular, deep learning algorithms for imaging require an enormous quantity of data to capture the variety of real-world images.[36] These include both static images (still pictures) and video recordings of colonoscopies, considering positive images, and quality of labeling. The labeling quality is considered to be the most important aspect, simply because models area data dependent and operate under a "garbage in, garbage out" framework and require expert endoscopist evaluation.[24] Current models used in colonoscopy are "supervised" machine learning models, which requires that all data used to train the models have had "ground truth" or labels attached to each of the datapoints. However, the expense and effort required to label images and video frames is prohibitive, particularly due to the need for specialized expertise.

FUTURE DIRECTIONS

Enhancements or additional algorithms could include automatic polyp sizing, evaluation of polyp borders that could be used to gauge the depth of invasion for large polyps, and clinical decision support to guide method of tumor removal.

Endoscopic tissue resection in particular is an emerging area in which the depth of tumor invasion in the esophagus, stomach and colon may help guide management decisions. Several deep learning–based CADx tools have been developed to detect very low risk lesions for esophageal squamous cell, early gastric, and colorectal cancer with similar criteria that have very low risk for lymph node spread.[37] In particular, computer-aided diagnosis platforms can help determine whether squamous cell carcinoma of the esophagus is classified as confined to the submucosa (SM1). SM1 lesions have very low risk for spread to lymph nodes and in the absence of high-risk features should undergo curative endoscopic resection.[38] Further work could provide real-time guidance that determines the extent of intervention needed (for example, endoscopic mucosal resection vs endoscopic submucosal dissection vs surgical intervention).

AI also has the potential to adjudicate when endoscopic assessment of diminutive colorectal polyps do not agree with pathologic diagnosis. A recent study provides reliminary evidence that an AI clinical decision support solution; for discordant diagnoses, the clinical decision support services provided additional analysis to suggest that endoscopic diagnoses were correct (90.3% of lesions).[39] The role for AI in clinical decision support to adjudicate discordant endoscopic and pathologic diagnosis could help future planning for surveillance colonoscopies.

The potential for misclassification rate for deep learning models in CADe exists with limited understanding of the neural network architecture. Increased interpretability of neural architectures could be achieved through unsupervised machine learning techniques that examine the presence of important or redundant images. By understanding how the neural network classifies polyps, a misclassified polyp image could be compared to see if there is a deficiency in the dataset or architecture that may have accounted for the error. Another limitation to deep learning–based model is the bottleneck of labeled images. Emerging work in unsupervised machine learning techniques to create autoencoders that could be used to generate synthetic datasets for training deep learning models may augment existing datasets to improve model performance.

In the future, imaging data could be integrated in context with other biological and electronic health record data to create a more nuanced and personalized risk assessment. For patients at particular risk (eg, patients with inflammatory bowel disease), the integration of other clinical risk scores could be used to modify the threshold accordingly for polyp detection.

DISCLOSURE

D.L. Shung: Grant Support through the National Institutes of Health T32 DK007017; M.F. Byrne: CEO and shareholder, Satisfai Health; founder of AI4GI joint venture. Co-development agreement between Olympus America and AI4GI in artificial intelligence and colorectal polyps.

REFERENCES

1. Zauber AG, Winawer SJ, O'Brien MJ, et al. Colonoscopic polypectomy and long-term prevention of colorectal-cancer deaths. N Engl J Med 2012;366(8):687–96.

2. Winawer SJ, Zauber AG, Ho MN, et al. Prevention of colorectal cancer by colonoscopic polypectomy. The National Polyp Study Workgroup. N Engl J Med 1993; 329(27):1977–81.

3. Ambulatory surgery centers database. 2018. Available at: https://www.definitivehc.com/product/our-databases/ambulatory-surgery-centers. Accessed: November 20, 2019.

4. Naik AD, Hinojosa-Lindsey M, Arney J, et al. Choosing Wisely and the perceived drivers of endoscopy use. Clin Gastroenterol Hepatol 2013;11(7):753–5.

5. Abu-Mostafa YS. Learning from data: a short course 2012. Available at: http://amlbook.com/. Accesses November 20, 2019.

6. Porter ME, Lee TH. From volume to value in health care: the work begins. JAMA 2016;316(10):1047–8.

7. Corley DA, Jensen CD, Marks AR, et al. Adenoma detection rate and risk of colorectal cancer and death. N Engl J Med 2014;370(14):1298–306.

8. Rex DK, Kahi C, O'Brien M, et al. The American Society for Gastrointestinal Endoscopy PIVI (Preservation and Incorporation of Valuable Endoscopic Innovations) on real-time endoscopic assessment of the histology of diminutive colorectal polyps. Gastrointest Endosc 2011;73(3):419–22.

9. Ahmad OF, Soares AS, Mazomenos E, et al. Artificial intelligence and computer aided diagnosis in colonoscopy: current evidence and future directions. Lancet Gastroenterol Hepatol 2019;4(1):71–80.

10. Wang P, Xiao X, Glissen Brown JR, et al. Development and validation of a deep learning algorithm for the detection of polyps during colonoscopy. Nat Biomed Eng 2018;2(10):741–8.

11. Misawa M, Kudo SE, Mori Y, et al. Artificial intelligence-assisted polyp detection for colonoscopy: initial experience. Gastroenterology 2018;154(8):2027–9.e3.

12. Urban G, Tripathi P, Alkayali T, et al. Deep learning localizes and identifies polyps in real time with 96% accuracy in screening colonoscopy. Gastroenterology 2018; 155(4):1069–78.e8.

13. Kominami Y, Yoshida S, Tanaka S, et al. Computer-aided diagnosis of colorectal polyp histology by using a real-time image recognition system and narrow-band imaging magnifying colonoscopy. Gastrointest Endosc 2016;83(3):643–9.

14. Chen PJ, Lin MC, Lai MJ, et al. Accurate classification of diminutive colorectal polyps using computer-aided analysis. Gastroenterology 2018;154(3):568–75.

15. Mori Y, Kudo SE, Berzin TM, et al. Computer-aided diagnosis for colonoscopy. Endoscopy 2017;49(8):813–9.

16. Rath T, Tontini GE, Vieth M, et al. In vivo real-time assessment of colorectal polyp histology using an optical biopsy forceps system based on laser-induced fluorescence spectroscopy. Endoscopy 2016;48(6):557–62.

17. Kuiper T, Alderlieste YA, Tytgat KM, et al. Automatic optical diagnosis of small colorectal lesions by laser-induced autofluorescence. Endoscopy 2015;47(1): 56–62.

18. Aihara H, Saito S, Inomata H, et al. Computer-aided diagnosis of neoplastic colo rectal lesions using 'real-time' numerical color analysis during autofluorescence endoscopy. Eur J Gastroenterol Hepatol 2013;25(4):488–94.

19. Byrne MF, Chapados N, Soudan F, et al. Real-time differentiation of adenomatous and hyperplastic diminutive colorectal polyps during analysis of unaltered videos of standard colonoscopy using a deep learning model. Gut 2019;68(1):94–100.

20. Karnes W, Requa J, Dao T, et al. Automated documentation of multiple colonos copy quality measures in real-time with convolutional neural networks: 2761. Am J Gastroenterol 2018;113:S1532.

21. Guizard N, Ghalehjegh SH, Henkel M, et al. 256 – Artificial intelligence for real time multiple polyp detection with identification, tracking, and optical biopsy dur ing colonoscopy. Gastroenterology 2019;156(6). S-48–S-49.

22. Shortliffe EH, Sepulveda MJ. Clinical decision support in the era of artificial intel ligence. JAMA 2018;320(21):2199–200.

23. Gellad ZF, Thompson CP, Taheri J. Endoscopy unit efficiency: quality redefined. Clin Gastroenterol Hepatol 2013;11(9):1046–9.e1.

24. Vinsard DG, Mori Y, Misawa M, et al. Quality assurance of computer-aided detec tion and diagnosis in colonoscopy. Gastrointest Endosc 2019;90(1):55–63.

25. Steyerberg EW, Vickers AJ, Cook NR, et al. Assessing the performance of predic tion models: a framework for traditional and novel measures. Epidemiology 2010; 21(1):128–38.

26. Justice AC, Covinsky KE, Berlin JA. Assessing the generalizability of prognostic information. Ann Intern Med 1999;130(6):515–24.

27. Leggett CL, Wang KK. Computer-aided diagnosis in GI endoscopy: looking into the future. Gastrointest Endosc 2016;84(5):842–4.

28. Wang F, Casalino LP, Khullar D. Deep learning in medicine-promise, progress, and challenges. JAMA Intern Med 2019;179(3):293–4.

29. Food and Drug Administration. Proposed Regulatory Framework for Modifications to Artificial Intelligence/Machine Learning (AI/ML)-Based Software as a Medical Device (SaMD). Available at: https://www.fda.gov/medical-devices/software-medical-device-samd/artificial-intelligence-and-machine-learning-software-medical-device. Accessed: October 27, 2019.

30. Food and Drug Administration. Proposed Regulatory Framework for Modifications to Artificial Intelligence/Machine Learning (AI/ML)-Based Software as a Medical Device (SaMD). Available at: https://www.fda.gov/medical-devices/software-medical-device-samd/artificial-intelligence-and-machine-learning-software-medical-device. Accessed: October 27, 2019.

31. Food and Drug Administration. Clinical Decision Support Software Draft Guidance for Industry and Food and Drug Administration Staff. Available at: https://www.fda.gov/regulatory-information/search-fda-guidance-documents/clinical-decision-support-software. Accessed: November 10, 2019.

32. Canada H. Draft Guidance Document - Software as a Medical Device (SaMD). In: Canada H, ed2019.

33. Chinzei K, Shimizu A, Mori K, et al. Regulatory science on AI-based medical devices and systems. Advanced Biomedical Engineering 2018;7:118–23.

34. Ahmad OF, Stoyanov D, Lovat LB. Barriers and pitfalls for artificial intelligence in gastroenterology: ethical and regulatory issues. Tech Gastrointest Endosc 2019;150636.

35. Lyell D, Coiera E. Automation bias and verification complexity: a systematic review. J Am Med Inform Assoc 2016;24(2):423–31.

36. Beam AL, Kohane IS. Big data and machine learning in health care. JAMA 2018;319(13):1317–8.

37. Shahidi N, Bourke MJ. Can artificial intelligence accurately diagnose endoscopically curable gastrointestinal cancers? Tech Gastrointest Endosc 2019;150639.

38. Pimentel-Nunes P, Dinis-Ribeiro M, Ponchon T, et al. Endoscopic submucosal dissection: European Society of Gastrointestinal Endoscopy (ESGE) guideline. Endoscopy 2015;47(9):829–54.

39. Shahidi NC, Rex DK, Kaltenbach T, et al. Use of endoscopic impression, artificial intelligence, and pathologist interpretation to resolve discrepancies from endoscopy and pathology analyses of diminutive colorectal polyps. Gastroenterology 2020;158(3):783–5.e1.

Evidenced-Based Screening Strategies for a Positive Family History

Jennifer M. Kolb, MD[a],*, Dennis J. Ahnen, MD[a],
N. Jewel Samadder, MD, MSc[b,c]

KEYWORDS

- Advanced adenoma • First-degree relative • Second-degree relative
- Colorectal cancer • Colon cancer screening

KEY POINTS

- Common familial colorectal cancer refers to the associated risk to family members from a sporadic colorectal cancer in probands.
- Individuals with a first-degree relative with colorectal cancer are at a 2-fold or higher risk of colorectal cancer and advanced neoplasia.
- Individuals with a first-degree relative with advanced adenoma have an increased risk of colorectal cancer and advanced neoplasia.
- Professional gastroenterology and oncology society guidelines recommend starting colorectal cancer screening by age 40 in high-risk groups with a positive family history.

INTRODUCTION

Successful implementation and uptake of colorectal cancer (CRC) screening in the United States have had a meaningful impact toward decreasing the incidence and mortality of CRC.[1] However, CRC remains the fourth most common cause of cancer in the United States and the second leading cause of cancer death with 51,020 deaths estimated to occur in 2019.[2] Because colon cancer is preventable, identifying those who might benefit most from screening has the greatest potential to decrease disease burden.

Funding Support: J.M. Kolb is supported in part by the NIH Gastrointestinal Diseases Training Grant (T32-DK007038).
[a] Division of Gastroenterology & Hepatology, University of Colorado Hospital, Anschutz Medical Campus, Aurora, CO, USA; [b] Division of Gastroenterology & Hepatology, Mayo Clinic, 5881 East Mayo Boulevard, Phoenix, AZ 85054, USA; [c] Department of Clinical Genomics, Mayo Clinic, Phoenix, AZ, USA
* Corresponding author. Division of Gastroenterology & Hepatology, University of Colorado Hospital, Anschutz Medical Campus, 1635 Aurora Court, F735, Aurora, CO 80045.
E-mail address: jennifer.m.kolb@cuanschutz.edu

The most commonly recognized high-risk group for CRC is individuals with a positive family history. It is generally recognized that those with a first-degree relative (FDR) with CRC are at a 2-fold or higher risk of CRC or advanced neoplasia. FDRs of patients with advanced adenomas (AAs) have a similarly increased risk. Accordingly, all major US guidelines recommend starting CRC screening by age 40 in these groups.[3-5] Recommendations on screening interval and type of examination are more nuanced and vary between guidelines.

The aims of this paper are to (1) define high-risk populations with a positive family history, (2) describe the risk in those with a positive family history, (3) review the current guidelines for screening and the strength of the recommendations, (4) review the evidence for earlier screening, and (5) discuss challenges and strategies to screening this group.

IDENTIFYING HIGH-RISK PATIENTS WITH A POSITIVE FAMILY HISTORY

In any patient with CRC, it is important to assess family history to see if the individual meets clinical criteria for genetic testing. The National Comprehensive Cancer Network (NCCN) recommends genetics evaluation in anyone with CRC under the age of 50 or with an FDR (parent, sibling, or child) with CRC under the age of 50.[6] In the most extreme situations, such as heritable, monogenic syndromes, such as Lynch syndrome or polyposis syndromes, the risk of CRC can approach 80% to 100%. These patients undergo specialized screening protocols that are beyond the scope of this article and are summarized elsewhere.[6,7]

In the present review, the authors focus on sporadic CRC in probands and the associated risk to family members often referred to as *common familial* CRC. In addition, the authors focus on a family history of AA as a risk factor. AAs are traditionally defined as large ($\geq$1 cm) tubular adenomas or any adenoma with high-grade dysplasia or villous histology. AAs are high-risk polyps that confer an increased risk of future colorectal neoplasia to the affected individual[8-11] and are considered the immediate precursors to CRC and the target of CRC screening.[12,13] Family history in the setting of advanced serrated polyps (ASPs), the analogous, potentially high-risk lesions in the serrated pathway, are also discussed.

RISK IN INDIVIDUALS WITH A POSITIVE FAMILY HISTORY OF COLORECTAL CANCER

The lifetime risk of CRC in average risk individuals is approximately 4.5% and approximately double in individuals with a positive family history.[14] Familial CRC may have some component that is genetic in origin or may be an effect of shared environmental exposures. It is estimated that approximately 10% of the general population aged 30 to 70 years old have an FDR affected by CRC,[15] and up to 30% will have an FDR or second-degree relative (SDR) with CRC.[16]

Numerous studies dating back to the 1980s and incorporated into screening guidelines provided data supporting an increased risk of CRC in patients with FDRs with CRC.[17] One of the first prospective studies by Fuchs and colleagues[18] with greater than 100,000 people using self-reported family history questionnaires demonstrated increased risk among those with affected FDRs compared with no family history (relative risk [RR] 1.72, 95% confidence interval [CI] 1.34–2.19) and even higher risk in younger patients less than 45 years (RR 5.37, 95% CI 1.98–14.6). Most other original studies were retrospective case control or cohort studies with inherent study limitations (did not control for confounders and were limited by self-reported family history); however, they still provided meaningful data on the increased familial risk outside of genetic syndromes.[19-21] These data have been summarized in meta-analyses that indicate a more than 2-fold higher risk of CRC (RR 2.24–2.81) in those with an FDR with CRC (**Table 1**).[22–24] In 2013, Johnson and colleagues[25] evaluated 12 different risk factors for CRC and identified an FDR with CRC as a significant factor associated with increased risk (RR 1.80, 95% CI 1.61–2.02). More recent studies from the authors' group in Utah using the specialized resources of the Utah Population Database, which houses genealogic data in association with linked cancer records, provides robust estimates of familial CRC risk without the family history recall bias of past studies. These data reported a 1.8-fold (95% CI 1.59–2.03) risk of CRC in those with an FDR with CRC and importantly demonstrated that the risk of CRC remains elevated no matter the age of the affected relative.[26,27]

ADDITIONAL FACTORS THAT INFLUENCE RISK IN INDIVIDUALS WITH A POSITIVE FAMILY HISTORY OF COLORECTAL CANCER

Several additional factors related to family history also influence the risk of CRC, including (1) proband age, (2) number of affected family members, (3) type of relative, and (4) site of cancer.

All relatives of individuals with CRC are at increased risk regardless of the age of the affected patient, but in general, the risk appears to be higher the younger the proband. A 2015 systematic review and meta-analysis reported the highest risk in those with an FDR who had CRC at age less than 50 (pooled risk 3.55, 95% CI 1.84–6.83).[28] Since that publication, data from the Utah Population Database and linked cancer registry showed highest risk when index CRC patients were diagnosed at age less than 40 years (hazard ratio 2.53, 95% CI 1.7–3.79).[27] This study and 2 others were included in a meta-analysis for the Banff consensus statement that reported a pooled RR of 2.35 (95% CI 1.92–2.86) for individuals with an FDR with CRC diagnosed at less than 60 years compared with no family history, and for FDR with CRC at ≥60 years, the RR was 1.79 (95% CI 1.58–2.03) (P = .02).[4] A more recent analysis similarly showed significantly elevated risk if the FDR had CRC at age less than 50 (RR 3.57,

Table 1		
Risk estimates for family history of colorectal cancer in meta-analyses		
Metaanalysis	**RR for FDR (95% CI)**	**RR for FDR According to Proband Age (95% CI)**
Johns et al,[22] 2001	2.25 (2.00–2.53)	<45: 3.87 (2.40–6.22) 45–59: 2.25 (1.85–2.72) >60: 1.82 (1.47–2.25)
Baglietto et al,[23] 2006	2.26 (1.86–2.73)	
Butterworth et al,[24] 2006	2.24 (2.06–2.43)	<50: 3.55 (1.84–6.83) >50: 2.18 (1.56–3.04)
Johnson et al,[25] 2013	1.80 (1.61–2.02)	—
Wong et al,[70] 2018	1.76 (1.57–1.97)	<50: 2.81 (1.94–4.07) >50: 1.47 (1.28–1.69)
Leddin et al,[4] 2018	1.31 (1.11–1.55)	<60: 2.35 (1.92–2.86) >60: 1.79 (1.58–2.03)
Mehraban Far et al,[71] 2019	1.87 (1.68–2.09)	
Roos et al,[29] 2019	1.92 (1.53–2.41)[a] 1.37 (0.76–2.46)[b]	<50: 3.57 (1.07–11.85)[a] >50: 3.25 (2.82–3.77)[b]

[a] For case-control studies (n = 42).
[b] For cohort studies (n = 20).

95% CI 1.73–4.55 for case control studies and RR 3.26, 95% CI 2.82–3.77 for cohort studies).[29]

The number of affected family members also impacts the risk of CRC. In a constellation approach using the Utah statewide cancer records linked to genealogy whereby the RR of CRC with ≥1 affected FDR with CRC was consistent with published estimates (2.05, 95% CI 1.96–2.14), the RR was modestly increased for 1 affected FDR, 1 affected SDR, and 0 affected third-degree relatives (TDR) (RR 1.88, 95% CI 1.59–2.20).[30] Risk significantly increased with the addition of affected relatives (RR 3.28, 95% CI 2.44–4.31 for 1 FDR, 1 SDR, and ≥3 TDRs affected). In the absence of an affected FDR, risk remained elevated compared with no family history when 1 SDR and 2 TDRs were affected (RR 1.33, 95% CI 1.13–1.55). More recent pooled risk estimates suggest a nearly 4-fold increase in risk for 2+ affected FDRs compared with no family history (RR 3.97, 95% CI 2.60–6.06).[28] The risk of CRC in more distant relatives is modestly increased,[14,28] but likely does not meet the need for clinical screening.[31]

There also appears to be a differential risk according to the type of FDR, whereby multiple studies demonstrate higher CRC risk in siblings versus parents,[32–34] although this finding may be limited to individuals greater than 50 years old.[31] Finally, the site of cancer (colon vs rectum) may also impact familial risk. Earlier studies suggest higher risk with colon versus rectal cancer,[35] but a large population-based study in Utah reported no difference according to the subsite of primary cancer.[36]

RISK IN INDIVIDUALS WITH A POSITIVE FAMILY HISTORY OF ADVANCED ADENOMAS

There is evidence of an increased CRC risk in those with an FDR with an AA, although the risk estimates may be less than having a relative with CRC (**Table 2**). Of note, although earlier studies suggested higher risk with family history of non-AA,[22,37] more recent analyses have shown that the presence of a non-AA does not significantly impact risk for AA or CRC.[38]

Many of the studies evaluating familial risk with AA focus only on a subtype of AA (advanced by size vs by polyp histology) and also are designed to report varying outcomes (advanced neoplasia, CRC). A large cross-sectional study from Hong Kong reported that siblings with AA had a 6-fold higher risk of having an AA than siblings of those with a normal colonoscopy (odds ratio [OR] 6.05, 95% CI 2.74–13.36) and even higher for adenoma with high-grade dysplasia (OR 19.98,

Table 2
Level of risk for family member of patients with advanced colorectal polyps

Pathology in Proband	Risk in FDR, OR/RR (95% CI)	
	AA	CRC
Advanced Adenoma	6.05 (2.74–13.36)[39,a]	—
Tubular adenoma ≥10 mm	8.59 (3.4–21.45)[39]	3.9 (0.89–17.01)[40]
	2.27 (1.01–5.09)[40,b]	
Adenoma with villous histology	1.65 (1.28–2.14)[37,c]	1.68 (1.29–2.18)[37]
	6.28 (2.02–19.53)[39]	
Adenoma with high-grade dysplasia	19.98 (2.03–1.97)[39]	—

[a] In siblings.
[b] For composite endpoint of large adenoma and/or CRC.
[c] For adenoma with villous histology only (not advanced by size or high-grade dysplasia).

5% CI 2.03–19.7).[39] A French case control study showed that FDRs of those with large adenomas were at least 2 times more likely to develop a composite endpoint of CRC and large adenomas (OR 2.27, 95% CI 1.01–5.09).[40] A nested case control study from Utah showed 1.7 times higher risk of CRC in those with an FDR with a villous adenoma (RR 1.65, 95% CI 1.28-2.18).[37]

Recognition of the serrated pathway contributing to up to 30% of CRC has prompted consideration for analogous lesions referred to as ASPs.[41,42] Similar to conventional AA, these are defined as sessile serrated polyp (SSP) $\geq$1 cm, SSP with any degree of cytologic dysplasia, or traditional serrated adenoma (TSA). TSAs of any size are considered advanced as related to surveillance (3-year interval recommended)[43] but only TSA $\geq$1 cm are considered advanced as related to the recommendation for earlier screening for FDRs.[3] There are no studies on familial risk with ASP, and therefore, the magnitude of risk is unknown, although presumed to be elevated.

CURRENT SCREENING GUIDELINES FOR POSITIVE FAMILY HISTORY

US guidelines recommending earlier screening for those with an FDR with CRC have been in place for nearly 30 years, with slight modifications over time. The US Multi-Society Task Force (US-MSTF), made up by the 3 major gastrointestinal societies, including the American Gastroenterological Association (AGA), the American Society for Gastrointestinal Endoscopy, and the American College of Gastroenterology, last released CRC screening guidelines in 2017.[3] The NCCN updates their CRC screening guidelines annually, although the 2019 recommendations are largely the same as previous years.[5] In 2018, the Canadian Association for Gastroenterology (CAG) in conjunction with the AGA released the Banff consensus statement for CRC screening in those with nonhereditary family history of CRC.[4] The US-MSTF, NCCN, and Banff statement all provide recommendations for screening individuals with a family history of CRC (**Table 3**) and a family history of AA (**Table 4**).

The US-MSTF recommends that individuals who have a single FDR with CRC at less than 60 years old (or in 2 FDRs of any age) start screening at age 40, or 10 years before the age of the youngest affected relative (whichever is earlier). Colonoscopy is the preferred screening test (with a 5-year interval), and if declined, fecal immunochemical test (FIT) should be offered. If the affected relative was $\geq$60 years old, screening should commence at age 40 with the same tests and intervals as average-risk individuals. The US-MSTF recommends the exact same approach whether the relative had CRC or AA. In addition, the US-MSTF suggests that individuals with FDR with ASPs can be treated similarly to those with conventional AA. All of these statements for family history of CRC/AA are noted to be weak recommendations based on low- or very-low-quality evidence.

The NCCN is largely similar to the US-MSTF with the 1 major difference being that age of the proband affected by CRC or AA/ASP is not taken into account in screening recommendations for FDRs. The other nuance is that the NCCN recommends commencing screening at age 40, or at the age of diagnosis of AA in the FDR. That means if the AA was diagnosed at age 45, the time to start screening would differ between the US-MSTF (age 35) and NCCN (age 40). The Banff consensus statement used robust methodology (systematic review and meta-analysis with the GRADE system) to evaluate the quality of the evidence and strength of the recommendation. Like the NCCN, there is no distinction according to age of the affected relative. Normal average risk approach is recommended for those with a family history of non-AAs or only SDRs with CRC. Most of these statements are conditional recommendations based on low- or very-low-quality evidence. Of note, the American Cancer Society

Table 3
Colorectal cancer screening guidelines and strength of recommendation for individuals with a family history of colorectal cancer

	Family History	Age to Initiate Screening	Preferred Test, Interval
Banff Consensus Statement (CAG/AGA)[4]	CRC in 1 FDR[a]	Age 40–50, or 10 y younger than age of diagnosis of FDR[b] *GRADE: conditional recommendation, very-low-quality evidence*	Colonoscopy preferred every 5–10 y or FIT[c] every 1–2 y
	CRC in ≥2 FDR	Age 40, or 10 y younger than age of diagnosis of FDR[b] *GRADE: conditional recommendation, very-low-quality evidence*	Colonoscopy[d] every 5 y
US-MSTF[3]	CRC in 1 FDR <60 y or in 2 FDRs with CRC (any age) *Weak recommendation, low-quality evidence*	Age 40, or 10 y younger than age of diagnosis of FDR[b]	Colonoscopy[e] every 5 y
	CRC in 1 FDR ≥60 y *Weak recommendation, very-low-quality evidence*	Age 40	Same as for average-risk persons (colonoscopy every 10 y or FIT annually)
NCCN[5]	≥1 FDR with CRC at any age	Age 40, or 10 y younger than age of diagnosis of FDR *Category 2A recommendation*	Colonoscopy every 5 y

[a] Recommend screening over no screening (*GRADE: strong recommendation, moderate-quality evidence*).
[b] Whichever is earlier.
[c] FIT as second-line screening option (*GRADE: conditional recommendation, moderate-quality evidence*).
[d] Colonoscopy as the preferred screening test over no screening or all other modalities (*GRADE: strong recommendation, very-low-quality evidence*).
[e] Persons should be offered annual FIT if they decline colonoscopy (*GRADE: strong recommendation, moderate-quality evidence*).

and US Preventive Services Task Force only provide recommendations on CRC screening for average-risk individuals.[44]

EVIDENCE THAT EARLIER SCREENING IS EFFECTIVE IN THOSE WITH A FAMILY HISTORY

The increased RR of CRC in individuals with an FDR with CRC (or AA) has been shown in many studies, but it is more difficult to study the benefit that has been appreciated from earlier screening in this group. The main reason to start screening earlier is that individuals with a positive family history of CRC have an earlier median age of CRC compared with those without a family history. Although there are no randomized controlled trials to guide the optimal interval for CRC screening in this group, the effectiveness of screening and the shorter screening interval were demonstrated in a large cohort study examining the incidence of CRC after a negative colonoscopy.[45] In the first 5 years after a negative colonoscopy, the incidence of

Table 4
Colorectal cancer screening guidelines and strength of recommendation for individuals with a family history of advanced colorectal polyp

	Family History	Age to Initiate Screening	Preferred Test, Interval
Banff Consensus Statement (CAG/AGA)[4]	*Documented* AA in >1 FDR (any age)[a]	Age 40–50, or 10 y younger than age of diagnosis of FDR[b]	Colonoscopy every 5–10 y or FIT every 1–2 y
		GRADE: conditional recommendation, very-low-quality evidence[c]	
US-MSTF[3]	Documented AA in 1 FDR <60 or in 2 FDRs with AA (any age)	Age 40, or 10 y younger than age of diagnosis of FDR[b]	Colonoscopy[d] every 5 y
		Weak recommendation, low-quality evidence	
	AA in 1 FDR ≥60 y	Age 40	Same as for average-risk persons (colonoscopy every 10 y or FIT annually)
		Weak recommendation, very-low-quality evidence	
	Documented ASL in >1 FDR	According to recommendations for family history of documented AA	
		Weak recommendation, very-low-quality evidence	
NCCN[5]	*Confirmed* AA or ASL in 1 FDR (any age)	Age 40, or at age of diagnosis of AA in FDR[b]	Colonoscopy every 5–10 y
		Category 2A recommendation	

Abbreviation: ASL, advanced serrated lesions.
  [a] Recommend screening over no screening (*GRADE: strong recommendation, moderate-quality evidence*).
  [b] Whichever is earlier.
  [c] Consensus group was not able to make a recommendation (neither for or against) the use of colonoscopy as the preferred screening test over no screening or all other screening modalities.
  [d] Persons should be offered annual FIT if they decline colonoscopy (*GRADE: strong recommendation, moderate-quality evidence*).

CRC was significantly lower in those with an FDR with CRC (standardized incidence ratio [SIR] 0.39, 95% CI 0.13–0.64), but not when the interval was greater than 5 years (SIR 0.74, 95% CI 0.32–1.16). Thus, a negative colonoscopy in individuals with an FDR with CRC confers a 45% lower reduction in CRC risk compared with those without family history, supporting a shorter interval in this high-risk group.

INTERNATIONAL APPROACHES TO FAMILY-BASED COLORECTAL CANCER SCREENING

Outside of the United States, many countries have tried to implement updates to their CRC screening programs that incorporate family history. In 2008 in Canada, a population-based screening program for individuals with a family history was introduced, and a microsimulation modeling study examined the potential impact of this new strategy over the following 30 years.[46] Compared with a regular guaiac fecal occult blood program, a family history–based program was projected to prevent 40% additional deaths while requiring 93% additional colonoscopies. In the Netherlands, where they have population-based FIT screening, they evaluated the impact of offering colonoscopy to a target group who were both FIT positive and had an FDR with CRC.[47] This strategy would increase the yield of advanced neoplasia from 3.2% to 4.8%, with a number needed to scope to detect 1 subject with advanced neoplasia of 5.0 compared with 2.8.

In Ireland, they implemented a special CRC screening service where they used family history questionnaires to stratify patients into risk categories (low risk, moderate risk, Lynch syndrome suspected or diagnosed).[48] Moderate risk was defined as 1 FDR with CRC diagnosed less than 60 years, or 2 FDR with CRC or 2 SDR with CRC diagnosed less than 60 years. At index colonoscopy in this group, they detected adenomas in 16.4% and AA in 4.4%. Interestingly, they did not find any difference in adenoma or AA yield according to risk category, although overall, they had low adenoma detection rate (18%). A US study evaluating screening computed tomographic colonography found no significant difference in rates of AA, non-AA, or cancer in patients with an FDR with CRC versus no family history.[49]

COST-EFFECTIVENESS OF SCREENING IN THOSE WITH FAMILY HISTORY

The cost-effectiveness of screening individuals with positive family history earlier and more frequently has been evaluated and appears to vary according to the number of affected FDRs.[50] Naber and colleagues[51] used the Microsimulation Screening Analysis model to determine the impact of various screening intervals for this high-risk group using a cost-effectiveness ratio less than $100,000 per quality-adjusted life-year as a threshold. Their results showed that the most cost-effective strategy for individuals with 1 affected FDR was to begin screening at age 40 and continue every 3 years, then to gradually extend the interval to 5 years (at age 45) and then 7 years (at age 55) if no adenomas are found. These results lend credence to current guidelines recommending initiation of screening at an earlier age from the perspective of societal cost. The finding that it is cost-effective to gradually increase the screening interval after a negative colonoscopy is important; however, cost is not currently factored into screening guidelines in the United States.

BARRIERS TO USE OF FAMILY CANCER HISTORY IN PRACTICE

The challenges to CRC screening for individuals with a positive family history are multifactorial and include patient level factors, provider limitations in collecting family history, and insufficient application of guidelines resulting in inadequate screening practices.

In general, patients have poor knowledge of their family history of cancer and know even less about their family history of colon polyps. When surveyed, almost a quarter of patients did not know which family members had polyps, and a large proportion of patients did not know the age at diagnosis (43%), polyp type (71%), number of polyps found (91%), or polyp size (97%).[52] With limited knowledge of polyps in relatives, it is nearly impossible to identify those with AA and incorporate this information into practice. On the provider side, physicians may not take comprehensive family histories[53] and may lack the knowledge to assess risk.[54] Multiple different online family history questionnaires have been developed to overcome these barriers, although most of them have failed to facilitate enrolling additional relatives in screening or surveillance programs for CRC.[55] In conjunction with the National Colorectal Cancer Roundtable, the authors' group has provided a guide for endoscopists to appreciate guideline recommendations for CRC screening in individuals with a family history of AA and tools to implement these recommendations in routine clinical practice.[56]

Adherence to screening in individuals with family history of CRC is suboptimal, although may be higher than the general population.[57,58] One study using National Health Interview Survey data revealed that FDRs were nearly twice as likely as those without family history to get a colonoscopy (adjusted odds ratio 1.7, 95% CI 1.5–1.9), but still only 46% of this at-risk group completed a colonoscopy.[59–61] Multiple interventions have been tried to improve colonoscopy utilization in this high-risk group. A tailored telephone counseling intervention for individuals with a positive family history who were due for colonoscopy within 24 months achieved 32% increase in screening adherence compared with a mailed packet with general information about screening.[62]

Recent literature shows the success and cost-effectiveness of state-wide patient navigation (PN) programs to target priority patients for CRC screening.[63,64] PN has also been studied in high-risk patients with a positive family history. Paskett and colleagues[65] assessed adherence to screening recommendation in a randomized clinical trial comparing a Web site intervention (survey and personal CRC screening recommendation) versus the Web site plus the addition of a PN intervention via telephone in patients with an FDR with CRC. Overall adherence was 79% (similar in both groups), and PN was only useful in cases whereby screening was needed immediately. Even in high-risk groups with targeted interventions, adherence to screening recommendations still falls short.

IMPACT OF FAMILY HISTORY ON THE INCREASE OF EARLY-ONSET COLORECTAL CANCER

There has been an unprecedented increase in the incidence of early onset (EO) CRC in young adults less than 50 years old worldwide with ongoing studies to identify the drivers of increasing disease. Although reports in the literature identify the majority of this young cohort as not having a positive family history, still an FDR with CRC has been shown to be associated with EO-CRC (OR 8.61, 95% CI 4.83–15.75) outside of hereditary cancers.[66,67] As we search for markers to indicate which young adults may be at increased risk, at a minimum, those with FDR with CRC or AA should be targeted for earlier screening.

FUTURE DIRECTIONS

Risk stratification for CRC is primarily driven by family history. More, and better, data are needed to more clearly understand the risk to family members and to help guide screening practices. Efforts should focus on improving acquisition of family history and better adherence to guidelines. New approaches for familial risk assessment include prediction algorithms through computation analyses and artificial neural networks to accurately stratify risk.[68,69] Perhaps genomic analysis may add to or replace family history information. However, most of these technologies still rely on self-reported family history, which requires individuals to be knowledgeable about their family members' colonoscopy findings (polyp and CRC). Providers should make a conscious effort to ascertain family history of cancer or polyps in all of their patients, inform their patients of colonoscopy findings and to share these with their relatives, and follow guidelines for earlier screening for those with a positive family history.

DISCLOSURE

None.

REFERENCES

1. Ansa BE, Coughlin SS, Alema-Mensah E, et al. Evaluation of colorectal cance incidence trends in the United States (2000-2014). J Clin Med 2018;7(2) [pii:E22

2. Siegel RL, Miller KD, Jemal A. Cancer statistics, 2019. CA Cancer J Clin 2019 69(1):7–34.

3. Rex DK, Boland CR, Dominitz JA, et al. Colorectal cancer screening: recommer dations for physicians and patients from the U.S. Multi-Society Task Force o colorectal cancer. Gastroenterology 2017;153(1):307–23.

4. Leddin D, Lieberman DA, Tse F, et al. Clinical practice guideline on screening fc colorectal cancer in individuals with a family history of nonhereditary colorect cancer or adenoma: the Canadian Association of Gastroenterology Ban Consensus. Gastroenterology 2018;155(5):1325–47.e3.

5. National Comprehensive Cancer Network. Colon Cancer. Version 2, 2019. https: www.nccn.org/professionals/physician_gls/pdf/colon.pdf. Accessed November 2019.

6. National Comprehensive Cancer Network. Genetic/Familial High-Risk Assessmen Colorectal. Version 3, 2019. https://www.nccn.org/professionals/physician_gls/pd genetics_colon.pdf. Accessed November 1, 2019.

7. Kastrinos F, Samadder NJ, Burt RW. Use of family history and genetic testing t determine risk of colorectal cancer. Gastroenterology 2020;158(2):389–403.

8. Click B, Pinsky PF, Hickey T, et al. Association of colonoscopy adenoma finding with long-term colorectal cancer incidence. JAMA 2018;319(19):2021–31.

9. Cottet V, Jooste V, Fournel I, et al. Long-term risk of colorectal cancer after ade noma removal: a population-based cohort study. Gut 2012;61(8):1180–6.

10. Leung K, Pinsky P, Laiyemo AO, et al. Ongoing colorectal cancer risk despite su veillance colonoscopy: the Polyp Prevention Trial Continued Follow-up Study Gastrointest Endosc 2010;71(1):111–7.

11. Lieberman DA, Weiss DG, Harford WV, et al. Five-year colon surveillance afte screening colonoscopy. Gastroenterology 2007;133(4):1077–85.

12. Toll AD, Fabius D, Hyslop T, et al. Prognostic significance of high-grade dysplasi in colorectal adenomas. Colorectal Dis 2011;13(4):370–3.

13. Fearon ER, Vogelstein B. A genetic model for colorectal tumorigenesis. Cell 1990 61(5):759–67.

14. Tian Y, Kharazmi E, Sundquist K, et al. Familial colorectal cancer risk in half sib lings and siblings: nationwide cohort study. BMJ 2019;364:l803.

15. Weigl K, Tikk K, Hoffmeister M, et al. Prevalence of a first-degree relative with colorectal cancer and uptake of screening among persons 40 to 54 years old Clin Gastroenterol Hepatol 2019. [Epub ahead of print].

16. Mitchell RJ, Campbell H, Farrington SM, et al. Prevalence of family history of colo rectal cancer in the general population. Br J Surg 2005;92(9):1161–4.

17. Levin B, Murphy GP. Revision in American Cancer Society recommendations fc the early detection of colorectal cancer. CA Cancer J Clin 1992;42(5):296–9.

18. Fuchs CS, Giovannucci EL, Colditz GA, et al. A prospective study of family histor and the risk of colorectal cancer. N Engl J Med 1994;331(25):1669–74.

19. Ponz de Leon M, Antonioli A, Ascari A, et al. Incidence and familial occurrence c colorectal cancer and polyps in a health-care district of northern Italy. Cance 1987;60(11):2848–59.

20. Lovett E. Family studies in cancer of the colon and rectum. Br J Surg 1976 63(1):13–8.

21. St John DJ, McDermott FT, Hopper JL, et al. Cancer risk in relatives of patients with common colorectal cancer. Ann Intern Med 1993;118(10):785–90.
22. Johns LE, Houlston RS. A systematic review and meta-analysis of familial colorectal cancer risk. Am J Gastroenterol 2001;96(10):2992–3003.
23. Baglietto L, Jenkins MA, Severi G, et al. Measures of familial aggregation depend on definition of family history: meta-analysis for colorectal cancer. J Clin Epidemiol 2006;59(2):114–24.
24. Butterworth AS, Higgins JP, Pharoah P. Relative and absolute risk of colorectal cancer for individuals with a family history: a meta-analysis. Eur J Cancer 2006;42(2):216–27.
25. Johnson CM, Wei C, Ensor JE, et al. Meta-analyses of colorectal cancer risk factors. Cancer Causes Control 2013;24(6):1207–22.
26. Samadder NJ, Curtin K, Tuohy TM, et al. Increased risk of colorectal neoplasia among family members of patients with colorectal cancer: a population-based study in Utah. Gastroenterology 2014;147(4):814–21.e5 [quiz: e815-816].
27. Samadder NJ, Smith KR, Hanson H, et al. Increased risk of colorectal cancer among family members of all ages, regardless of age of index case at diagnosis. Clin Gastroenterol Hepatol 2015;13(13):2305–11.e1-2.
28. Lowery JT, Ahnen DJ, Schroy PC, et al. Understanding the contribution of family history to colorectal cancer risk and its clinical implications: a state-of-the-science review. Cancer 2016;122(17):2633–45.
29. Roos VH, Mangas-Sanjuan C, Rodriguez-Girondo M, et al. Effects of family history on relative and absolute risks for colorectal cancer: a systematic review and meta-analysis. Clin Gastroenterol Hepatol 2019;17(13):2657–67.e9.
30. Taylor DP, Burt RW, Williams MS, et al. Population-based family history-specific risks for colorectal cancer: a constellation approach. Gastroenterology 2010;138(3):877–85.
31. Kim NH, Yang HJ, Park SK, et al. The risk of colorectal neoplasia can be different according to the types of family members affected by colorectal cancer. J Gastroenterol Hepatol 2018;33(2):397–403.
32. Hemminki K, Chen B. Familial risks for colorectal cancer show evidence on recessive inheritance. Int J Cancer 2005;115(5):835–8.
33. Boardman LA, Morlan BW, Rabe KG, et al. Colorectal cancer risks in relatives of young-onset cases: is risk the same across all first-degree relatives? Clin Gastroenterol Hepatol 2007;5(10):1195–8.
34. Carstensen B, Soll-Johanning H, Villadsen E, et al. Familial aggregation of colorectal cancer in the general population. Int J Cancer 1996;68(4):428–35.
35. Yu H, Hemminki A, Sundquist K, et al. Familial associations of colon and rectal cancers with other cancers. Dis Colon Rectum 2019;62(2):189–95.
36. Samadder NJ, Smith KR, Mineau GP, et al. Familial colorectal cancer risk by subsite of primary cancer: a population-based study in Utah. Aliment Pharmacol Ther 2015;41(6):573–80.
37. Tuohy TM, Rowe KG, Mineau GP, et al. Risk of colorectal cancer and adenomas in the families of patients with adenomas: a population-based study in Utah. Cancer 2014;120(1):35–42.
38. Ng SC, Kyaw MH, Suen BY, et al. Prospective colonoscopic study to investigate risk of colorectal neoplasms in first-degree relatives of patients with non-advanced adenomas. Gut 2019;69(2):304–10.
39. Ng SC, Lau JY, Chan FK, et al. Risk of advanced adenomas in siblings of individuals with advanced adenomas: a cross-sectional study. Gastroenterology 2016;150(3):608–16 [quiz: e616–7].

40. Cottet V, Pariente A, Nalet B, et al. Colonoscopic screening of first-degree relatives of patients with large adenomas: increased risk of colorectal tumors. Gastroenterology 2007;133(4):1086–92.

41. Kolb JM, Soetikno RM, Rao AK, et al. Detection, diagnosis, and resection of sessile serrated adenomas and polyps. Gastroenterology 2017;153(3):646–8.

42. Noffsinger AE. Serrated polyps and colorectal cancer: new pathway to malignancy. Annu Rev Pathol 2009;4:343–64.

43. Lieberman DA, Rex DK, Winawer SJ, et al. Guidelines for colonoscopy surveillance after screening and polypectomy: a consensus update by the US Multi-Society Task Force on Colorectal Cancer. Gastroenterology 2012;143(3):844–57.

44. Wolf AMD, Fontham ETH, Church TR, et al. Colorectal cancer screening for average-risk adults: 2018 guideline update from the American Cancer Society. CA Cancer J Clin 2018;68(4):250–81.

45. Samadder NJ, Pappas L, Boucherr KM, et al. Long-term colorectal cancer incidence after negative colonoscopy in the state of Utah: the effect of family history. Am J Gastroenterol 2017;112(9):1439–47.

46. Goede SL, Rabeneck L, Lansdorp-Vogelaar I, et al. The impact of stratifying by family history in colorectal cancer screening programs. Int J Cancer 2015; 137(5):1119–27.

47. Kallenberg FGJ, Vleugels JLA, de Wijkerslooth TR, et al. Adding family history to faecal immunochemical testing increases the detection of advanced neoplasia in a colorectal cancer screening programme. Aliment Pharmacol Ther 2016;44(1): 88–96.

48. Walshe M, Moran R, Boyle M, et al. High-risk family colorectal cancer screening service in Ireland: critical review of clinical outcomes. Cancer Epidemiol 2017; 50(Pt A):30–8.

49. Pickhardt PJ, Mbah I, Pooler BD, et al. CT colonographic screening of patients with a family history of colorectal cancer: comparison with adults at average risk and implications for guidelines. AJR Am J Roentgenol 2017;208(4):794–800.

50. Wilschut JA, Steyerberg EW, van Leerdam ME, et al. How much colonoscopy screening should be recommended to individuals with various degrees of family history of colorectal cancer? Cancer 2011;117(18):4166–74.

51. Naber SK, Kuntz KM, Henrikson NB, et al. Cost effectiveness of age-specific screening intervals for people with family histories of colorectal cancer. Gastroenterology 2018;154(1):105–16.e120.

52. Elias PS, Romagnuolo J, Hoffman B. Poor patient knowledge regarding family history of colon polyps: implications for the feasibility of stratified screening recommendations. Gastrointest Endosc 2012;75(3):598–603.

53. Solomon BL, Whitman T, Wood ME. Contribution of extended family history in assessment of risk for breast and colon cancer. BMC Fam Pract 2016;17(1):126.

54. Schroy PC 3rd, Barrison AF, Ling BS, et al. Family history and colorectal cancer screening: a survey of physician knowledge and practice patterns. Am J Gastroenterol 2002;97(4):1031–6.

55. Kallenberg FGJ, Aalfs CM, The FO, et al. Evaluation of an online family history tool for identifying hereditary and familial colorectal cancer. Fam Cancer 2018;17(3): 371–80.

56. Molmenti CL, Kolb JM, Karlitz JJ. Advanced colorectal polyps on colonoscopy: a trigger for earlier screening of family members. The Am J Gastroenterol 2020; 115(3):311–4.

7. Dillon M, Flander L, Buchanan DD, et al. Family history-based colorectal cancer screening in Australia: a modelling study of the costs, benefits, and harms of different participation scenarios. PLoS Med 2018;15(8):e1002630.

8. Henrikson NB, Webber EM, Goddard KA, et al. Family history and the natural history of colorectal cancer: systematic review. Genet Med 2015;17(9):702–12.

9. Tsai MH, Xirasagar S, Li YJ, et al. Colonoscopy screening among US adults aged 40 or older with a family history of colorectal cancer. Prev Chronic Dis 2015; 12:E80.

0. Bronner K, Mesters I, Weiss-Meilnik A, et al. Do individuals with a family history of colorectal cancer adhere to medical recommendations for the prevention of colorectal cancer? Fam Cancer 2013;12(4):629–37.

1. Taylor DP, Cannon-Albright LA, Sweeney C, et al. Comparison of compliance for colorectal cancer screening and surveillance by colonoscopy based on risk. Genet Med 2011;13(8):737–43.

2. Lowery JT, Horick N, Kinney AY, et al. A randomized trial to increase colonoscopy screening in members of high-risk families in the colorectal cancer family registry and cancer genetics network. Cancer Epidemiol Biomarkers Prev 2014;23(4): 601–10.

3. Rice K, Sharma K, Li C, et al. Cost-effectiveness of a patient navigation intervention to increase colonoscopy screening among low-income adults in New Hampshire. Cancer 2019;125(4):601–9.

4. DeGroff A, Gressard L, Glover-Kudon R, et al. Assessing the implementation of a patient navigation intervention for colonoscopy screening. BMC Health Serv Res 2019;19(1):803.

5. Paskett ED, Bernardo BM, Young GS, et al. Comparative effectiveness of two interventions to increase colorectal cancer screening for those at increased risk based on family history: results of a randomized trial. Cancer Epidemiol Biomarkers Prev 2019;29(1):3–9.

6. Stoffel EM, Murphy CC. Epidemiology and mechanisms of the increasing incidence of colon and rectal cancers in young adults. Gastroenterology 2019; 158(2):341–53.

7. Gausman V, Dornblaser D, Anand S, et al. Risk factors associated with early-onset colorectal cancer. Clin Gastroenterol Hepatol 2019. [Epub ahead of print].

8. Rieger AK, Mansmann UR. A Bayesian scoring rule on clustered event data for familial risk assessment–an example from colorectal cancer screening. Biom J 2018;60(1):115–27.

9. Nartowt BJ, Hart GR, Roffman DA, et al. Scoring colorectal cancer risk with an artificial neural network based on self-reportable personal health data. PLoS One 2019;14(8):e0221421.

0. Wong MCS, Chan CH, Lin J, et al. Lower relative contribution of positive family history to colorectal cancer risk with increasing age: a systematic review and meta-analysis of 9.28 million individuals. Am J Gastroenterol 2018;113(12): 1819–27.

1. Mehraban Far P, Alshahrani A, Yaghoobi M. Quantitative risk of positive family history in developing colorectal cancer: a meta-analysis. World J Gastroenterol 2019;25(30):4278–91.

Moving?

Make sure your subscription moves with you!

To notify us of your new address, find your **Clinics Account Number** (located on your mailing label above your name), and contact customer service at:

Email: journalscustomerservice-usa@elsevier.com

800-654-2452 (subscribers in the U.S. & Canada)
314-447-8871 (subscribers outside of the U.S. & Canada)

Fax number: 314-447-8029

Elsevier Health Sciences Division
Subscription Customer Service
3251 Riverport Lane
Maryland Heights, MO 63043

*To ensure uninterrupted delivery of your subscription, please notify us at least 4 weeks in advance of move.

Printed and bound by CPI Group (UK) Ltd, Croydon, CR0 4YY

08/05/2025

01864691-0005